Dermatoses in Dark vs Light Skin

Diagnosis in dermatology is largely based on visual inspection of a lesion or a suspicious skin area; however, visual diagnosis and pattern recognition can vary according to patients' skin types, and the disorders themselves can have markedly different presentation profiles in different skin colors. This book provides succinct information to identify the differing clinical manifestations of skin diseases in darker skin and lighter skin, discussing 130 skin conditions with high-quality color illustrations, and will be an invaluable reference for even experienced professionals working on skin diseases in heterogeneous populations.

Dermatoses in Dark vs Light Skin

Differing Clinical Manifestations

Ranthilaka R. Gammanpila, MBBS, MD
Consultant Dermatologist
Teaching Hospital Kalutara
Lady Ridgeway Hospital for Children
Colombo, Sri Lanka

Eckart Haneke, MD, PhD
Inselspital, University of Bern, Switzerland
Dermatology Practice Dermaticum, Freiburg, Germany
Centro de Dermatología Epidermis, Instituto CUF, Porto, Portugal

CRC Press
Taylor & Francis Group
Boca Raton London New York

CRC Press is an imprint of the
Taylor & Francis Group, an **informa** business

Designed cover image: Authors

First edition published 2025
by CRC Press
2385 NW Executive Center Drive, Suite 320, Boca Raton, FL 33431

and by CRC Press
4 Park Square, Milton Park, Abingdon, Oxon, OX14 4RN

CRC Press is an imprint of Taylor & Francis Group, LLC

ISBN: 9781032766638 (hbk)
ISBN: 9781032762739 (pbk)
ISBN: 9781003479512 (ebk)

DOI: 10.1201/9781003479512

Typeset in Palatino
by Deanta Global Publishing Services, Chennai, India

CONTENTS

PREFACE

Since my residency, I have observed the differences in clinical manifestations in our patients (Fitzpatrick skin type [FST] 5, brown skin) compared to the textbook descriptions which are of white skin (FST 1–3). Although dark and light skin share many similarities, through 16 years as a consultant dermatologist, I have observed several unique characteristics in brown skin.

For example

- Erythema hidden in dark skin obscures the severity in erythroderma, toxic epidermal necrolysis, staphylococcal scalded skin syndrome, or psoriasis and may lead to distressing outcomes in inexperienced hands.
- Moreover, hypopigmented disorders – such as hypopigmented mycosis fungoides, polymorphic light eruption with hypopigmentation, lichen sclerosus, chemical depigmentation, and progressive macular hypomelanosis – are striking and present early to clinicians; therefore, they have a good prognosis.

It is interesting to note that we identified several variances in dark and white skin while completing this book,

We identified seven skin problems that are prevalent and cosmetically concerning in dark skin (FST5) but are not recognized in white skin: central centrifugal cicatricial alopecia (CCCA), seborrheic melanosis, hair dye melanosis, maturity melanosis, pigmented transverse nasal band, dermatosis papulosa nigra (DPN), and benign vitiliginous patches on shins.

There are some skin problems that are very common in FST5 but are rare in white skin, such as macular amyloidosis, acne keloidalis nuchae, Mongolian blue spots, and secondary ochronosis.

Moreover, some dermatoses are infrequent in dark skin but much rarer in white skin, such as tinea nigra and lichen planus pigmentosus.

In this book, both authors contributed to all the chapters with their clinical experiences, clinical photographs, and published data. Even though there are many more skin dermatoses we could discuss, we limited this book to 130 due to restraints in cost and time. Awareness of these differences is important in countries where the majority population is heterogeneous, to avoid delayed diagnoses and mismanagement of dark-skinned patients. Similarly, developing countries where the local population has dark skin but where Western texts are used to identify clinical presentations should also be aware of these differences.

Dr. Ranthilaka R. Gammanpila (Ranawaka) MBBS MD

Dark and light skin have much in common, but there are also important differences. Light skin is, above all, much more sensitive to the harmful effects of ultraviolet light, whereas the influence of pigmentation on the long-term effects of infrared have barely been investigated. This means that epidermal changes are more pronounced in light skin. Actinic damage is common in middle-aged and elderly persons with fair skin whereas dermal alterations are not fundamentally different. Further, except for Inuit in the Arctic regions, most light-skinned individuals live in temperate and cold climates although admittedly, there are tropical and subtropical regions where people with fair skin migrated centuries ago; from a biogeographical point of view, they might be called 'foreign bodies/people' in these regions where their ancestors had not lived.

There are more environmental factors playing a role. Moderate to cold climates do not usually require daily showering as sweating is much less common unless due to physical work and sports activities. The horny layer of fair skin takes over much of the sun protection task that pigment does in dark skin. In fact, red-haired freckled people have more pheomelanin, which does not provide good ultraviolet protection. The percentage of urban people is higher in Europe and North America, and outdoor work has become much less common. Skin cancer due to sun exposure is now recognized as an occupational disease in Germany, and outdoor workers like those in construction and agriculture are entitled to reimbursement if their basal and squamous cell carcinomas are beyond what is seen in vacation sunbathers. Although many regions of the world now make up the obesity pandemic, big and heavy people are more frequent among individuals of European descent than in South and East Asia, and this is associated with diseases like varicose veins, diabetes-associated conditions, intertrigo, etc. Genetic skin diseases are often seen in cultures where intermarriage is common: In Europe, they are frequently seen in immigrants from Asia and North Africa, whereas consanguinity is infrequent in Europe.

Fair skin exhibits different skin signs in inflammation and oncology. Dermatologists who have grown up with skin of color are not used to the sheer endless number of shades of red, whereas those used to seeing patients with light skin cannot see all the nuances of red in dark skin.

Thus, a comparison of skin diseases in light and dark skin is certainly necessary.

We hope this text helps readers to better diagnose dermatoses on skin of all colors.

Eckart Haneke

ACKNOWLEDGEMENTS

I take this opportunity to thank Prof. Haneke and members of the German Dermatological Society (Deutsche Dermatologische Gesellschaft) who have been contributing their immense knowledge in enhancing dermatology training in Sri Lanka.

Our sincere gratitude goes to Prof. Ian Coulson and Dr. Richard Ashton from the UK, Prof. Uwe Wollina from Germany, Prof. Nooshin Bagherani from Iran, Prof. Archana Singal and Dr. Daniel Henry from India, Prof. Osvaldo Correia from Portugal, Prof. Carlo Enrico Urbanii from Italy, and Dr. Ajith P. Kannangara from Sri Lanka for their generosity for sharing their clinical photos with us; special thanks are due to Prof. Coulson who took great trouble to complete the required white skin clinical photos.

Finally, we convey our sincere gratitude to our patients, who are the main source of inspiration for this book.

1
ACANTHOSIS NIGRICANS

Introduction

Acanthosis nigricans (AN) is an asymptomatic, symmetrical darkening affecting the skin of intertriginous areas, such as axillae, neck, submammary folds, and groin. The skin in those areas is thickened, velvety, hyperpigmented, and may be studded with skin tags. Benign AN is associated with obesity, hypothyroidism, acromegaly, polycystic ovary disease, insulin-resistant diabetes, Cushing and Addison diseases, and certain medications like systemic glucocorticoids and oral contraceptives. Paraneoplastic AN is clinically very similar but may also occur on the mucous membranes of the nose, oral cavity, esophagus, or larynx. Women may also develop lesions on the nipple. Rare cases of AN have been reported in the conjunctiva.

Epidemiology

AN occurs at any age and equally in both sexes. AN is more common in darker skins: Native Americans, African Americans (13.3%), and Hispanics when compared to Whites (1%).

Associated diseases

Obesity and insulin resistance are the most common associations with benign AN and can regress with weight loss. Many syndromes have been associated with AN; polycystic ovary syndrome (PCOS) is the most common in women. Malignant AN has been associated with many internal cancers, but over 90% are with gastrointestinal cancer, of which two-thirds are gastric. The familial form of AN is inherited in an autosomal dominant pattern.

Clinical characteristics in light skin (Fitzpatrick skin types I–III)

AN is generally divided into a benign form associated with obesity and other syndromes and a paraneoplastic form due to internal carcinomas, most of which are gastrointestinal. Clinically, the benign form has more skin tags and lacks mucosal involvement. As gastric cancer has dramatically dropped in prevalence, paraneoplastic AN is now even rarer.

In the benign form, the skin in the big folds becomes velvety, more pigmented, deep folds develop, and innumerable acrochordons grow where skin rubs against skin (Figures 1.1 to 1.3). The malignant or paraneoplastic AN is clinically similar; however, it is not necessarily associated with being overweight. Mucosal lesions are characteristic of paraneoplastic AN, particularly around the lips. Malignancy-associated AN was found to be associated with an increased transforming growth factor (TGF), which appears to act on epidermal tissue via the epidermal growth factor receptor. Familial AN is due to a mutation of the fibroblast growth factor receptor 3.

The rare hereditary variants are associated with fibroblast growth factor defects.

Clinical characteristics in dark skin (Fitzpatrick skin types IV–V)

The lesions of AN typically occur in areas of skin folds like the groin, axilla, decubital fossa, or posterior neck. Facial acanthosis is very common and a main cosmetic concern in middle-aged, obese men and women, aged 45 years or above. This mainly appears on the forehead, malar prominence of the face, and in front of and behind the ears. Facial acanthosis is the most common cause of facial melanosis in men and is associated with obesity (Gupta and Mahajan 2017). A significant association between male patients with positive oral glucose tolerance test (OGTT), increased waist-hip ratio (WHR), body mass index (BMI), and facial acanthosis nigricans (FAN) is reported (Figures 1.4 to 1.7).

Investigations

Diagnosis of AN is a clinical diagnosis.

However, further investigations are needed to assess associated diseases such as serum insulin for insulin resistance, hormonal assays, ultrasonography for PCOS, and screening for malignancy.

Treatments

- Management of AN is the management of the underlying condition.
- Benign AN can regress with weight loss.
- In familial AN or AN not associated with an underlying condition, treatment is aimed at improving the cosmetic appearance of the condition.
- Topical retinoids – may reduce the hyperkeratosis.
- Topical α-hydroxy acids and keratolytics such as salicylic acid may improve appearance by reducing hyperkeratosis.
- In extensive cases, oral isotretinoin has been used with some success.

Further reading

Das A, Datta D, Kassir M, et al. (2020). Acanthosis Nigricans: A Review. *J Cosmet Dermatol*;19(8):1857–1865.

Gupta M, Mahajan VK (2017). Clinical Profile of 300 Men with Facial Hypermelanosis. *J Dermatol Case Rep*;11(2):20–24.

Kong AS, Williams RL, Rhyne R, et al. (2010). PRIME Net Clinicians. Acanthosis Nigricans: High Prevalence and Association with Diabetes in a Practice-Based Research Network Consortium – A Primary-Care Multi-Ethnic Network (PRIME Net) Study. *J Am Board Fam Med*;23(4):476–485.

Ranawaka RR (2021). Facial Melanosis. In: Ranawaka RR, et al. (eds), *Atlas of Dermatoses in Pigmented Skin*. Springer, Singapore: 810–813.

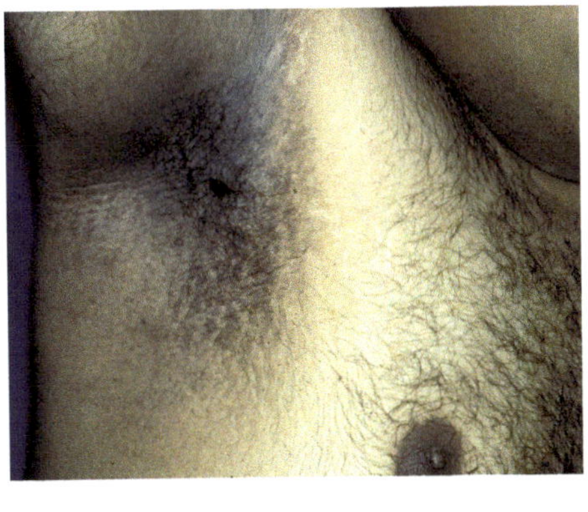

FIGURE 1.1 Acanthosis nigricans in axillae FST2. (Courtesy Prof. Ian Coulson, UK.)

DOI: 10.1201/9781003479512-1

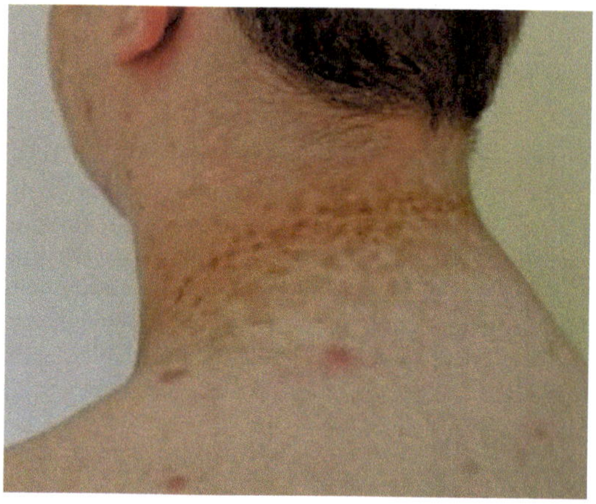

FIGURE 1.2 Acanthosis nigricans on the back of the neck FST1. (Courtesy Prof. Katerina Damevska, Macedonia.)

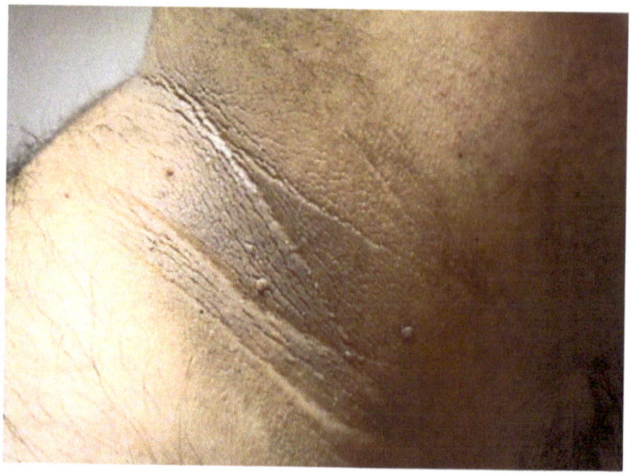

FIGURE 1.3 Acanthosis nigricans and skin tags on the neck FST3. (Courtesy Prof. Osvaldo Correia, Portugal.)

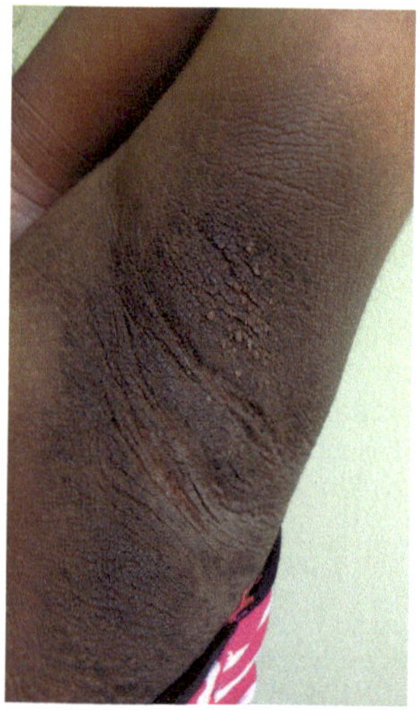

FIGURE 1.4 Acanthosis nigricans in axillae with skin tags in a 15-year-old obese girl FST5.

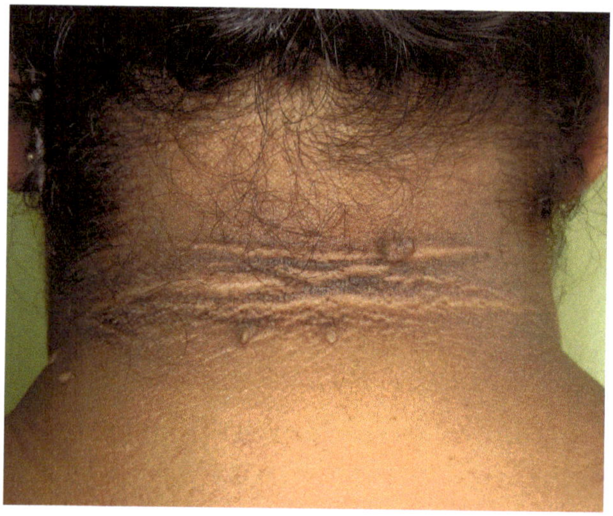

FIGURE 1.5 Acanthosis nigricans and skin tags on the back of the neck in a 37-year-old obese woman FST5.

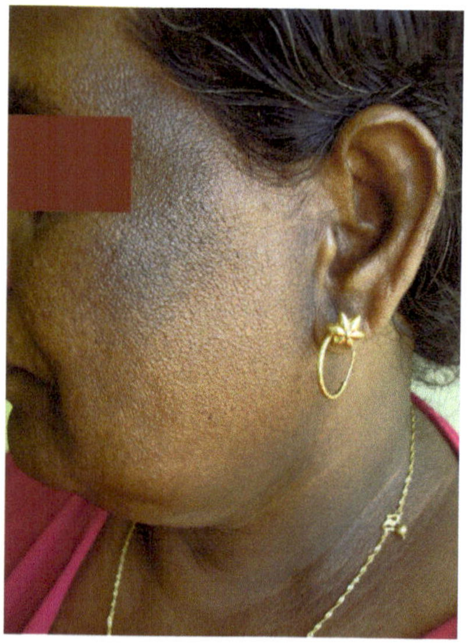

FIGURE 1.6 Facial AN in a 56-year-old obese (BMI 35) Sri Lankan (South Asian) woman FST5.

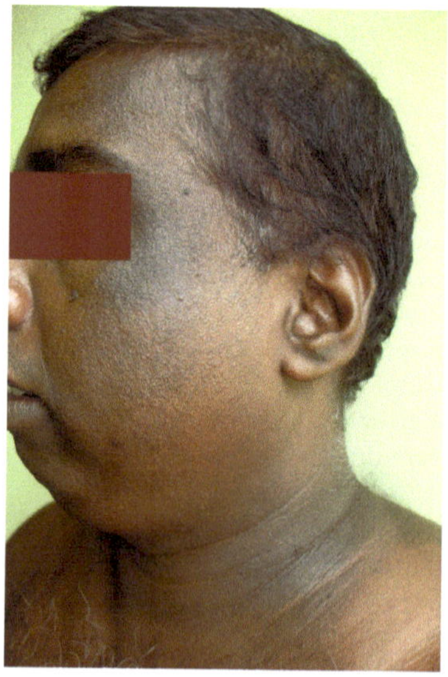

FIGURE 1.7 Facial acanthosis nigricans in a 47-year-old obese (BMI 34.5) man FST5.

2

ACNE KELOIDALIS NUCHAE/FOLLICULITIS KELOIDALIS

Introduction

Chronic inflammatory process involving the hair follicles at the nape of the neck leads to hypertrophic scarring in papules and plaques. It may extend into the scalp. Many patients have or have had significant acne. The observation of foreign body granulomas surrounding fragments of hair has led to the suggestion that the process begins with the penetration of cut hair into the skin, but this is not convincing. Associated keloids in other sites have not been reported.

Epidemiology

Occurs in males after puberty, between 14 and 25 years of age.

Associated diseases

Most affected men are either overweight or obese with Michelin tires on their necks.

Clinical characteristics in light skin (Fitzpatrick skin types I–III)

This condition is not true acne and is rare in light-skinned persons (Figure 2.1). It is virtually only seen in males with curly hair. Probably, it starts with the penetration of a hair shaft through the follicular epithelium, inciting a chronic foreign body reaction that tends to elicit a fibroblastic and finally keloidal response.

Pseudofolliculitis, also called *pili recurvati*, is a similar condition and is seen in men who have to shave regularly. The beard hairs grow at a very flat angle and curve in so that they also pierce the epidermis.

Clinical characteristics in dark skin (Fitzpatrick skin types IV–V)

This is a common skin problem in our setting, and almost all our patients are obese young men aged 20–35 years of age (Figure 2.2). Curly hair is not a constant finding in our patients. Follicular papules or pustules develop on the nape of the neck, just below and within the hairline. The papules may remain discrete or may fuse into horizontal bands or irregular plaques. The inflammatory changes are persistent and troublesome, with undermined abscesses and discharging sinuses.

Investigations

This is diagnosed clinically.

Treatments

- Close shaving of the hair on the nape of the neck and occipital scalp should be avoided.
- Intralesional or potent topical corticosteroids may reduce scarring and inflammation.
- Laser-assisted hair removal with the long-pulsed Nd:YAG laser causes miniaturization of the hair shafts, which is thought to reduce subsequent inflammatory episodes.
- Topical antiseptics, topical and oral antibiotics (tetracyclines).
- Oral isotretinoin.
- In troublesome cases, the affected area may be excised and grafted or excised and allowed to heal by secondary intention.

Further reading

Madura C, Kareddy S, Kusuma MR, et al. (2021). Multimodality Surgical Treatment Approach to Acne Keloidalis Nuchae Based on Lesion Morphology. *J Cutan Aesthet Surg*;14(2):256–259.

Michelen-Gómez EA, Chiesa Fuxench ZC, Cancel-Artau KJ, et al. (2023). Treatment of Acne Keloidalis Nuchae and Dissecting Cellulitis of the Scalp with Diclofenac Sodium Gel: A Case Series. *JAAD Case Rep*;42:113–116.

Umar S, Ton D, Carter MJ, et al. (2023). Unveiling a Shared Precursor Condition for Acne Keloidalis Nuchae and Primary Cicatricial Alopecias. *Clin Cosmet Investig Dermatol*;16:2315–2327.

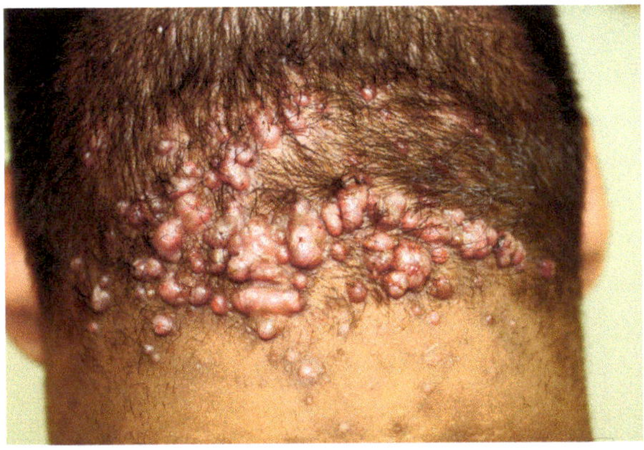

FIGURE 2.1 Acne keloidalis nuchae in FST3. (Courtesy Prof. Ian Coulson, UK.)

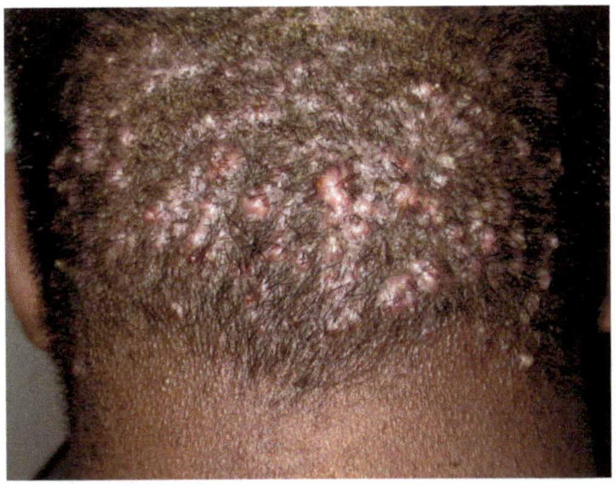

FIGURE 2.2 Acne keloidalis nuchae in an obese 29-year-old man FST5.

DOI: 10.1201/9781003479512-2

3
ACTINIC DERMATITIS, CHRONIC

Introduction

Chronic actinic dermatitis (CAD) is a rare persistent immunological photodermatitis mainly affecting photo-exposed sites, in association with abnormal photosensitivity. The classic features are a pruritic, recurrent, or persistent dermatitis predominantly affecting photo-exposed sites; it is worse in summer. Shading unexposed sites and clear demarcation at photo-protected sites are the key to differentiating it from other widespread dermatitis.

Epidemiology

CAD occurs worldwide in any skin type, although it is more common in temperate climates. It typically occurs in elderly males.

Associated diseases

Common in patients with multiple contact allergies.

Most patients have a history of atopic, contact allergic, seborrheic dermatitis, or endogenous hand eczema. CAD may be confused with photo-aggravated seborrheic dermatitis.

Clinical characteristics in light skin (Fitzpatrick skin types I–III)

CAD in light-skinned individuals is not frequent although the prevalence varies with the intensity and duration of sun exposure (Figures 3.1 to 3.4). The skin lesions are first red, as in chronic eczema; the lesional skin is infiltrated and indurated, then starts desquamating and often develops deep folds, particularly in the nape of the neck. The face may get coarse wrinkles and slowly take on the characteristics of a leonine face. Hyperpigmentation is typical in patients with skin type (2–)3. Chronic itching leads to rubbing and scratching, increasing the thickening of the skin. In severe cases, progression to erythroderma with palmoplantar hyperkeratosis, and in some instances, even transformation into cutaneous lymphoma, was observed. However, the exact pathophysiology is still not exactly known; a delayed-type hypersensitivity reaction to an endogenous photoinduced antigen, UV-altered DNA, was suggested. Ultraviolet A and B, as well as short-wave visible light, elicit the disease. In the Western world, people often self administer drgs of plant origin that may contain photoallergens.

Histopathology shows a dense lymphocytic infiltrate, which is mainly perivascular in the beginning and later gradually turns diffuse, simulating a lymphoma.

Clinical characteristics in dark skin (Fitzpatrick skin types IV–V)

CAD is not uncommon in our setting (Figures 3.5 to 3.7). Patients often present with widespread dermatitis, pseudo-lymphomatous (actinic reticuloid) changes, nodular prurigo-like changes, with unexplained erythroderma or exfoliative dermatitis. Almost all the patients we encounter are middle-aged men, farmers or manual laborers who work outdoors. Their main complaint is severe itching and an uncomfortable, irritable sensation on sunlight exposure. Post-inflammatory hyperpigmentation is common and persistent in chronic recurrent cases.

Investigations

This is a clinical diagnosis.

Photopatch testing in clinically doubtful cases and for confirmation.

Monochromator phototesting to UV and visible wavelengths across the solar spectrum is the investigation of choice. These tests can only be undertaken if there is sufficient clear skin on the back and should avoid potent topical corticosteroids to the back in the week prior to phototesting.

Treatments

- The most important thing is to identify and avoid allergens and photoallergens indefinitely.
- Photoprotection using behavioral modification, hats, clothing, and UV-absorbing window film should be advised.
- Use of high-factor, broad-spectrum, non-fragranced, low-allergenic sunscreens.
- If a patient is taking a photoactive drug such as thiazide or quinine, this should be stopped if feasible.
- Use of very potent/potent topical corticosteroids is the first line of drug management. Topical tacrolimus or pimecrolimus can be effective in some cases.
- If topical measures are inadequate, systemic glucocorticoids may be used in acute flare-ups.
- Azathioprine 150 mg/day can be used as a steroid-sparing agent. Hydroxychloroquine, azathioprine, mycophenolate mofetil, hydroxycarbamide, etretinate, danazol, thioguanine, topical nitrogen mustard, thalidomide, infliximab, and INF-α have been used with variable success.
- Recently, the Janus kinase inhibitor tofacitinib was used successfully.

Further reading

de Silva H (2021). Photodermatosis. In: Ranawaka RR, et al. (eds). *Atlas of Dermatoses in Pigmented Skin*. Springer, Singapore; 189.

Paek SY, Lim HW (2014). Chronic Actinic Dermatitis. *Dermatol Clin*;32(3):355–361, viii–ix.

Vesely MD, Imaeda S, King BA (2016). Tofacitinib Citrate for the Treatment of Refractory, Severe Chronic Actinic Dermatitis. *JAAD Case Rep*;3(1):4–6.

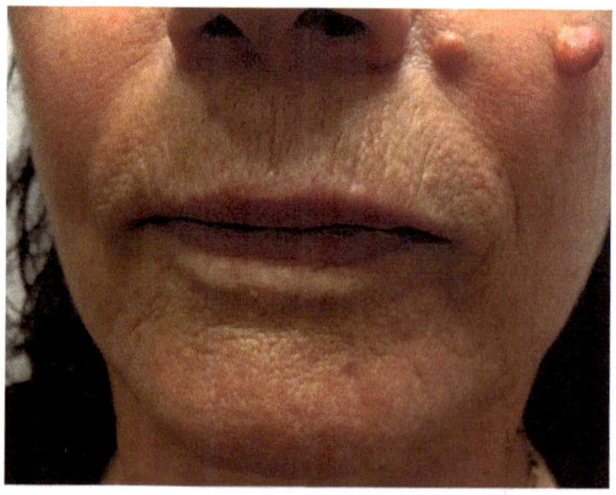

FIGURE 3.1 Solar elastosis on the upper lip in FST2. (Courtesy Prof. Eckart Haneke, Germany.)

DOI: 10.1201/9781003479512-3

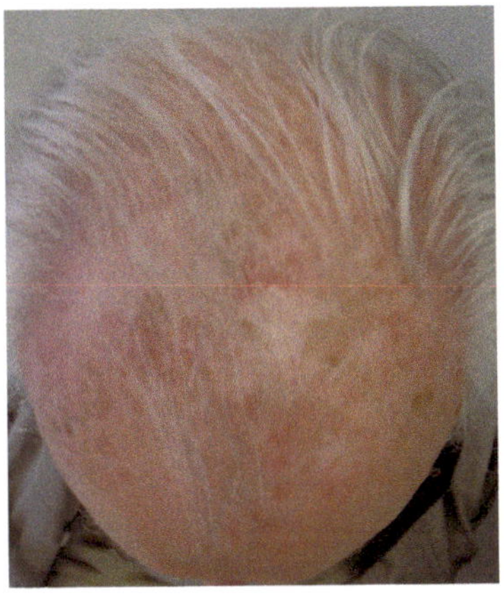

FIGURE 3.2 Actinic damage on the bald scalp in an 87-year-old man FST1. (Courtesy Prof. Eckart Haneke, Germany.)

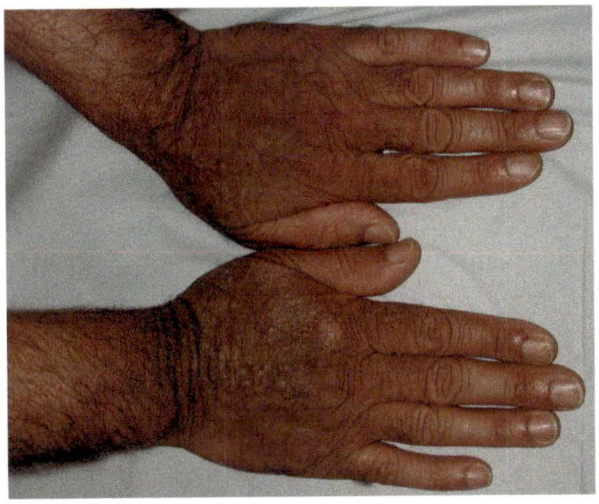

FIGURE 3.3 Chronic actinic dermatitis FST2. (Courtesy Prof. Ian Coulson, UK.)

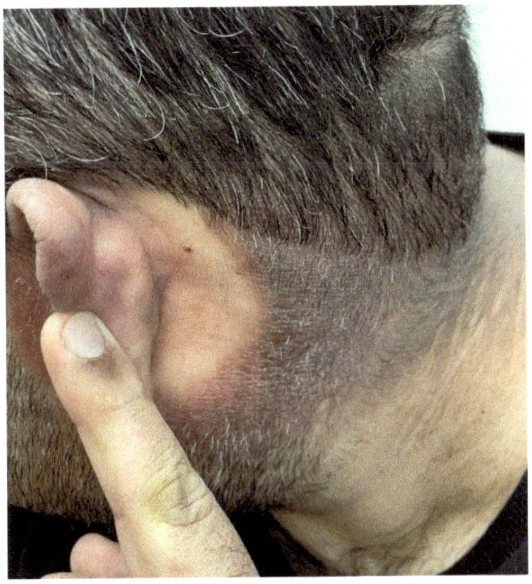

FIGURE 3.4 Chronic actinic dermatitis FST1. (Courtesy Prof. Ian Coulson, UK.)

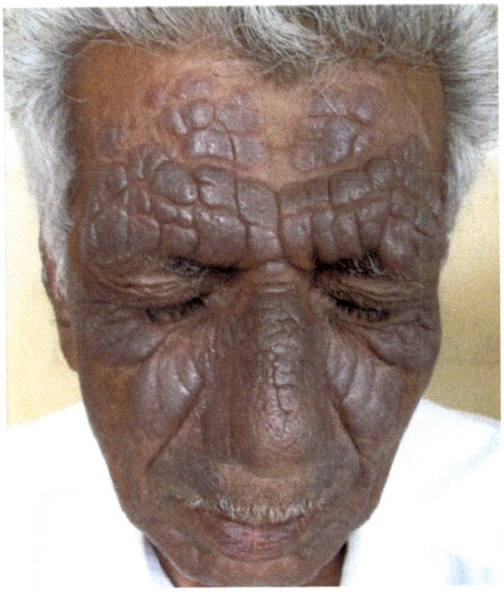

FIGURE 3.5 Pseudo-lymphomatous (actinic reticuloid) type in a 67-year-old farmer FST5.

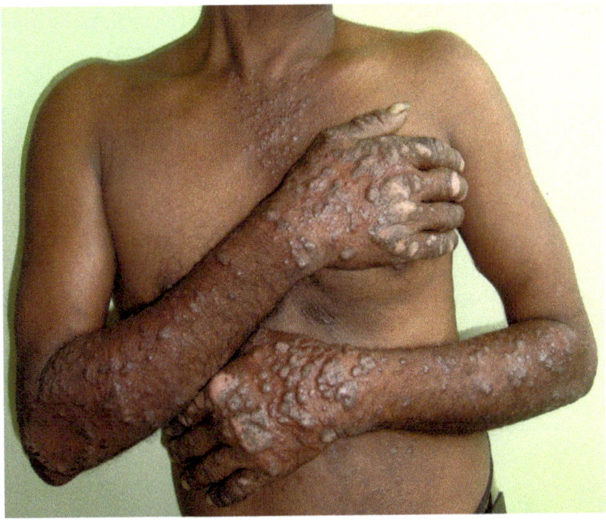

FIGURE 3.6 Nodular prurigo-like morphology in a 47-year-old farmer FST5.

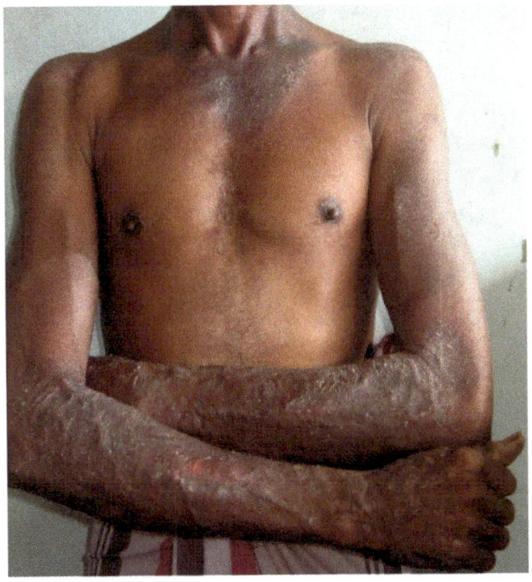

FIGURE 3.7 Eczematous dermatitis confined to sun-exposed areas in a 52-year-old postman FST5.

4
ALOPECIA AREATA

Introduction

Alopecia areata (AA) is a common autoimmune disorder attacking the hair and sometimes the nails. The hair loss is patchy and non-scarring; it commonly affects the scalp but may involve any hair-bearing region.

Epidemiology

Approximately 0.2% of the world population is affected, and the lifetime risk is 1.7%. There is no gender predilection. It often affects children, with a profound psychological impact on the quality of life. Familiarity is estimated at around 15% with variable expressivity.

Associated diseases

AA may be associated with atopic eczema, cataract, psoriasis, thyroid disease, and vitiligo. There are many other autoimmune phenomena, particularly autoantibodies against thyroid structure, cardiac muscle cells, stomach parietal cells, and hepatocytes; however, these autoantibodies usually remain clinically silent.

Clinical characteristics in light skin (Fitzpatrick skin types I–III)

AA may present in several different clinical forms with the patchy hair loss on the scalp being the most frequent one (Figures 4.1 and 4.2). These round hairless patches may merge to form polycyclic bald areas and finally involve the entire scalp hair (AA totalis). A special type is called ophiasis where the occipital hair is lost; this form is particularly chronic and recalcitrant. The hairless spots are white to pale in the beginning but tend to tan easily; however children, in particular, have to learn to protect their scalp against intense sun exposure. A rare form is alopecia areata diffusa where hair loss is not patchy; this type often goes unnoticed (AA incognita). Pigmented hair is more sensitive to the attack of the CD8-positive cells, and when hair regrows it is often non-pigmented before it slowly gets its normal color again. This is also the rationale for the so-called graying overnight when acute widespread AA causes loss of the pigmented hair and the white hair remains. AA may also affect the eyebrows, lashes, or beard region alone or in association with scalp involvement. Also, the body hair can be affected, usually in the course of universal hair loss (AA universalis), rarely without scalp involvement. Nail involvement occurs in about 10% and may present as rough nails (sandpaper nails, trachyonychia); the more extensive the alopecia the more likely are nail changes.

Clinical characteristics in dark skin (Fitzpatrick skin types IV–V)

AA manifestations in dark skin are the same as in white skin except for the absence of risks in sunlight exposure (Figures 4.3 to 4.6). The author has not seen any patients with AA totalis or AA universalis with increased incidence of skin cancers. Even though routine exposure to sunlight is the norm in tropical countries, sunbathing is not a custom in our setting.

Investigations

AA is diagnosed clinically in most cases, although the diagnosis of AA diffusa, as well as isolated hair loss in non-scalp areas, may require a biopsy.

Close inspection and trichoscopy of the bald spots may reveal black dots from so-called cadaver hairs. Exclamation sign hairs are short hairs that taper proximally.

Determination of thyroid values is generally recommended.

Skin biopsy for histopathology may be performed for confirmation: usually, a loose peribulbar lymphocytic infiltrate is seen around the deep hair follicle, the 'bee swarm' pattern. However, the histopathology is strongly dependent on the phase of the disease. Curiously, the histopathological pattern of hair and nail infiltrates are completely different, with an epitheliotropic lymphocytic infiltrate with exocytosis, spongiosis, and exoserosis in nails, which is not seen in the hair follicle.

Treatments

- Traditionally, high doses of systemic corticosteroids were given, but they were hardly able to positively influence the natural course. A breakthrough was achieved with topical immunotherapy via sensitization to an obligate contact allergen: First dinitrochlorobenzene, then squaric acid dibutyl ester, and finally diphenyl cyclopropenone which was shown in half-side experiments to be more effective than a placebo.
- Considerable progress has been achieved with the new biologics and small molecules. The pathogenesis of AA involves the breakdown of the immune privilege of the hair follicle (and nail matrix). Thus, Janus kinase (JAK) inhibitors can interfere with the JAK-mediated pathways. Of the many substances now on the market or under investigation, tofacitinib has been used as the first JAKi, followed by systemic ruxolitinib, baricitinib, ritlecitinib, and deuruxolitinib, as well as topical 2% tofacitinib ointment and 1% ruxolitinib ointment.

Further reading

Haneke E (2019). Nail disorders. In: Kang S, et al. (eds). *Fitzpatrick's Dermatology*, 9th ed. McGraw-Hill, New York; 91:1569–1609.

Muhammad A, Saleem S, Khan S, et al. (2024). Comparison of Efficacy of Autologous Platelet Rich Plasma Therapy with 5% Topical Minoxidil Spray in Treating Alopecia Areata: A Head-to-Head Assessment of Novel Approaches. *Cureus;*Jun7;16(6):e61878.

Otberg N, Shapiro J (2019). Alopecia areata. In: Kang S, et al. (eds). *Fitzpatrick's Dermatology*, 9th ed. McGraw-Hill, New York; 87:1517–1523.

Rudnicka L, Waskiel-Burnat A (2021). Disorders of Hair. In: Ranawaka RR, et al. (eds). *Atlas of Dermatoses in Pigmented Skin*. Springer, Singapore; 642–645.

DOI: 10.1201/9781003479512-4

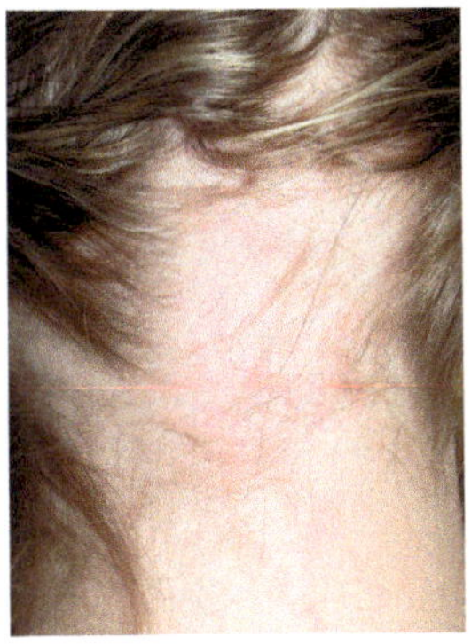

FIGURE 4.1 Alopecia areata occiput area FST1. (Courtesy Prof. Ian Coulson, UK.)

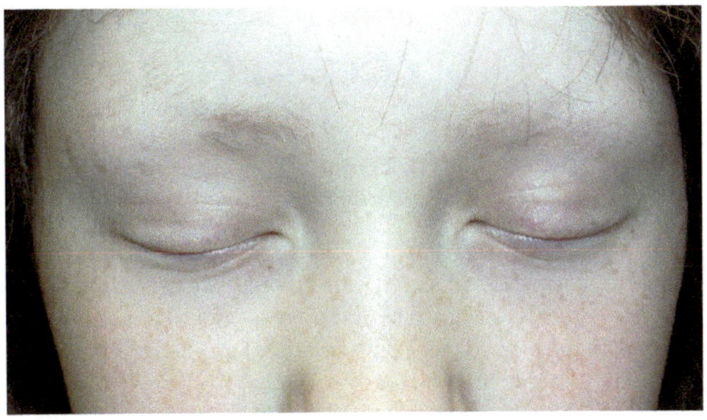

FIGURE 4.2 Alopecia areata Robert brow pattern FST1. (Courtesy Prof. Ian Coulson, UK.)

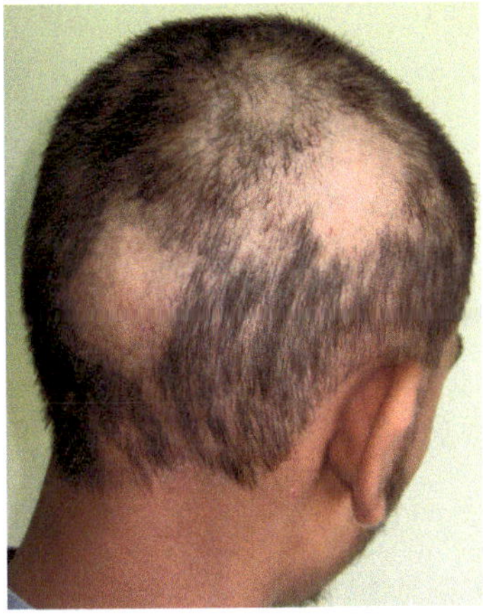

FIGURE 4.3 Alopecia areata in a 29-year-old man FST5. Hair pulling disorder is a differential diagnosis in easily accessible sites.

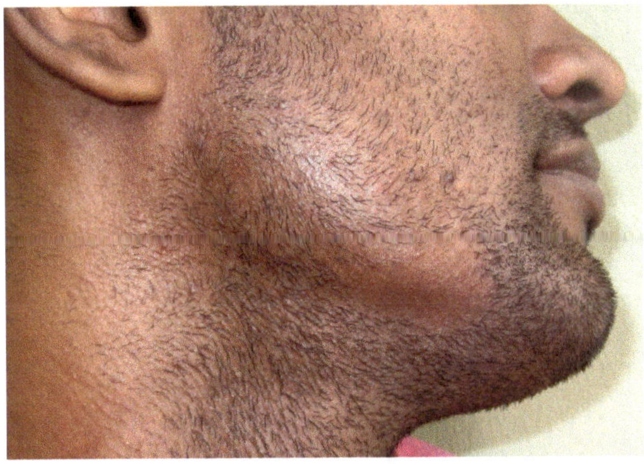

FIGURE 4.4 Alopecia areata in beard area FST5.

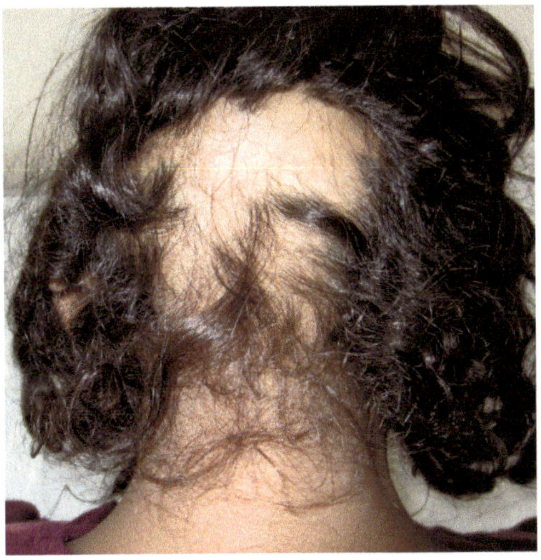

FIGURE 4.5 Alopecia areata in occiput (ophiasis pattern) in a 9-year-old girl FST5.

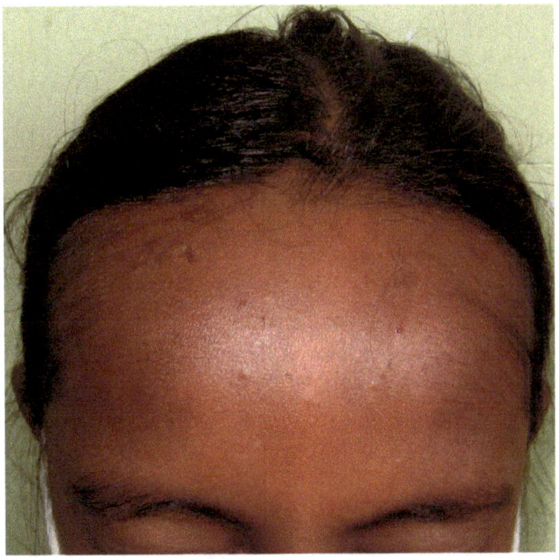

FIGURE 4.6 Alopecia areata reverse ophiasis pattern in an 11-year-old girl FST5.

5
CENTRAL CENTRIFUGAL CICATRICIAL ALOPECIA

Introduction

First described as hot comb alopecia over 50 years ago, central centrifugal cicatricial alopecia (CCCA) is a form of scarring alopecia that is mainly reported in women of African ethnicity. The etiopathogenesis of CCCA is unknown; however, it is assumed that genetic factors, heat, traction, and straightening chemicals work together in a detrimental way for the hair follicle. It begins as a single focus of cicatricial alopecia over the vertex of the scalp that gradually spreads outward in a centrifugal pattern but remains unifocal. The alopecia is slowly progressive and symmetrical. It is predominately centered on the crown with forward progression. There may be clinical evidence of inflammation at the advancing margin. The skin is smooth, shiny, non-inflamed, and often soft and supple to the touch. Usually asymptomatic, unusual sensations, such as pins and needles, itching, or tenderness may occur. The condition eventually burns out spontaneously.

Epidemiology

Almost exclusively in women (97%), with a median age of 46 years.

Associated diseases

None reported. These women are otherwise healthy and normal.

Clinical characteristics in light skin (Fitzpatrick skin types I–III)

CCCA is exceedingly rare in white people, with only 1.6% of 185 patients and no males at all.

Clinical characteristics in dark skin (Fitzpatrick skin types IV–V)

CCCA is not uncommon in our settings (Figures 5.1 and 5.2). It is reported only in women, of 30–45 years. They present to us with hair loss on the central scalp. On examination, scarring alopecia is noticed. The exact etiology of this scarring alopecia is not identified. Women in our culture do not use hot combs or have traumatic hair care practices. It is mostly asymptomatic, but unusual sensations, such as pins and needles, itching, or tenderness are reported by some. The skin is smooth, shiny, and non-inflamed. These women are not followed up long-term, therefore, progression is unknown.

Important differential diagnoses are scarring traction alopecia and pseudopelade of Brocq.

Investigations

Scarring is noticed in skin biopsies. But detailed histology on hair or hair root was not studied.

Published data show superficial perivascular and perifollicular lymphocytic infiltrate in active areas. Sebaceous glands are lost, but eccrine glands are spared. Hair follicle destruction is severe and widespread, leaving prominent concentric lamellar fibrosis.

Treatments

Currently, there is no definitive cure for the disease; however, multiple management options are available.

- Topical and intralesional steroids and tetracycline antibiotics are the mainstays of treatment.
- Refractory cases may be considered for hair transplantation.
- Emerging therapies using platelet-rich plasma, botanical formulas, and cosmetic procedures have shown promising results for the future management of CCCA.

Further reading

Alchorne MMA, Conceição KDC, Barraza LL, et al. (2024). Dermatology in Black Skin. *An Bras Dermatol*;99(3):327–341.

Fatima SZ (2024). Central Centrifugal Cicatricial Alopecia: A Deeper Insight into the Disease. *Wien Med Wochenschr*; Nov:174(15–16):323–327.

George EA, Matthews C, Roche FC, et al. (2023). Beyond the Hot Comb: Updates in Epidemiology, Pathogenesis, and Treatment of Central Centrifugal Cicatricial Alopecia from 2011 to 2021. *Am J Clin Dermatol*;24(1):81–88.

Miteva M, Tosti A (2014). Dermatoscopic Features of Central Centrifugal Cicatricial Alopecia. *J Am Acad Dermatol*;71(3):443–449.

Rathnayake D (2021). Trichoscopy: Dermoscopy Hair. In: Ranawaka RR, et al. (eds). *Atlas of Dermatoses in Pigmented Skin*. Springer, Singapore; 663–722.

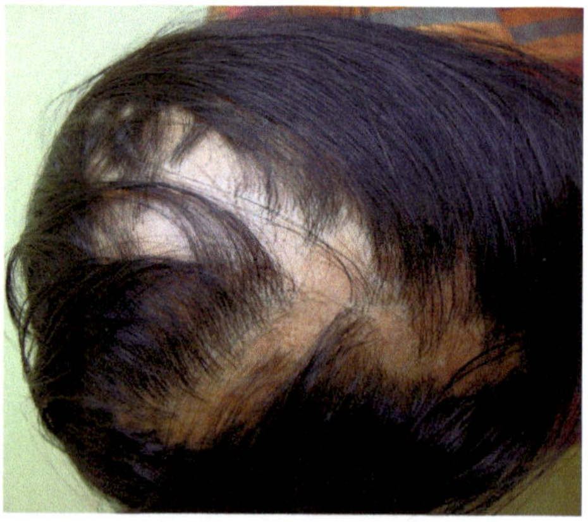

FIGURE 5.1 A 29-year-old woman with central centrifugal cicatricial alopecia FST5.

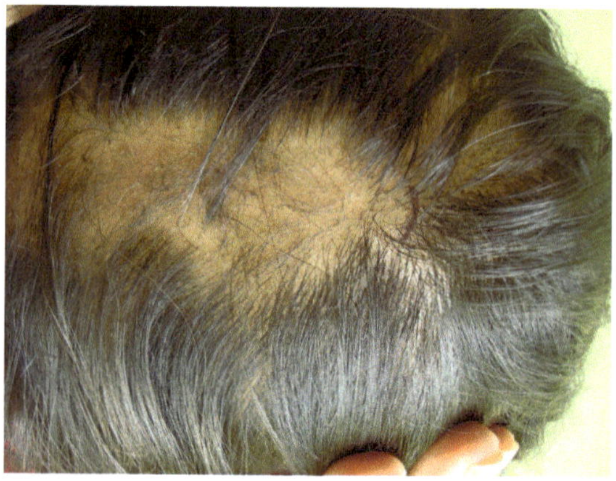

FIGURE 5.2 A 32-year-old woman with central centrifugal cicatricial alopecia FST5.

DOI: 10.1201/9781003479512-5

6
LICHEN AMYLOIDOSUS OR PAPULAR AMYLOIDOSIS

Introduction

The key feature of amyloidosis is the extracellular deposition of autologous proteins as morphologically characteristic amyloid fibrils. Amyloid can originate from various precursor proteins.

Amyloidosis may be acquired or hereditary. It is subclassified as:

1. *Primary localized cutaneous amyloidosis (PLCA)* – deposition is limited to the papillary dermis.
2. *Secondary localized cutaneous amyloidosis (SLCA)* – following skin tumors, photochemotherapy (PUVA) therapy or discoid lupus erythematosus (DLE).
3. *Primary systemic amyloidosis with cutaneous involvement* – deposition in deeper skin layers and in blood vessels.
4. *Cutaneous amyloidosis due to other systemic diseases* – presents with petechiae, ecchymosis, and non-healing ulcers.

Macular, papular, and mixed maculopapular PLCA account for the vast majority of localized cutaneous amyloidosis, whereas nodular (tumefactive) PLCA is very rare or may go unnoticed since it is asymptomatic and skin-colored. For cutaneous amyloidoses, pruritus is a typical symptom.

Epidemiology

Rare in Europe but more frequent in South Asia, South-East Asia, China, and South America. Both lichenoid and macular types are more common in women.

Associated diseases

Lichenoid PLCA is associated with the Koebner phenomenon.

Clinical characteristics in light skin (Fitzpatrick skin types I–III)

In light-skinned people, lichen amyloidosus is a fairly characteristic skin disease with insidious development of hard, follicular-appearing grouped papules predominantly over the shins. The involved skin is diffusely hyperpigmented and feels harder. Itching may be prominent. As the amyloid is of keratinocytic origin, rubbing and scratching will aggravate the condition (Figure 6.1).

Clinical characteristics in dark skin (Fitzpatrick skin types IV–V)

Lichen amyloidosis is a fairly common skin issue in our settings (Figure 6.2). Firm papules with blackish lichenoid glossiness that are intensely itchy are the most common presentation. Mostly middle-aged women seek treatment, but it is also not uncommon in middle-aged men. In most cases, it starts on the lower legs on the lateral aspects around the ankle, and gradually spreads upward, surrounding the whole leg. In extensive cases, they may appear on the extensor surfaces of the arms and forearms. Most women report a history of using rough clothes, pumice stones, or brushes to clean the skin on affected areas before and after the lesions.

Investigations

The most important diagnostic step is a lesion skin biopsy.

In papular (lichen) and macular cutaneous amyloidosis, amyloid is found in the papillary dermis directly below the basal epidermal layer. It stains light blue with toluidin blue and alkaline fuchsin, in H&E stain it appears as amorphous masses of eosinophilia (pink). Periodic acid–Schiff (PAS) is positive. Kresyl violet is metachromatic.

Using Congo red, amyloid exhibits characteristic apple-green birefringence when viewed under polarized light, a phenomenon called dichroism. Thioflavin T staining viewed under fluorescence microscopy with a blue light filter shows the bright yellow to green staining of amyloid whereas, when viewed with ultraviolet excitation, the fluorescence is bright light blue. This is actually the amyloid-specific fluorescence.

Treatments

- Antipruritic treatment for all to prevent itchiness and further precipitating deposition.
- Topical steroids under occlusion (occlusive dressings) or intralesional corticosteroid injections are the classic treatments.
- Topical potent steroids with salicylic acid combination give good results.
- In extensive cases, phototherapy (narrow-band UVB) and PUVA are helpful.
- Ablative CO_2 lasers
- Recently, alitretinoin has been used successfully.

Further reading

Ahramiyanpour N, Akbari Z, Sarasyabi MS, et al. (2022). The Therapeutic Role of Lasers in Primary Localized Cutaneous Amyloidosis: A Systematic Review. *Lasers Med Sci*;37(2):799–813.

Schreml S (2024). Cutaneous Amyloidoses. In: Griffiths C, et al. (eds). *Rook's Textbook of Dermatology*, 10th ed. John Wiley & Sons Ltd., UK; 56.6.

Tietze JK, Heppt MV, Flaig MJ, et al. (2016). Successful Treatment of Lichen Amyloidosus with Oral Alitretinoin. *J Eur Acad Dermatol Venereol*;30(5):884–885.

DOI: 10.1201/9781003479512-6

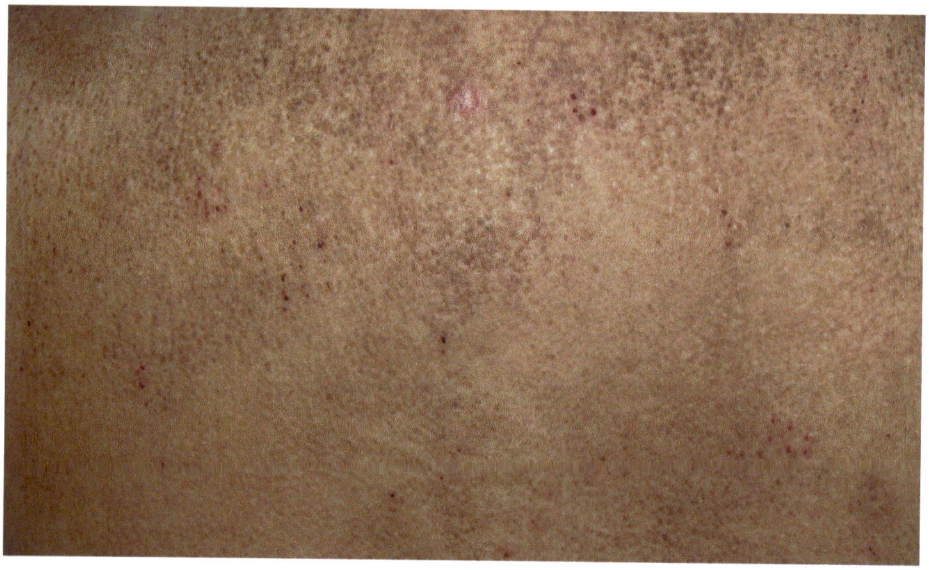

FIGURE 6.1 Lichen amyloidosis at the back of the upper trunk FST2. (Courtesy Prof. Ian Coulson, UK.)

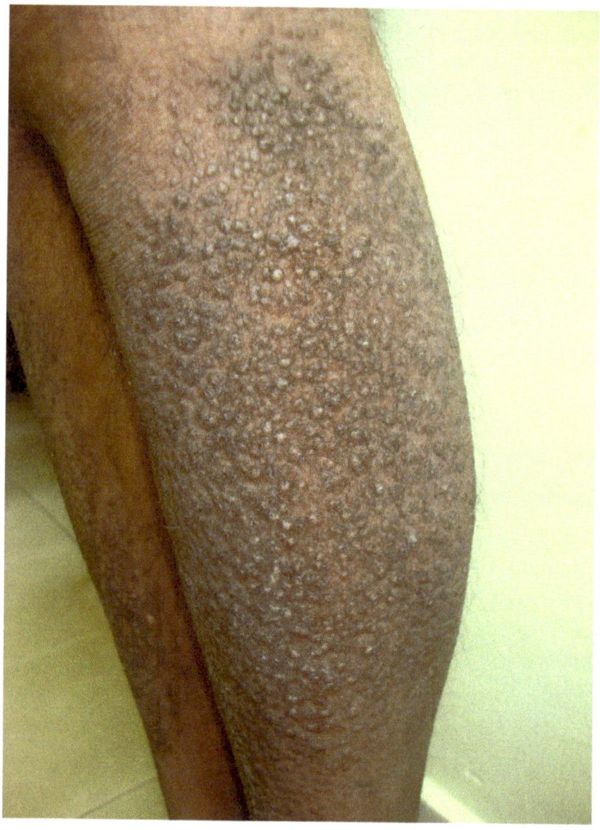

FIGURE 6.2 Lichen amyloidosis in a 40-year-old woman's legs FST5.

7
MACULAR AMYLOIDOSIS

Introduction

This is a common primary localized cutaneous amyloidosis (PLCA).

Epidemiology

Rare in Europe but more frequent in South Asia, South-East Asia, China, and South America. Both lichen and macular types are more common in women.

Associated diseases

Associations between macular PLCA, multiple endocrine neoplasia 2a (MEN2a), and primary biliary cirrhosis have been reported.

Clinical characteristics in light skin (Fitzpatrick skin types I–III)

Macular amyloidosis is a rare event in Caucasians, usually manifesting as slightly infiltrated and pigmented plaques (Figure 7.1). The diagnosis is made by histopathology.

Clinical characteristics in dark skin (Fitzpatrick skin types IV–V)

This is a very common skin condition among young to middle-aged women in our setting (Figures 7.2 and 7.3). Similar to lichen amyloidosus, most women give a history of using rough clothes, pumice stones, or brushes to clean the skin on affected areas before and after the start of the lesions. Macular amyloidosis presents as vaguely demarcated hyperpigmented, blackish, or dark brown macules on the extensor surfaces of the upper arms, upper back of the trunk, and anterior thighs. It is mostly asymptomatic but can be mildly itchy. A distinctive 'ripple' pattern is characteristic. Most patients present due to cosmetic concerns.

Investigations

This is diagnosed clinically.
If doubtful histopathology is obtained from the lesional skin.

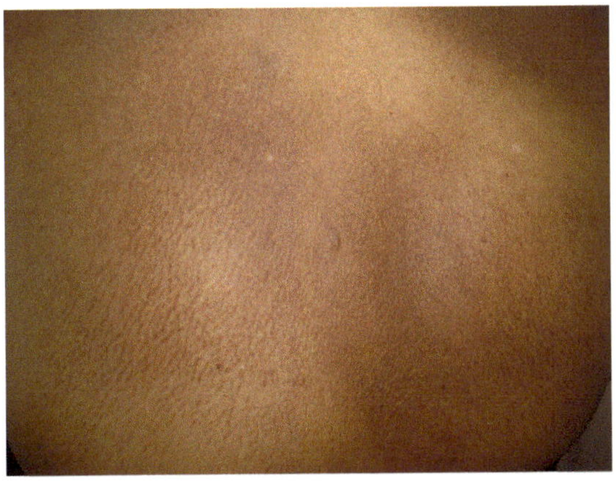

FIGURE 7.2 Macular amyloidosis in a 45-year-old woman's upper back FST5. Note the distinctive 'rippled' pattern.

Treatments

- Topical diluted corticosteroids over months give favorable results.
- Advice to stop rubbing is important.
- Laser therapy: Both fractional Nd:YAG laser alone and in combination with fractional erbium:YAG laser therapy have shown promising effects considering the reduction in melanin content. Carbon dioxide (CO_2) laser also gives promising effects.

Further reading

Ahramiyanpour N, Akbari Z, Sarasyabi MS, et al. (2022). The Therapeutic Role of Lasers in Primary Localized Cutaneous Amyloidosis: A Systematic Review. *Lasers Med Sci.* Mar;37(2):799–813.

Esmat SM, Fawzi MM, Gawdat HI, et al. (2015). Efficacy of Different Modes of Fractional CO_2 Laser in the Treatment of Primary Cutaneous Amyloidosis: A Randomized Clinical Trial. *Lasers Surg Med*;47(5):388–895.

Gakkhar A, Mehendale AM, Mehendale S (2024). An Interesting Case of Macular Amyloidosis with No Significant Etiology. *Cureus*;Mar 16(3):e56248.

Rajendiran P (2021). Hyperpigmentary Disorders. In: Ranawaka RR, et al. (eds). *Atlas of Dermatoses in Pigmented Skin.* Springer, Singapore; 860–861.

Schreml S (2024). Cutaneous Amyloidoses. In: Griffiths C, et al. (eds). *Rook's Textbook of Dermatology,* 10th ed. John Wiley & Sons Ltd., UK; 56.6.

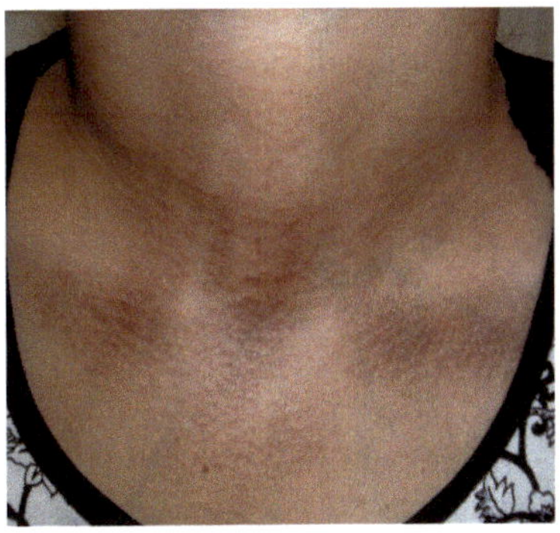

FIGURE 7.1 Macular amyloidosis in anterior chest FST3. (Courtesy Prof. Ian Coulson, UK.)

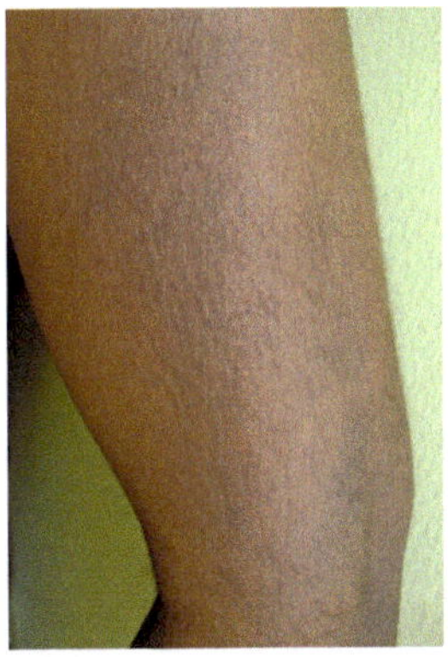

FIGURE 7.3 Macular amyloidosis in a 40-year-old woman's extensor surface of upper arm FST5. Note the distinctive 'rippled' pattern.

DOI: 10.1201/9781003479512-7

8
CHERRY ANGIOMAS

Introduction

Very common, benign, cherry-red papules are seen in the skin due to abnormal capillary proliferations. They begin to appear at the age of 25 years and increase in number with age. Cherry angioma, cherry hemangioma, Campbell de Morgan spots, and senile angiomas are synonyms.

Epidemiology

Common in old age. Equal in both sexes.

Associated diseases

Reported to appear during pregnancy.

Exposure to chemicals such as bromides, solvents, and mustard gas has been associated with the development of cherry angiomas.

Clinical characteristics in light skin (Fitzpatrick skin types I–III)

Senile or cherry angiomas are extremely common (prevalence 50–75%) and present as small dome-shaped papules of intense purple-red color (Figures 8.1 and 8.2). The earlier the first one appears, the more the patient will develop over time, so that many patients may present with hundreds if not thousands of them distributed all over the trunk and the proximal part of the extremities. They remain asymptomatic but may cause cosmetic embarrassment. Treatment is easy (different lasers), although only needed if they bleed.

Clinical characteristics in dark skin (Fitzpatrick skin types IV–V)

Cherry angiomas are not notable in darker skin and are mostly seen among fairer-skinned individuals (Figure 8.3). Therefore, this is not a common complaint among our patients.

Round to oval, dome-shaped papules and pinpoint macules vary from less than 1 mm in diameter to several millimeters in diameter; single or multiple lesions on the upper trunk and arms. In darker skin, these appear blackish red rather than bright red.

Investigations

This is diagnosed clinically.

Treatments

- No treatment is needed in most cases; reassurance is adequate.
- For lesions that are bleeding or cosmetically troubling, treatment options include shave excision, hyfrecation, cryotherapy, and a variety of different lasers, including pulsed dye laser and intense pulsed light.
- The pulsed dye laser has extremely selective absorption by blood, which means that it does not penetrate deep enough for these angiomas; that's why non-selective lasers are better for this indication.

Further reading

Goldsmith PG, George C (2024). Dermatoses Resulting from Disorders of the Veins and Arteries. In: Griffiths C, et al. (eds). *Rook's Textbook of Dermatology*, 10th ed. John Wiley & Sons Ltd., UK; 101.12.

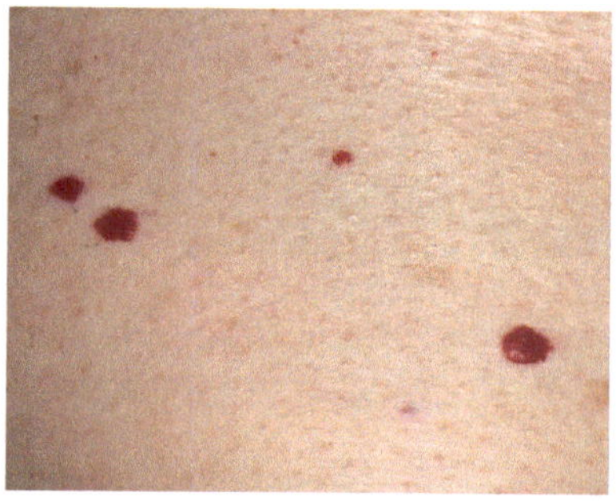

FIGURE 8.1 Campbell de Morgan spots/cherry angiomas FST1. (Courtesy Dr. Richard Ashton, UK.)

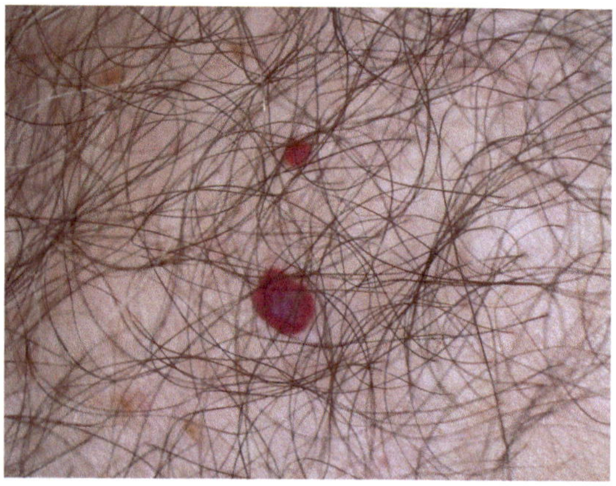

FIGURE 8.2 Campbell de Morgan spots FST1. (Courtesy Prof. Ian Coulson, UK.)

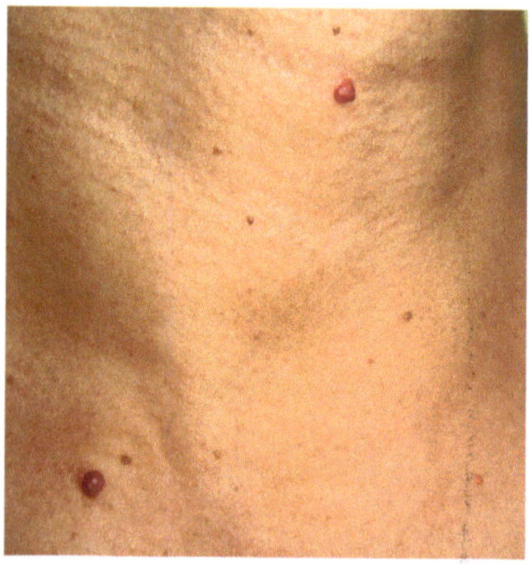

FIGURE 8.3 Multiple cherry angiomas in a fairer-skinned woman FST4.

DOI: 10.1201/9781003479512-8

9
ASHY DERMATOSIS

Introduction

Ashy dermatosis is an idiopathic hypermelanotic disorder characterized by bluish-gray macules, mostly symmetrical, usually affecting the face, arms, neck, and trunk in healthy individuals. Dark-colored individuals are most affected in their second decade of life. Mucosa is rarely involved.

Its etiology is unknown; however, drug ingestion, infection, and genetic factors have been suggested to elicit ashy dermatosis. No gold standard treatments have been established yet.

Epidemiology

Most frequent in young adults, but can occur at any age. Mostly reported in Central and South America, South Asia, or East Asia.

Associated diseases

None reported.

Clinical characteristics in light skin (Fitzpatrick skin types I–III)

Light-skinned individuals have a much lower risk of developing pigmentation after inflammation (Figure 9.1). Skin types 1 and 2 are usually spared. Bluish-gray macules are seen on the trunk, neck, limbs, and rarely in the face. They are commonly symptomless. A pre-pigmentary stage has been claimed but is virtually never seen.

Histopathology shows very mild pigmentary incontinence. Whether there is a relation to pigmented lichen planus is not clear.

Clinical characteristics in dark skin (Fitzpatrick skin types IV–V)

Author has never seen an inflammatory phase with erythema in darker skin patients. Therefore, ashy dermatosis is a more appropriate term for our brown-skinned patients. This is rather common in both children and adults of any age in our setting (Figures 9.2 to 9.4). They present with ashy-gray macules on the trunk, neck, face, or limbs, initially discrete macules that later coalesce into larger areas of ashy-gray, shiny hyperpigmentation. Mostly asymptomatic.

Investigations

This is diagnosed clinically.

Skin biopsy for histopathology is performed for confirmation; the epidermis contains much pigment, and there is pigmentary incontinence. The dermal vessels are sleeved with an infiltrate of lymphocytes and histiocytes, and there is pigmentary incontinence and many melanophages in the deep dermis.

Treatments

- There is no consistently effective treatment.
- Diluted topical corticosteroids have been used with favorable response in some patients, lightening the patches. In most patients, the pigmentation is persistent, with a tendency to extend gradually over years.
- Drug of choice is clofazimine 100 mg/day for 3 months in inflammatory cases (response rate of 66–87%). However, clofazimine itself has a certain risk to cause pigmentation in inflamed skin.

Further reading

Nguyen K, Khachemoune A (2019). Ashy dermatosis: A review. *Dermatol Online J*;25(5):13030/qt44f462s8.

Rajendiran P (2021). Hyperpigmentary Disorders. In: Ranawaka RR, et al. (eds). *Atlas of Dermatoses in Pigmented Skin*. Springer, Singapore; 851–853.

Ranawaka RR (2021) Facial melanosis. In: Ranawaka RR, et al. (eds). *Atlas of Dermatoses in Pigmented Skin*. Springer, Singapore; 808–811.

Rutnin S, Udompanich S, Pratumchart N, et al. (2019). Ashy Dermatosis and Lichen Planus Pigmentosus: The Histopathological Differences. *Biomed Res Int*. 2019;2019:5829185.

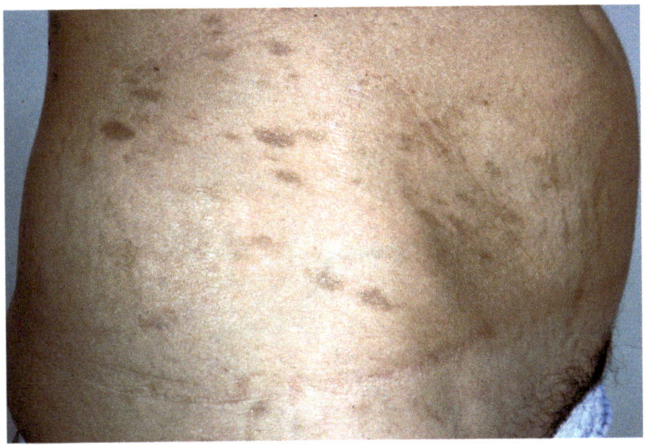

FIGURE 9.1 Ashy dermatoses FST1. (Courtesy Dr. Richard Ashton, UK.)

DOI: 10.1201/9781003479512-9

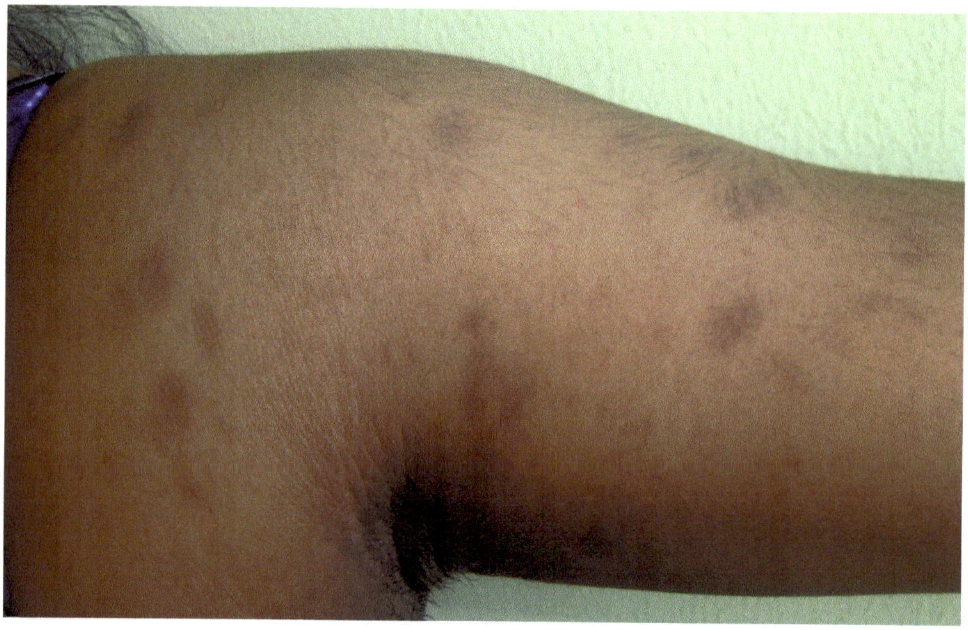

FIGURE 9.2 Ashy dermatoses in a 21-year-old woman FST5.

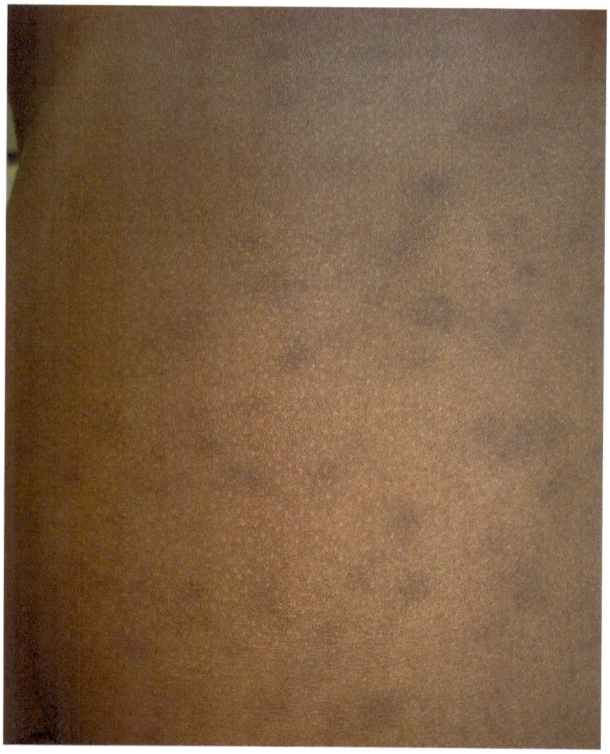

FIGURE 9.3 Ashy dermatoses on the trunk FST5.

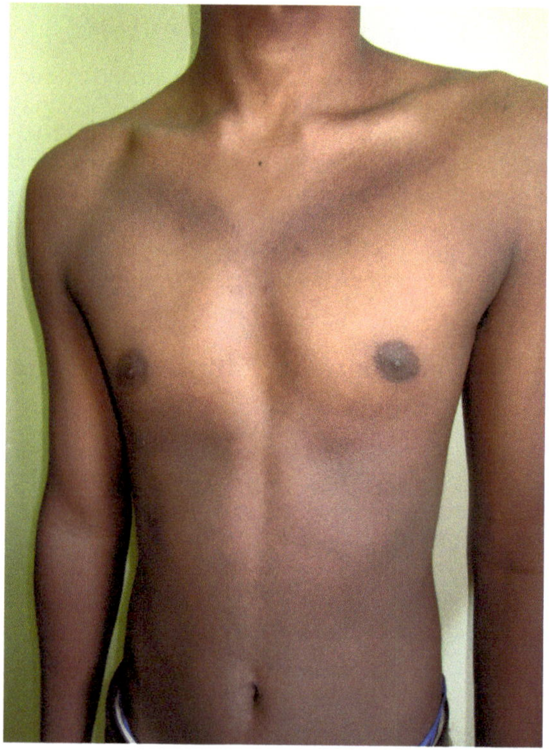

FIGURE 9.4 Generalized ashy dermatoses on the trunk, limbs and face in a 17-year-old boy FST5. His normal skin color is seen in the upper torso.

10
BASAL CELL CARCINOMA

Introduction

Basal cell carcinoma (BCC) is the most common human cancer. Approximately 80% of BCCs occur on the head and neck, and clinical diagnosis is relatively straightforward.

Epidemiology

Worldwide, the incidence of BCC varies widely, with the highest rates in Australia (>1000/100,000 person years) and the lowest rates in parts of Africa (<1/100,000 person years). The incidence increases with advancing age, with almost equal sex incidence.

Associated diseases

Higher incidence of BCC is detected in immunosuppressed patients, transplant recipients, and albinos. Exposure to inorganic arsenic through drinking water, UVB phototherapy, and ionizing radiation are high-risk factors.

Clinical characteristics in light skin (Fitzpatrick skin types I–III)

BCC is the most frequent malignancy in light-skinned persons (Figures 10.1 to 10.8) (except when you count actinic keratoses as early squamous cell carcinoma [SCC] then this would be the most frequent), it outnumbers in fact all other carcinomas taken together. In general, BCCs are slow growing tumors with a high potential to infiltrate but rarely to metastasize. Subclinical growth is frequent, the longer it exists and the bigger its diameter the bigger is its true extension.

There are many different clinical and even more histopathologically different types.

- ***Nodular BCC***: This is a skin-colored to slightly yellowish small papule that insidiously grows to the size of several centimeters in diameter. It may enlarge asymmetrically to take on a multinodular appearance. Cystic degeneration in the tumor mass may lead to superficial erosion and ulceration with a subsequent decrease in size, often erroneously taken by the patient as spontaneous healing. At its margin, it may show small pearly papules with a transparent appearance, allowing the characteristic arborizing vessels to be seen. If untreated, it may reach an enormous size.
- ***Superficial BCC***, also called ***truncal skin BCC***, is very common. It presents as a patch or flat plaque with a pearly margin and a reddish center in which small crusts may be seen as a sign of tiny ulcerations. They often occur in multitude or may reach diameters of more than 20 cm. In skin type III with brown eyes, there may be some pigment in the marginal tiny papules, which is virtually never seen in blue-eyed individuals.
- ***Morpheic, sclerodermiform, or cicatricial BCC*** is a characteristic tumor of the face, particularly the nose and temple. It usually grows insidiously for years and is diagnosed late. Clinically, it appears as an infiltrated skin- to ivory-colored firm plaque with ill-defined borders. Small ulcers are a late sign.
- ***Fibroepithelial tumor of Pinkus*** is mainly localized in the lumbar region. It has a plaque-like early stage which can be identified as such by histopathology. Finally, it grows as an exophytic lesion resembling a giant acrochordon. It runs a benign course but may become invasive and ulcerate after years.
- Particular ***BCCs may ulcerate*** after a certain time and reach deep structures; then it is called ulcus rodens. This type is often seen around and threatening the eyes. BCCs invading the bone down and through the calvarium are called **ulcus terebrans.**
- ***Advanced BCC*** is a term for neglected BCCs with horrifying extension and tissue destruction. Their occurrence is now less frequent, but they still continue to exist, predominantly in remote mountainous regions and in mentally debilitated individuals. Their size may render them inoperable.
- ***Metastasizing BCC*** is a rare event and was denied for a long time. It has to be differentiated from extension *per continuitatem* to lymph nodes and other underlying structures.

Histopathology of all BCC types is diagnostic. Margin control is recommended.

Clinical characteristics in dark skin (Fitzpatrick skin types IV–V)

Even though BCC is the most common skin carcinoma in pigmented skin, BCC and other skin cancers are not common in dark skin. All types of BCCs in dark skin are pigmented and appear black (Figures 10.9 to 10.13).

Investigations

This is diagnosed clinically and confirmed histopathologically; islands of atypical proliferation of basaloid cells in the dermis are observed.

Treatments

Both tumor (clinical and histological nature, size, and site) and patient factors determine the choice of treatment for BCC. Other factors dictating the choice of treatment include local experience and availability of treatments, which may indirectly depend upon the cost.

- Surgery is the mainstay of treatment for BCC in most countries with fair-skinned populations. This allows the diagnosis to be made with certainty and helps control the excision margins for complete resection.
- Excision with margin (4–5 mm surgical margin).
- Mohs micrographic surgery.
- 'Blind methods' are second line.
- Topical imiquimod.
- Photodynamic therapy.

DOI: 10.1201/9781003479512-10

- Curettage and electrodesiccation.
- Cryosurgery – the application of liquid nitrogen.
- Superficial and electron beam radiotherapy.
- Carbon dioxide laser.

The risk of recurrence after treatment is highest in tumors with aggressive growth patterns, in tumors located in the facial H-zone and in recurrent tumors. The optimal treatment of high-risk BCCs is surgical excision or radiotherapy.

Further reading

Bertozzi N, Simonacci F, Greco MP, et al. (2019). Single Center Evidence for the Treatment of Basal Cell Carcinoma of the Head and Neck. *Acta Biomed*;90(1):77–82.

Fukumoto T, Fukumoto R, Oka M, et al. (2019). Comparing Treatments for Basal Cell Carcinoma in Terms of Long-Term Treatment-Failure: A Network Meta-Analysis. *J Eur Acad Dermatol Venereol*;33(11):2050–2057.

Glud M, Omland SH, Gniadecki R (2016). Basal Cell Carcinoma Surgery. *Ugeskr Laeger*;178(20):V07150603.

Rasulić LG, Jovanović MD (2014). Surgical Treatment and Dilemmas in the Treatment of Basal Cell Carcinomas with Intracranial Propagation. *Vojnosanit Pregl*;71(11):1045–1048.

Salavastru C, Tiplica GS, Fritz K (2018). Laser Treatment of Basal Cell Carcinoma. *Hautarzt.*;69(1):10–16.

Tourli I, Langner D, Haroske G, et al. (2016). Basal Cell Carcinoma of the Head-and-Neck Region: A Single Center Analysis of 1,750 Tumors. *Georgian Med News*;2016(250):33–39.

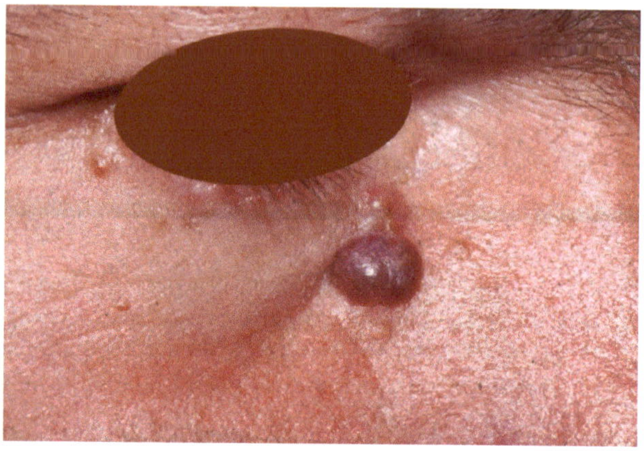

FIGURE 10.1 Nodulocystic basal cell carcinoma on the lower lid FST1. (Courtesy Prof. Eckart Haneke, Germany.)

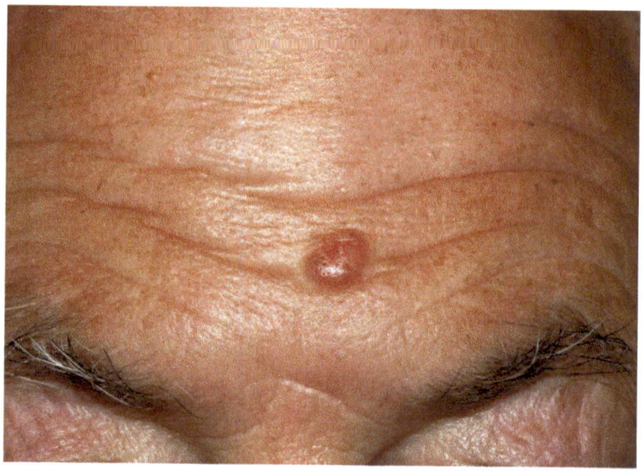

FIGURE 10.2 Nodular basal cell carcinoma on the forehead FST3. (Courtesy Prof. Ian Coulson, UK.)

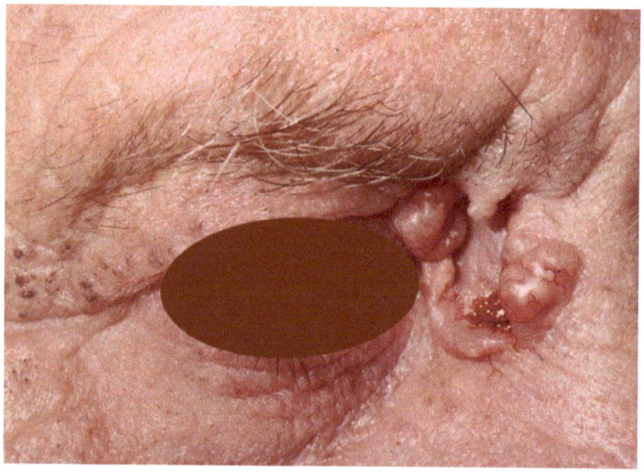

FIGURE 10.3 Basal cell carcinoma of the inner canthus. Note the actinic comedones at the canthus lateralis. (Courtesy Prof. Eckart Haneke, Germany.)

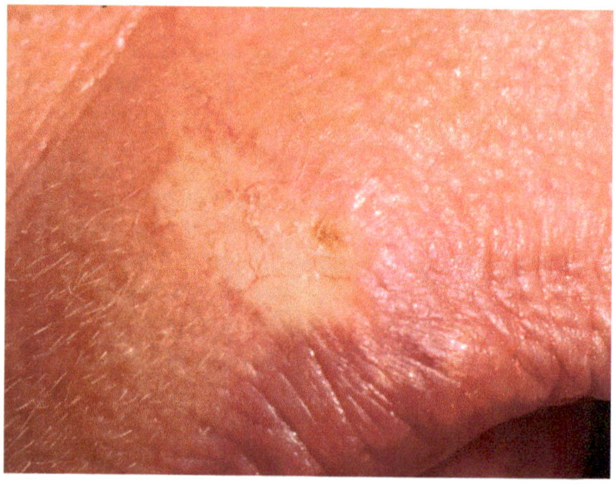

FIGURE 10.4 Morpheaform basal cell carcinoma on the upper lip FST1. (Courtesy Prof. Ian Coulson, UK.)

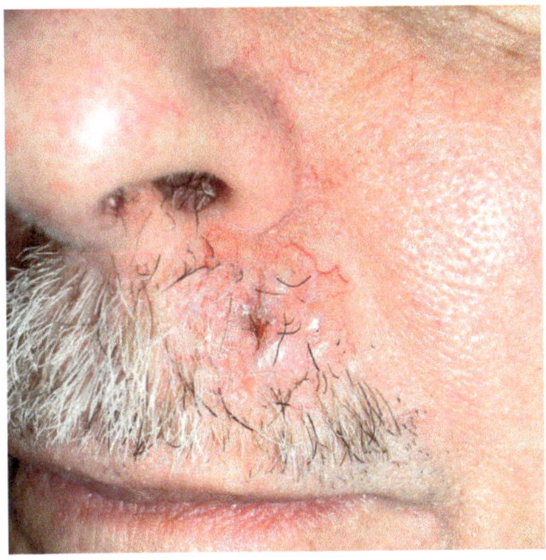

FIGURE 10.5 Morpheaform basal cell carcinoma on the upper lip FST1. (Courtesy Prof. Ian Coulson, UK.)

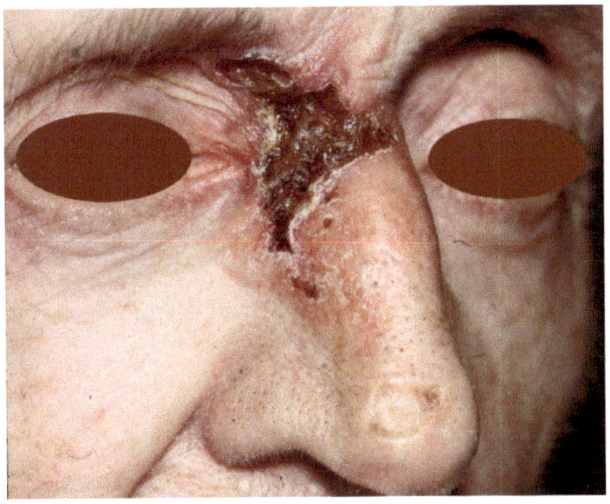

FIGURE 10.6 Large basal cell carcinoma on the bridge of the nose and inner canthus with subclinical extension to the tip of the nose. (Courtesy Prof. Eckart Haneke, Germany.)

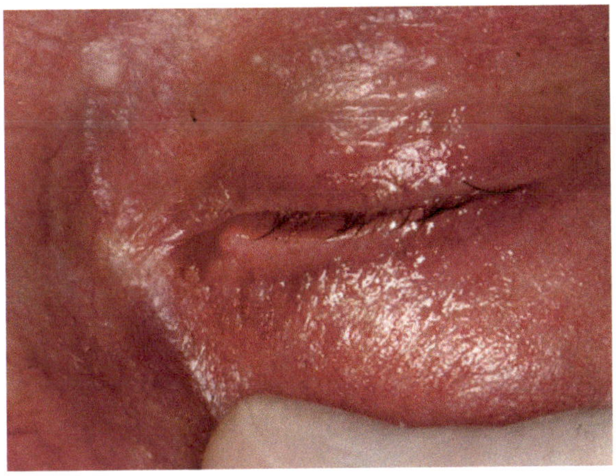

FIGURE 10.7 Ulcerating basal cell carcinoma medial of the punctum lacrimale. (Courtesy Prof. Eckart Haneke, Germany.)

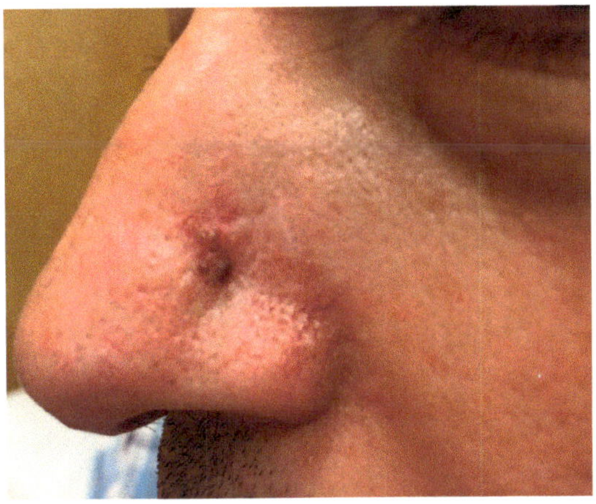

FIGURE 10.8 Basal cell carcinoma in FST 2. (Courtesy Prof. Eckart Haneke, Germany.)

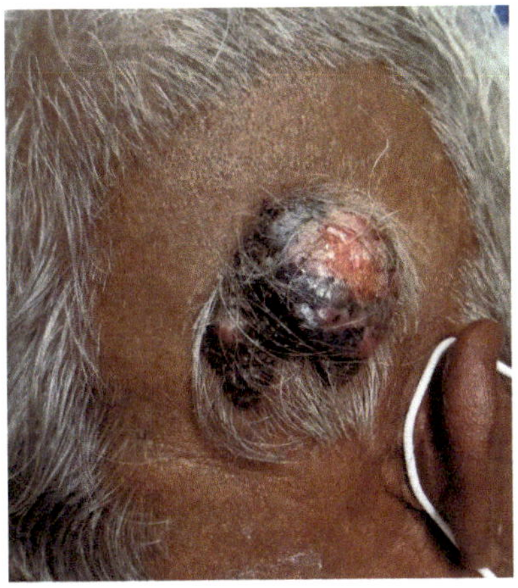

FIGURE 10.9 Nodular basal cell carcinoma arising on an untreated nevus sebaceous in an 86-year-old man FST5.

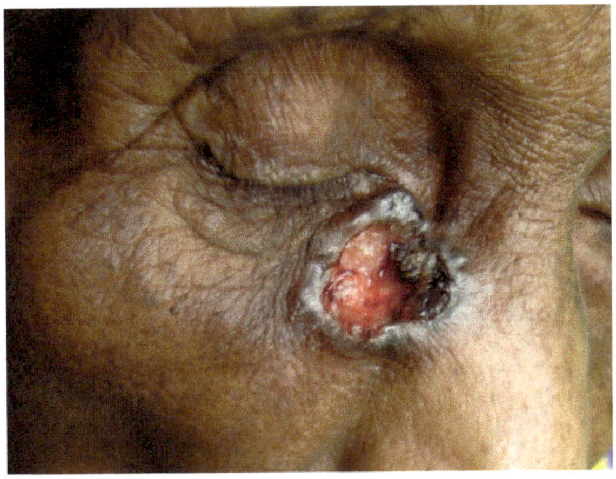

FIGURE 10.10 Ulcerated basal cell carcinoma of the inner canthus in an 85-year-old woman.

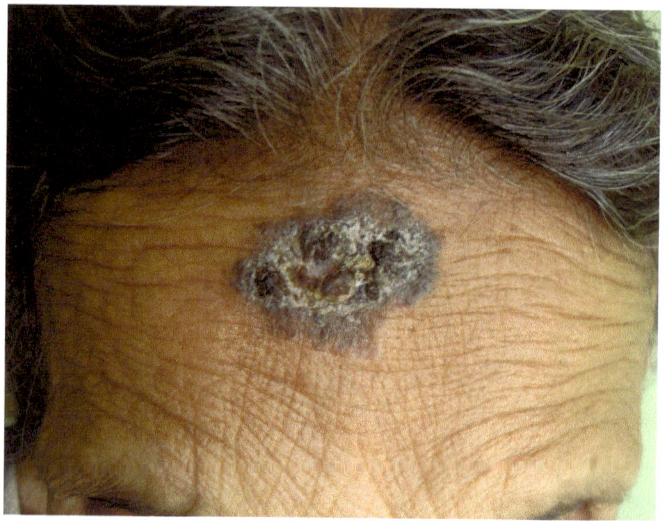

FIGURE 10.11 Morpheic basal cell carcinoma in a 76-year-old woman.

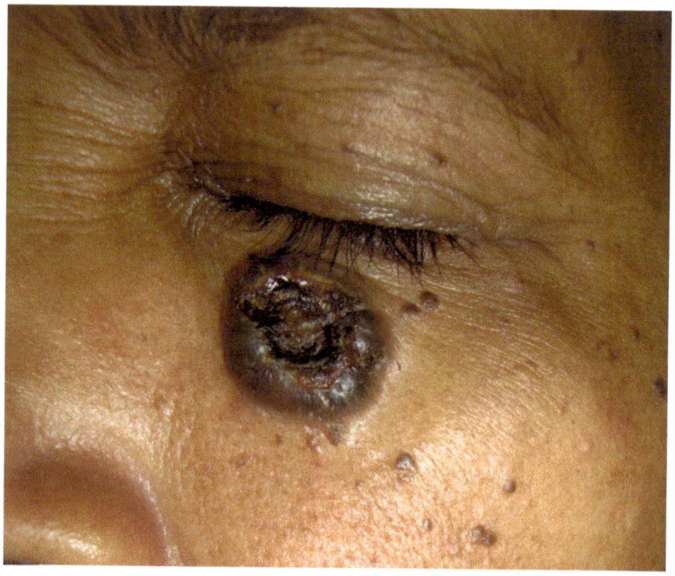

FIGURE 10.12 Rodent ulcer in a 39-year-old woman. She has multiple dermatosis papulosa nigra too.

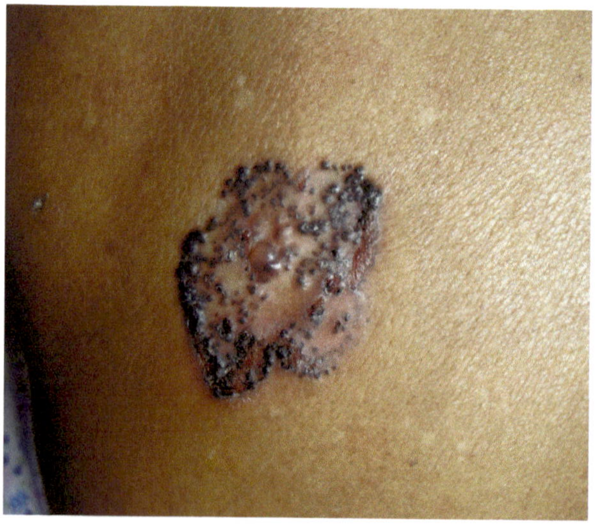

FIGURE 10.13 Superficial basal cell carcinoma on the trunk in a 73-year-old man FST5.

11
BECKER NEVUS

Introduction

Becker nevus (or Becker melanosis), a relatively common hyperpigmented, hairy epidermal nevus, is a hamartoma (hamartoma is a local malformation made up of an abnormal mixture of cells and tissue). It is only rarely congenital, with the majority of lesions appearing in the first two decades. It appears classically at puberty and slowly enlarges in size up to 25 years of age, then remains static. It is frequently, but not always hypertrichotic, and is most common on the upper trunk. Spontaneous clearance is unlikely.

Epidemiology

An incidence of around 0.25%, and it is more common in males than females.

Associated diseases

When this is associated with extracutaneous abnormalities, it is termed Becker nevus syndrome, which can involve underlying structures, namely aplasia or hypoplasia of the underlying breast tissue or pectoralis major muscle (or sometimes shoulder muscles) or lipoatrophy. Other extracutaneous associations described are ipsilateral limb growth disturbance, supernumerary nipples, and scoliosis.

Clinical characteristics in light skin (Fitzpatrick skin types I–III)

In light-skinned persons, melanosis naeviformis of Becker is a light-brown spot with an irregular outline, often resembling an archipelago (Figure 11.1). It is often hairy, with the hair having a darker color and being thicker. It is apparently androgen-dependent. Most Becker nevi enlarge over the course of some years and then remain stable. Some respond to external stimuli with slight contraction, as they are a hamartoma with an increased number of smooth muscle cells.

Clinical characteristics in dark skin (Fitzpatrick skin types IV–V)

Becker nevus is blackish-brown or black in darker-skinned individuals (Figure 11.2).

Investigations

This is diagnosed clinically.

Histopathology shows hyperpigmentation of the basal layer, mild acanthosis, elongation of the rete ridges, numerous melanophages in the upper dermis, and a marked increase of smooth muscle bundles in the dermis.

Treatments

- Pulsed dye lasers (PDL), Er:YAG lasers, and intense pulsed light (IPL) 550 nm have been used with variable success. These cannot permanently eradicate the condition, but they can reduce its pigmentation and therefore visual prominence.
- Intense pulsed light 615 nm, Q-switched ruby laser 694 nm, long-pulsed alexandrite laser 755 nm, and Q-switched Nd:YAG 1064 nm have been effective in the treatment of hypertrichosis.

Further reading

Anannya S, Wahab AJ, Jacob SM, et al. (2024). Follicular Becker's Nevus: A Case Report of an Uncommon Clinical Variant. *Cureus*;16(4):e58264.

Haneke E (1979). The Dermal Component in Melanosis Naeviformis Becker. *J Cutan Pathol*;6:53–58.

Patrizi A, Medri M, Raone B, et al. (2012). Clinical Characteristics of Becker's Nevus in Children: Report of 118 Cases from Italy. *Pediatr Dermatol*;29(5):571–574.

Ranawaka RR (2021). Congenital Naevi and Melanocytic Maevi. In: Ranawaka RR, et al. (eds). *Atlas of Dermatoses in Pigmented Skin*. Springer, Singapore; 54–57.

Wulkan AJ, McGraw T, Taylor M (2018). Successful Treatment of Becker's Nevus with Long-Pulsed 1064-nm Nd:YAG and 755-nm Alexandrite Laser and Review of the Literature. *J Cosmet Laser Ther*;20(4):211–214.

Zhong Y, Yang B, Huang L, et al. (2019). Lasers for Becker's nevus. *Lasers Med Sci*;34(6):1071–1079.

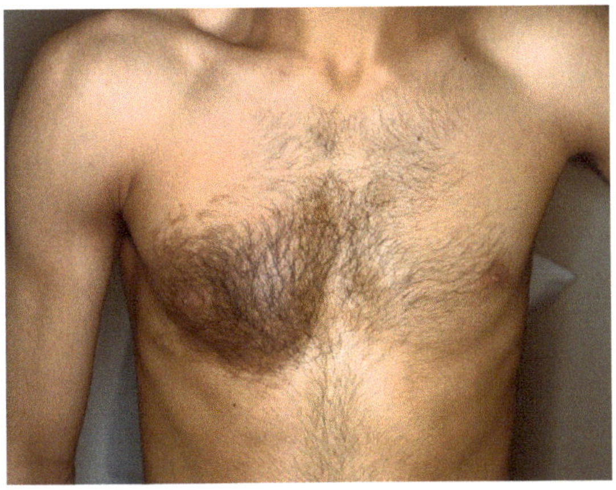

FIGURE 11.1 Becker nevus in a man FST3. (Courtesy Prof. Ian Coulson, UK.)

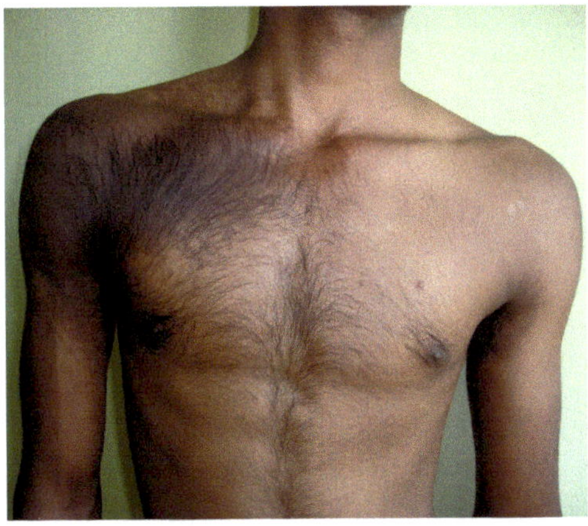

FIGURE 11.2 Becker nevus in a 17-year-old boy FST5.

DOI: 10.1201/9781003479512-11

12
CAFÉ-AU-LAIT MACULES

Introduction

Café-au-lait macules (CALMs) are uniformly hyperpigmented, asymptomatic, well-demarcated macules with regular, distinct borders that appear since birth. Cafe-au-lait (milky coffee) spots are usually the earliest manifestation in children with the syndromes below.

CALMs appear in many neurocutaneous syndromes.

Neurofibromatosis I (NF1), characteristically, café-au-lait spots are present at birth or, more commonly, develop in early childhood and increase in number throughout life. NF1 is the most common neurocutaneous syndrome we encounter.

Segmental neurofibromatosis is characterized by café-au-lait spots, cutaneous neurofibromas, and sometimes visceral neurofibromas, limited to a circumscribed body segment.

Legius syndrome presents as a mild form of neurofibromatosis with many café-au-lait spots (CLS) but without neurofibromas.

Fanconi anemia is also sometimes associated with pigmentation anomalies including reticulate or patchy hyper- or hypopigmentation and café-au-lait spots.

Watson syndrome, CALMs are associated with pulmonary stenosis, low intelligence, and freckling in the axillae and perineum. Café-au-lait spots are present in about 60% of patients with this syndrome.

In ***Cowden syndrome***, café-au-lait spots have been identified occasionally.

Bloom syndrome, rare autosomal recessive disorder with a characteristic appearance: narrow, slender, delicate facies with a relatively prominent nose and small jaw. The limbs tend to be long with large hands and feet, and there may be reduced subcutaneous fat. They also have café-au-lait patches, clinodactyly, syndactyly, congenital heart disease, annular pancreas, and a high-pitched voice.

Von Hippel–Lindau disease is an autosomal dominantly inherited condition that carries a high risk of internal malignancy and is associated with non-specific cutaneous manifestations, such as hemangiomas and café-au-lait spots.

About 35% of patients with ***McCune–Albright syndrome*** have CALMs.

Leukocyte adhesion deficiency-III (LAD-III) is a rare autosomal recessive genetic syndrome with bleeding disorder of the Glanzmann type and life-threatening infections due to a mutation of the FERMT3 gene, which encodes kindlin-3. CLS may be present.

Epidemiology

CALMs are present in 10–20% of normal individuals. There is no sex predilection.

Associated diseases

Associated with many syndromes, although the commonest in NF1, CALMs are not pathognomonic of NF1.

Clinical characteristics in light skin (Fitzpatrick skin types I–III)

Café-au-lait spots are common and an almost obligatory sign of neurofibromatosis 1 (Figures 12.1 and 12.2), but they occur in other genodermatoses and also sporadically, although in lesser numbers.

They are uniformly brown macules of variable size, some measuring more than 10 cm in diameter. They are asymptomatic and remain hairless. The lighter the skin, the more obvious the CLS are.

Clinical characteristics in dark skin (Fitzpatrick skin types IV–V)

CALM are dark brown or black in darker skin (Figure 12.3). They are uniformly pigmented, asymptomatic, well-demarcated macules with regular, distinct borders. They usually appear in multiples.

Investigations

This is diagnosed clinically.

In café-au-lait spots and ephelides, melanocytes are normal in number. In neurofibromatosis, in both café-au-lait spots and clinically unaffected skin, giant pigment granules are occasionally found in epidermal cells and melanocytes.

Treatments

- None for CALM; however, picosecond lasers have proven to improve the cosmetic appearance of CALM.
- Manage the associated syndrome appropriately.

Further reading

Brems H, Pasmant E, Van Minkelen R, et al. (2012). Review and Update of SPRED1 Mutations Causing Legius Syndrome. *Hum Mutat*;33(11):1538–1546.

Fernandez JK, Guo EL, Richmond H, et al. (2024). The 730-nm Picosecond Titanium Sapphire Laser for Treatment of Café-au-lait Macules in All Skin Types. *Lasers Surg Med*;56(3):257–262.

Padeniya A, Lebbe F (2021). Neurocutaneous Syndromes. In: Ranawaka RR, et al. (eds). *Atlas of Dermatoses in Pigmented Skin*. Springer, Singapore; 82–84.

Rajan N, Mellerio JE, Irvine AD (2024). Inherited Skin Tumour Syndromes. In: Griffiths C, et al. (eds). *Rook's Textbook of Dermatology*, 10th ed. John Wiley & Sons Ltd., UK; 78.3.

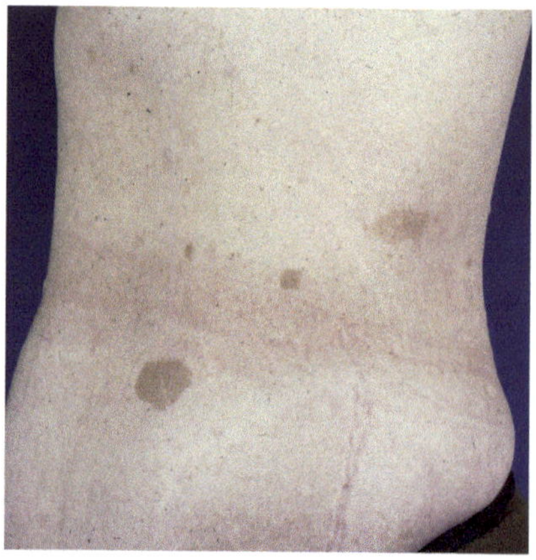

FIGURE 12.1 Multiple café-au-lait macules FST1. (Courtesy Prof. Ian Coulson, UK.)

DOI: 10.1201/9781003479512-12

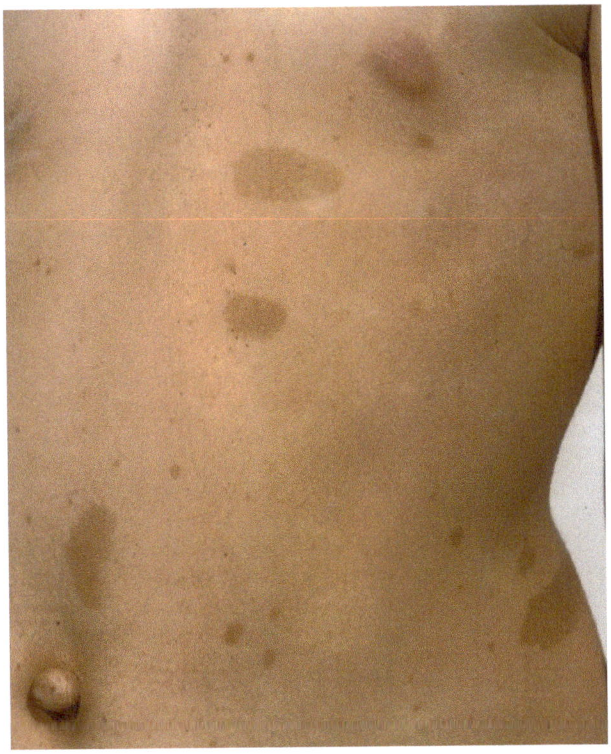

FIGURE 12.2 Multiple café-au-lait macules FST2. (Courtesy Dr. Richard Ashton, UK.)

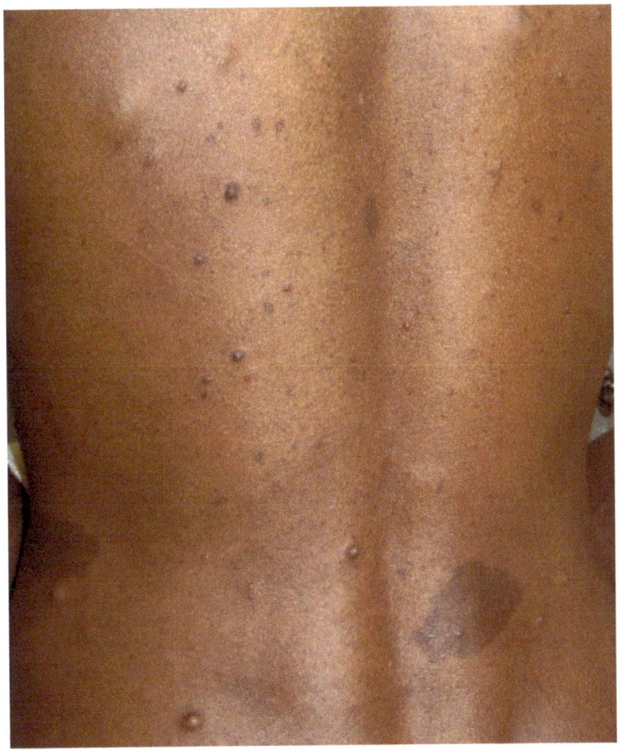

FIGURE 12.3 Multiple café-au-lait macules and neurofibromas in a 24-year-old man with NF1 FST5.

13
CHEMICAL DEPIGMENTATION/CHEMICAL VITILIGO

Introduction

Chemical leukoderma denotes an acquired vitiligo-like depigmentation triggered by repeated exposure to specific chemical compounds, independent of their sensitizing potential. These chemicals are toxic to melanocytes only in subjects having a specific genetic susceptibility to vitiligo. This entity is distinctly separate from post-inflammatory depigmentation and Koebnerization in vitiligo.

A number of chemicals can produce cutaneous depigmentation when applied to the skin: *p*-tertiary butylphenol (in detergents, disinfectants, sealant, adhesive), monobenzylether of hydroquinone (MBEH) (in rubber), monomethylether of hydroquinone (in cosmetic creams), and several phenolic germicidal preparations. Other chemicals that are known to cause chemical leucoderma are *p*-phenylenediamine (PPD), certain azo dyes, sulfhydryls, mercurials, and arsenic.

Monobenzyl ether of hydroquinone is used in the treatment of hypermelanosis and can produce confetti-like areas of depigmentation in the treated areas. The chemical 4-*tert*-butylphenol (4-TBP) was the suspected culprit in patients who presented with depigmentation under their bindi, where adhesive glue contains this phenol compound (in India and Sri Lankan Tamils, married women apply bindi on the forehead). 4-*tert*-amylphenol (4-TAP) in detergents and disinfectants caused depigmentation in hospital workers. Rhododendrol contained in a skin-lightening cream marketed by a Japanese cosmetic company led to 16,000 users developing vitiligo.

P-phenylenediamine (PPD) in hair dyes, 'black henna,' or hair rinses may induce depigmentation. Patients may develop hair dye-induced depigmentation on the scalp or face, depending on the site of application. PPD is often used as a dye or antioxidant in various consumer and industrial products such as fur, textiles, leather, rubber, paints, nylon stockings, and industrial printing inks. Chemical depigmentation on the glans penis from rubber condoms is extremely difficult to differentiate from vitiligo. Perioral depigmentation was reported using cinnamic aldehyde-containing toothpaste.

Associated diseases

Nowadays, monobenzylether of hydroquinone (MBEH) is used to achieve complete depigmentation of patients with universal vitiligo. MBEH as a depigmenting agent was first reported in a 1939 case series of workers in a leather manufacturing company who wore rubber gloves containing MBEH.

Clinical characteristics in light skin (Fitzpatrick skin types I–III)

As in dark-skinned patients, chemical leukoderma is clinically indistinguishable from vitiligo. It is much less obvious and may even occur in skin types I and II. A Wood's lamp may be necessary to find the depigmented spots and characterize their outlines.

Vitiligo-like depigmentation appears to be a relatively frequent adverse effect of the treatment of melanoma with immune checkpoint inhibitors (7.2%).

Clinical characteristics in dark skin (Fitzpatrick skin types IV–V)

Chemically induced vitiligo or depigmentation is not uncommon in our settings. Depigmentation limited to the contact area, with a clear imprint of the culprit on the skin, helps differentiate this from vitiligo. However, repigmentation after withdrawal of the offending agent may take months to years. Common items from which synthetic leather-/rubber-related leucoderma has been reported are rain shoes, rubber slippers, synthetic leather wallets (particularly when held directly against the skin), condoms, watch straps, hearing aid, and rubber gloves. Culprit chemical in these is monobenzyl ether of hydroquinone. Vitiligo appearing on the lips in betel chewers is not uncommon in Sri Lanka and South India. They develop oral submucous fibrosis (OSF), which is a premalignant condition; however, only some patients develop vitiligo on the lips. The etiology of OSF is proven to be due to alkaloids in areca nut, namely arecoline, arecaidine, guvacine, and guvacoline. Nevertheless, the etiology of vitiligo appearing on the lips in only some OSF patients is not explained.

Investigations

Patch testing for the suspected chemical ingredient.

Treatments

- When the chemical ingredient is removed, repigmentation is usual in most cases but not in all. This may take months to years.
- Topical 0.1% tacrolimus ointment may hasten the repigmentation in some.

Further reading

Bajaj AK, Saraswat A, Srivastav PK (2010). Chemical Leucoderma: Indian Scenario, Prognosis, and Treatment. *Indian J Dermatol*;55(3):250–254.

Damevska K, Peev I, Ranawaka RR, et al. (2020). Hypopigmentation from Chemical and Physical Agents. In Nicolaidou E, et al. (eds). *Hypopigmentation*. CRC Press, USA; 159–164.

Ghosh S (2020). Chemical Vitiligo: A Subset of Vitiligo. *Indian J Dermatol*;65(6):443–449.

Harris JE (2017). Chemical-Induced Vitiligo. *Dermatol Clin*;35(2):151–161.

Medri M, Savoia F, Foca F, et al. (2023); IMI, Italian Melanoma Intergroup. A Retrospective Observational Study on Cutaneous Adverse Events Induced by Immune Checkpoint Inhibitors. *Ital J Dermatol Venerol*;158(6):437–444.

Ranawaka RR (2021). Allergic and Irritant Contact Dermatitis. In: Ranawaka RR, et al. (eds). *Atlas of Dermatoses in Pigmented Skin*. Springer, Singapore; 161–163.

Tilakaratne WM, Jayasinghe RD. (2021). Oral Potentially Malignant Disorders. In: Ranawaka RR, et al. (eds). *Atlas of Dermatoses in Pigmented Skin*. Springer, Singapore; 890–891.

DOI: 10.1201/9781003479512-13

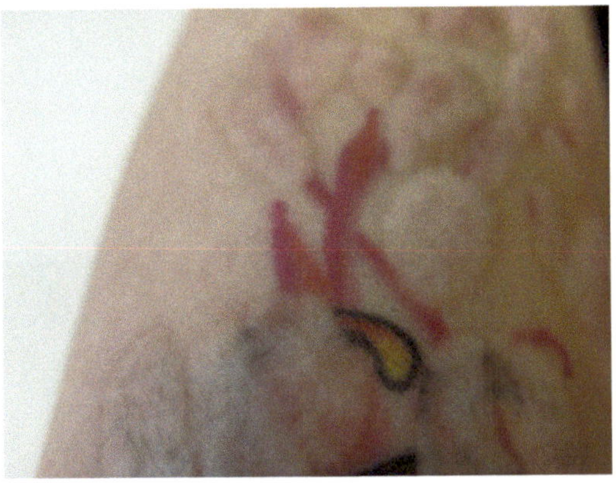

FIGURE 13.1 Chemical depigmentation after lactic acid injection for tattoo removal. (Courtesy Prof. Uwe Wollina, Germany.)

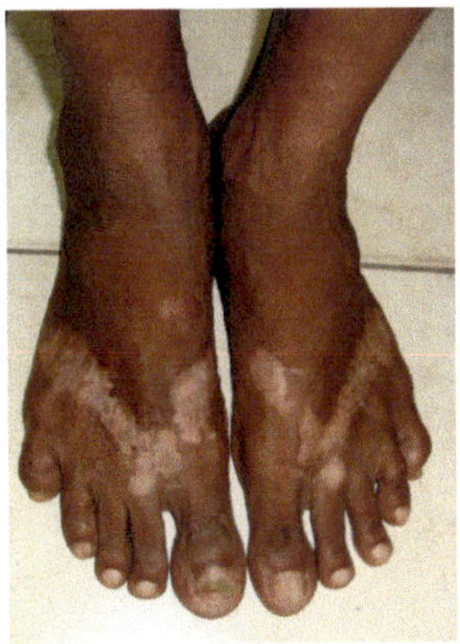

FIGURE 13.2 Chemical depigmentation to rubber footwear FST5.

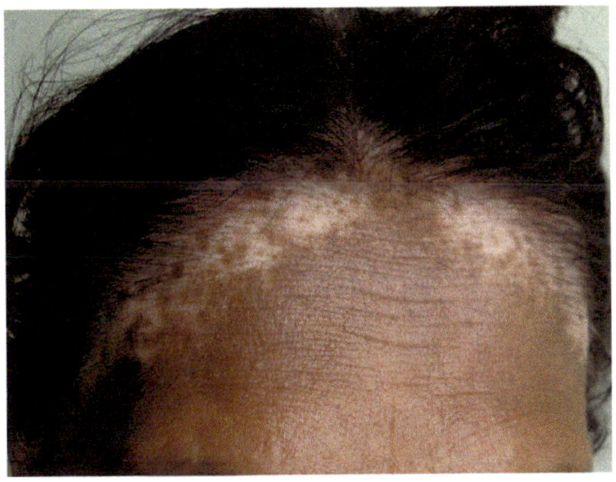

FIGURE 13.3 Chemical depigmentation to black hair dye containing PPD in FST5.

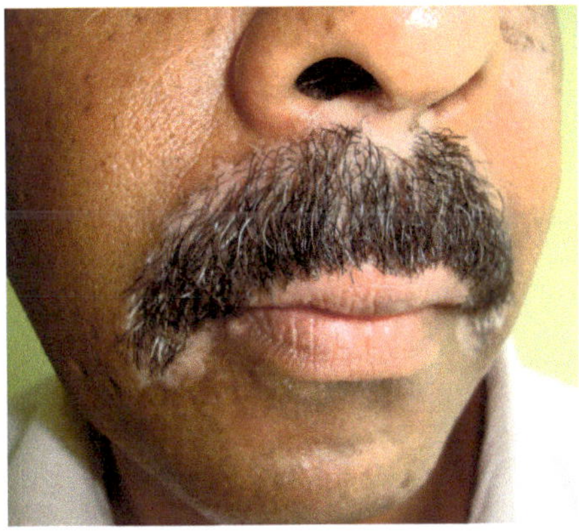

FIGURE 13.4 Chemical depigmentation to black hair dye containing PPD applied on the beard FST5.

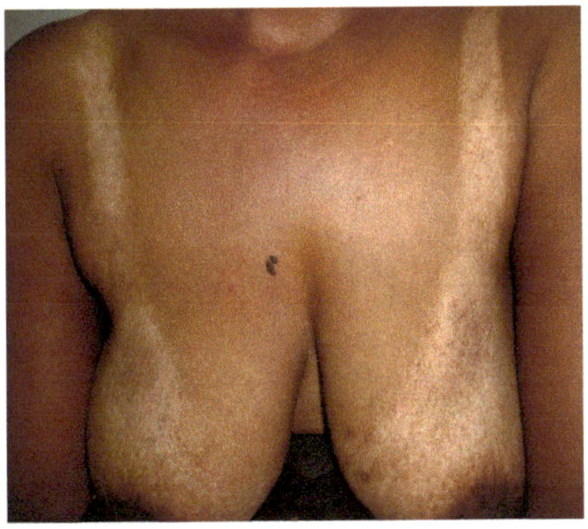

FIGURE 13.5 Chemical depigmentation to black dye or synthetic fabric in the brassiere FST5. This woman used to only wear black-colored brassieres.

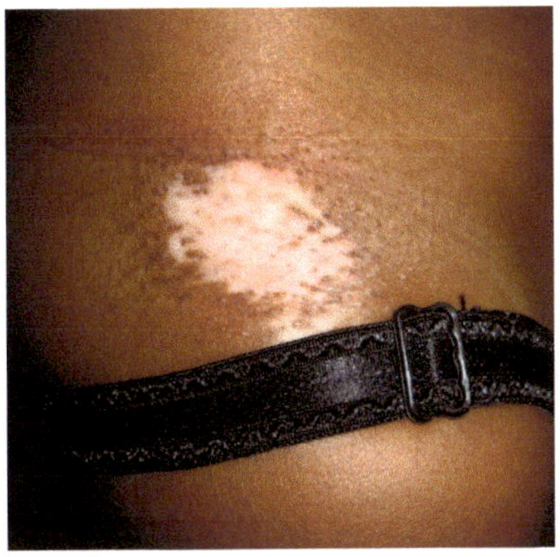

FIGURE 13.6 Chemical depigmentation due to plastics FST5.

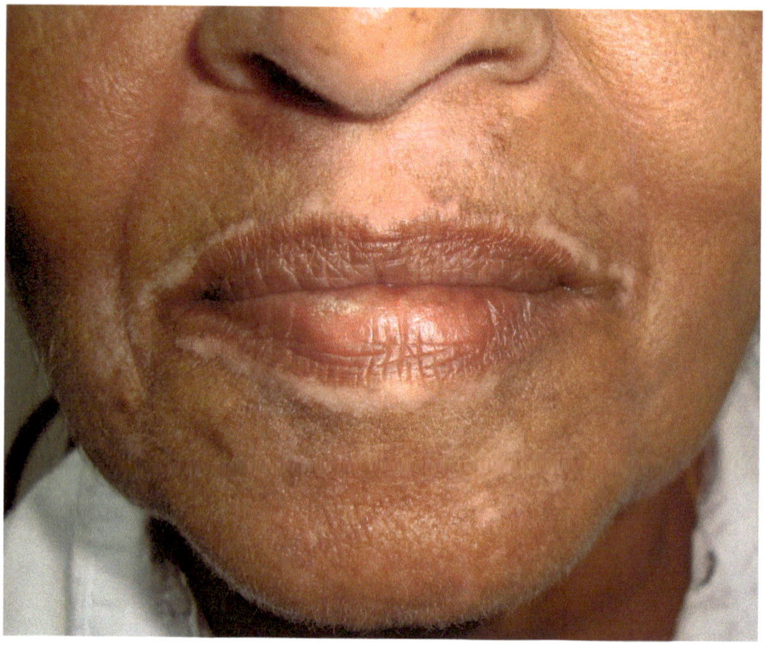

FIGURE 13.7 Perioral depigmentation in a woman using cinnamic aldehyde-containing toothpaste FST5.

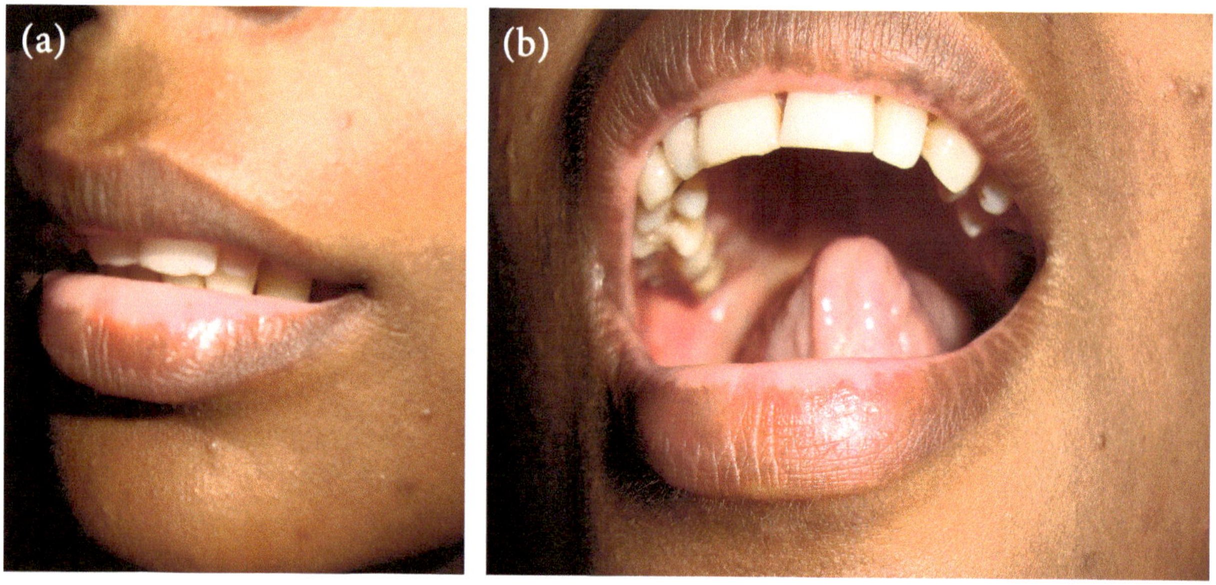

FIGURE 13.8 A 30-year-old woman with oral submucous fibrosis FST5. She presented with a complaint that she was getting (a) vitiligo on lips. On direct inquiry she admitted a burning sensation of the mouth and (b) restricted tongue movements and restricted mouth opening.

14
CONFLUENT AND RETICULATED PAPILLOMATOSIS

Introduction

Confluent and reticulated papillomatosis (CARP), also known as Gougerot–Carteaud syndrome, is an uncommon disorder of epidermal keratinization. The pathogenesis of CARP is poorly understood. It is thought to be an abnormal host reaction to *Malassezia* organisms, and it is currently suggested that infection with Dietzia papillomatosis, a gram-positive aerobic actinomycete bacterium, may play a role. However, diabetes, obesity, ultraviolet light, amyloidosis, and K16 mutation were also seen as causes, not just associated diseases.

CARP first appears as pigmented, 1–2 mm diameter hyperkeratotic papules on the trunk. These coalesce to form pigmented plaques that are confluent at the center but become reticular toward the periphery of the plaques. These initial stages may go unnoticed in most patients.

Epidemiology

CARP is identified in young adults; the mean age of onset is 19 years, with a reported predominance of women.

Associated diseases

CARP has been associated with obesity and insulin resistance, as well as thyroid dysfunction and Cushing's disease.

Clinical characteristics in light skin (Fitzpatrick skin types I–III)

CARP is a rare condition starting with small papules on the upper trunk that extend and coalesce to form large plaques, the borders of which are reticulated. In light skin, the lesions are definitely darker than the normal surrounding skin, often a bit velvety (Figures 14.1 and 14.2). Thus, there is much in common with benign acanthosis nigricans from a clinical point of view.

Clinical characteristics in dark skin (Fitzpatrick skin types IV–V)

CARP is not uncommon in our settings, and the initial stages may go unnoticed in dark skin. Most patients have extensive lesions at presentation (Figures 14.3 and 14.4).

Asymptomatic dark brown to blackish plaques of CARP are located mainly on the trunk, especially in the interscapular area extending to the whole back, presternal, and epigastric areas. Patients first notice a dirty skin area that does not wash off. Then it spreads over weeks and months and becomes darker. CARP is a chronic disease with remissions and exacerbations leading to much distress for the patient due to the 'dirty skin' appearance.

Investigations

This is a clinical diagnosis.

Histopathology from a skin biopsy is performed for confirmation.

There is hyperkeratosis and papillomatosis, with a decrease in the thickness or disappearance of the granular cell layer. There may be increased melanin in the basal cell layer and in the stratum corneum, and this is reflected in the color of the plaques. The dermis shows at most a mild non-specific inflammatory infiltrate.

Treatments

This is purely a cosmetic problem. Even if CARP responds to treatment, it often relapses when treatment is withdrawn.

The following therapies have been beneficial in some patients:

- The first-line therapy is minocycline.
- Topical mupirocin ointment.
- Topical and systemic antifungal agents, including selenium sulfide shampoo.
- Topical retinoids and vitamin D analogues.
- Oral isotretinoin in both high and low doses.

Further reading

David A, Srivastava D (2023). Confluent and Reticulated Papillomatosis Resembling Pityriasis Versicolor and Acanthosis Nigricans: Case Report. *JMIR Dermatol*;6:e41245.

Enwereji N, Mallett J (2023). Concomitant Confluent and Reticulated Papillomatosis and Acanthosis Nigricans in Patients with Skin of Color and Need for Early Interventions for Insulin Resistance. *Int J Womens Dermatol*;9(4):e119.

Rajendiran P (2021). Hyperpigmentary Disorders. In: Ranawaka RR, et al. (eds). *Atlas of Dermatoses in Pigmented Skin*. Springer, Singapore; 862.

DOI: 10.1201/9781003479512-14

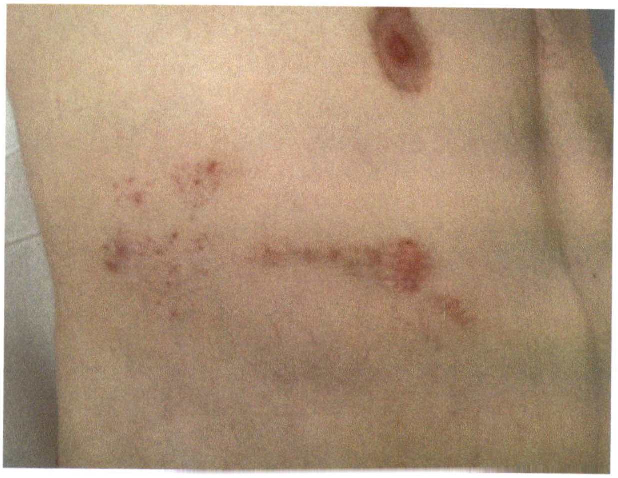

FIGURE 14.1 Confluent and reticulated papillomatosis FST2. (Courtesy Prof. Carlo Enrico Urbani, Italy.)

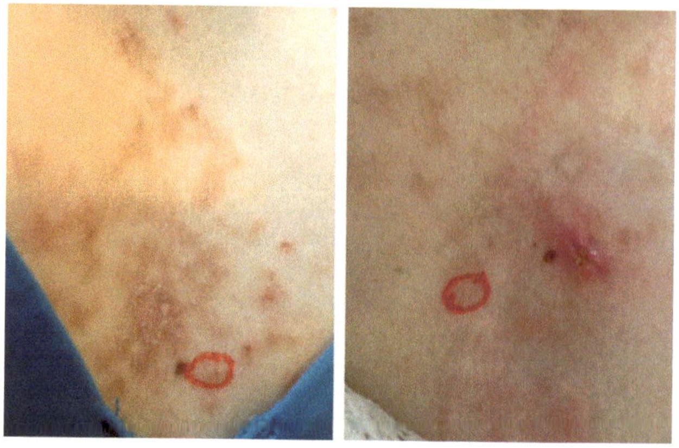

FIGURE 14.2 Confluent and reticulated papillomatosis FST1. (Courtesy Prof. Carlo Enrico Urbani, Italy.)

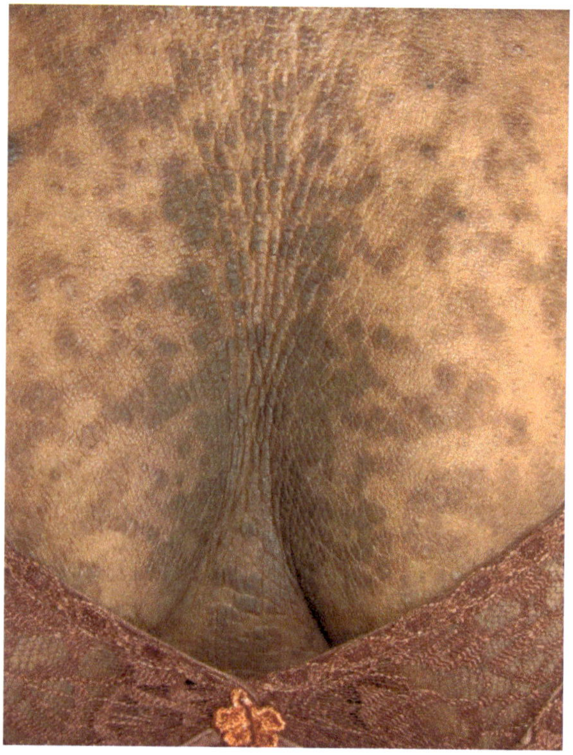

FIGURE 14.3 Confluent and reticulated papillomatosis involving the pre-sternal area extending to breasts and anterior chest in a 19-year-old woman FST5.

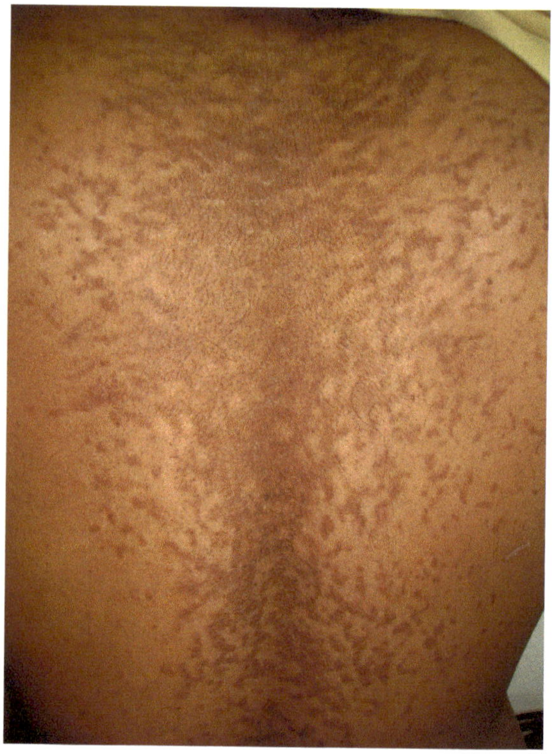

FIGURE 14.4 Confluent and reticulated papillomatosis involving the interscapular area extending to back of the trunk in a 21-year-old man FST5.

15
DARIER DISEASE

Introduction

Darier disease (DD) is an autosomal dominant genodermatosis caused by mutations in the *ATP2A2* gene and characterized by a chronic eruption of keratotic papules, the histology of which shows acantholysis and dyskeratosis. Penetrance is complete in adults, although phenotypic expression may be variable. There is considerable variation in the severity of the disease, even within families, ranging from subtle palmar or nail changes to widespread involvement.

DD is characterized by chronic and recurrent focal and aggregated keratotic papules, predominantly in seborrheic areas. The rash usually first appears in the early teenage years, but may appear in infancy or in old age. Acrokeratosis verruciformis (plane wart-like lesions most common on the dorsal hands), typical nail changes (red and white longitudinal bands terminating in V-shaped nicks), focal palmoplantar pits or keratosis, diffuse keratoderma, filiform keratosis, mucosal involvement (presents with white umbilicated or cobblestone papules commonly on the labial mucosa and soft palate), and ocular manifestations (hyperkeratotic plaques and seborrheic debris at the eyelid margin) are other frequent manifestations.

Epidemiology

Men and women are equally affected.

Associated diseases

Impetiginization and eczematization are common, and patients have an increased susceptibility to infections with herpes simplex.

Clinical characteristics in light skin (Fitzpatrick skin types I–III)

The skin may take on a dirty, rough appearance due to aggregated reddish to light brown keratotic papules developing in so-called seborrheic and intertriginous areas, usually starting on the upper trunk (Figures 15.1 and 15.2). Mild cases are often diagnosed by gentle sliding palpation of the temple and observing the inner side of the lower lip, where the papules give a characteristic interruption of light reflexes. The lesions intensify with age and may become very extensive. Sweating may cause malodorous lesions that tend to fissure. They are often exacerbated by sunlight, heat, infections, and friction.

Clinical characteristics in dark skin (Fitzpatrick skin types IV–V)

Keratotic papules are discrete or confluent, rough, greasy, dark brown to black in color and are commonest on the seborrheic and intertriginous areas (Figure 15.3).

Investigations

This is diagnosed clinically and confirmed histopathologically.

Histology of the keratotic lesions shows suprabasal acantholysis and many dyskeratoses (corps ronds).

Treatments

Treatment of this autosomal dominant condition is challenging. Oral retinoids are often used with variable effects. A new drug developed for Gaucher and Niemann–Pick disease was found to increase the intercellular bonds in the epidermis of Darier disease.

- Avoid aggravating factors such as friction, heat, sweating, and sunlight or UVB.
- Symptomatic therapy in mild to moderate cases.
- Oral retinoids are the mainstay of management in severe cases; oral acitretin 0.25–0.5 mg/kg/day or isotretinoin 0.5 mg/kg/day are commonly used.

Further reading

Leonart LP, Fachi MM, Böger B, et al. (2023). A Systematic Review and Meta-Analyses of Longitudinal Studies on Drug Treatments for Gaucher Disease. *Ann Pharmacother*;57(3):267–282.

Munro CS, Cox NH (1992). An Acantholytic Dyskeratotic Epidermal Naevus with Other Features of Darier's Disease on the Same Side of the Body. *Br J Dermatol*;127(2):168–71.

Zamiri M (2024). Inherited Acantholytic Disorders. In: Griffiths C, et al. (eds). *Rook's Textbook of Dermatology*, 10th ed. John Wiley & Sons Ltd., UK; 64.1.

DOI: 10.1201/9781003479512-15

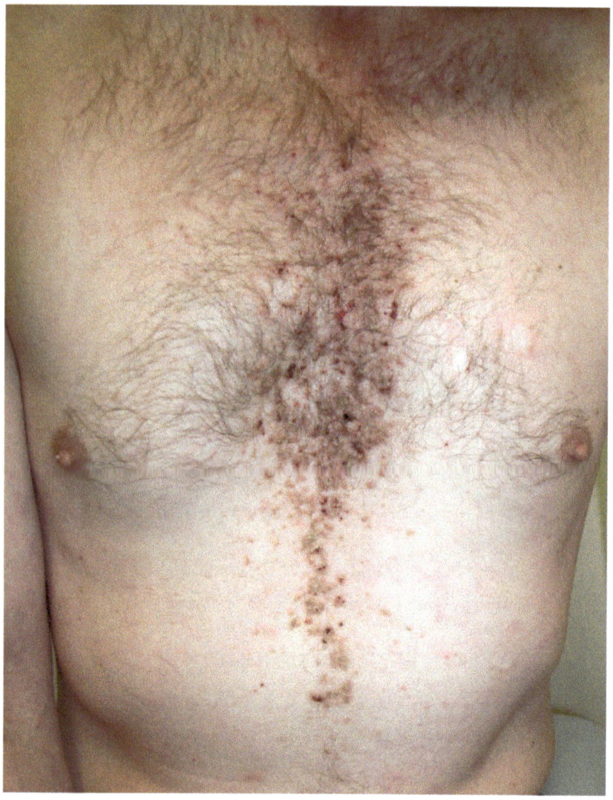

FIGURE 15.1 Darier disease FST2. (Courtesy Prof. Ian Coulson, UK.)

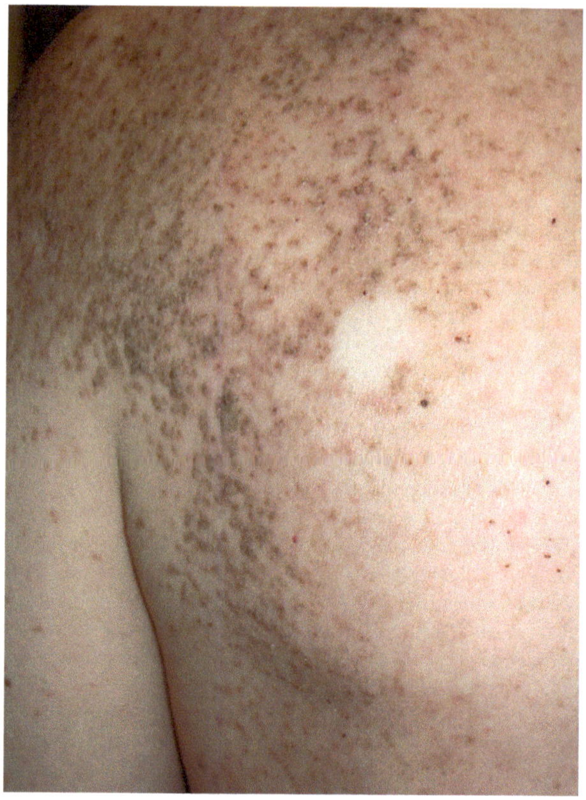

FIGURE 15.2 Darier disease close-up view FST2. Note the absence of lesions in the superficial scar. (Courtesy Prof. Ian Coulson, UK.)

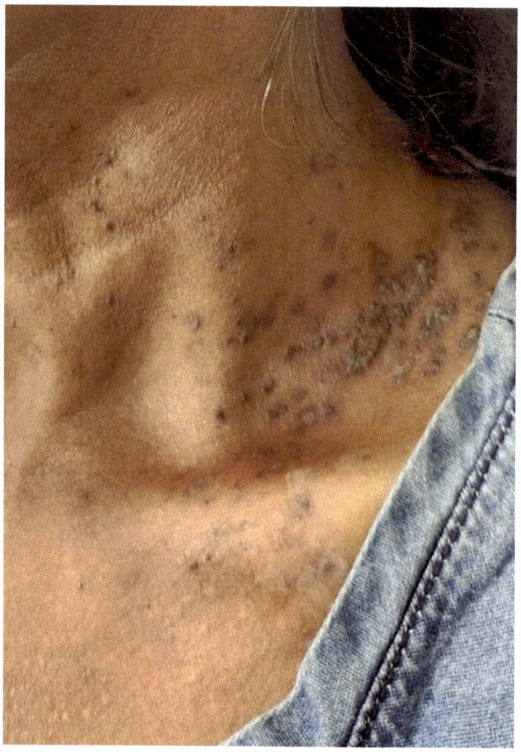

FIGURE 15.3 Darier disease in a 67-year-old woman FST5 showing focal and aggregated dark brown to black keratotic papules in the neck. (Courtesy Dr. Ajith P. Kannangara, Sri Lanka.)

16
DERMATOMYOSITIS

Introduction

Dermatomyositis (DM) is an autoimmune disorder predominantly affecting the skin and skeletal muscle. It is classified alongside polymyositis in the idiopathic inflammatory myopathies (IIMs). According to the Bohan and Peter classification in 1975, the typical skin rash of DM is essential to diagnose DM, and the skin rash is absent in polymyositis. Symmetrical proximal muscle weakness (proximal myopathy), muscle biopsy evidence of myositis, elevation in serum skeletal muscle enzymes, and characteristic electromyography pattern of myositis are the other four features shared with polymyositis.

There are subsets of DM introduced later: Amyopathic DM (no clinical evidence of proximal muscle weakness and no serum muscle enzyme abnormalities) and hypomyopathic DM (if these investigations are positive or abnormal). At one end of the spectrum, myopathy predominates; at the other end, skin disease is prominent with minimal or absent myositis (amyopathic DM). Mortality is increased in DM, with a 10-year survival of up to 90%. The main causes of death are cardiac and respiratory diseases and malignancy.

Anti-melanoma differentiation-associated gene 5 (anti-MDA5) positive dermatomyositis carries a high risk for interstitial lung disease and has a grave prognosis.

Epidemiology

Idiopathic inflammatory myopathies, including DM, are rare. The peak incidence is around 50–60 years of age and is twice as high in women. Juvenile DM is very rare and is not associated with malignancies.

Associated diseases

There is a strong association between internal malignancy and adult DM: Adenocarcinomas, carcinomas of the breast and ovary, lung cancer, and nasopharyngeal cancer.

Clinical characteristics in light skin (Fitzpatrick skin types I–III)

The most typical skin lesion is a violaceous, often edematous rash around the eyes, called the heliotropic rash. This may slowly or sometimes rapidly spread to the entire face, which then usually looks extremely tired. The neck and upper trunk follow. Sunlight worsens the exanthem. The nail folds may show small hemorrhages, and capillary changes can be seen with the dermatoscope. Specifically, on the dorsa of the fingers, small reddish to whitish papules may be seen, known as Gottron papules, which may also occur on the elbows and knees (Figures 16.1 to 16.4).

A subtype of DM is positive for the anti-MDA5 antibody, which is representative of rapidly progressive interstitial pneumonia. Muscle weakness is typical, with the proximal arm and leg muscles being particularly involved. The patient cannot stand up again after squatting down or is not able to raise both arms above the horizontal.

Clinical characteristics in dark skin (Fitzpatrick skin types IV–V)

The facial rash, which is the initial presenting feature in over 50% of DM cases, may be very subtle in dark skin (Figure 16.5). Even though the edema of the upper eyelids and periorbital skin is marked and characteristic, an erythema that is lilac (or heliotropic) in color, even pathognomonic of DM, is not seen in dark skin. Fixed macular erythema commonly appears on the upper torso, both the V of the chest and across the shoulders, where it is termed the 'shawl sign,' may be mistaken for a photosensitive rash in a tropical climate. Therefore, identification of DM without myositis (amyopathic or hypomyopathic DM) is extremely difficult in our settings. Gottron papules are either skin-colored or mildly erythematous in dark skin and appear on typical sites, the dorsa of finger joints. Nail fold changes, ragged cuticles, linear red streaks on the skin overlying the extensor tendons, and calcinosis cutis may present in variable degrees.

Investigations

Patients with suspected DM should have a full biochemical profile, full blood count, inflammatory markers, and muscle enzymes (creatine kinase levels).

Electromyography is pathological in affected muscle groups (proximal arm and leg muscles), and a muscle biopsy should be taken from such an area.

Muscle biopsy: Histopathology shows lymphocytic infiltrates in the skeletal muscle, loss of striation, and finally lysis of the muscle cells.

Skin biopsy: The dermatopathology of DM is often subtle. A lichenoid tissue reaction with vacuolar changes in the basal layer and occasional Civatte bodies are typical.

Treatments

- Multidisciplinary care with specialists in dermatology, rheumatology, cardiology, and respiratory medicine.
- Systemic corticosteroid is the primary treatment for DM when both skin and muscles are involved. Oral prednisolone, given at a dose of 0.5–1.0 mg/kg, improves the rash and muscle weakness within 1–2 weeks.
- Pulsed IV methylprednisolone 0.5–1.0 g/day on three consecutive days (for severe life-threatening disease) followed by oral prednisolone 0.5–1 mg/kg/day.
- Disease-modifying antirheumatic drug (DMARD) after pulsed methyl prednisolone, such as methotrexate, azathioprine, or ciclosporin.
- Consider IVIg, particularly if the patient has dysphagia.
- For skin-limited disease, potent topical corticosteroid ointment or topical tacrolimus 0.1% ointment plus hydroxychloroquine (with or without mepacrine).
- Mycophenolate mofetil, oral tacrolimus, tofacitinib, or rituximab are second-line therapies.

DOI: 10.1201/9781003479512-16

Further reading

Goradia S, Holper S, Lim YZ, et al. (2024). Anti-Melanoma Differentiation-Associated Gene 5 (Anti-MDA5) Positive Dermatomyositis: Early Detection Is Crucial. *BMJ Case Rep*;17(6):e259338.

Gordon P, Creamer D (2016). Dermatomyositis. In: Griffiths C, et al. (eds). *Rook's Textbook of Dermatology*, 10th ed. John Wiley & Sons Ltd., UK; 52.1.

Pandya R, Kleitsch J, Lim D, et al. (2024). Clinical Characteristics and Symptom Progression of Dermatomyositis Subtypes: A Retrospective Analysis of a Prospective Database. *J Am Acad Dermatol*;S0190-9622(24)00312-8.

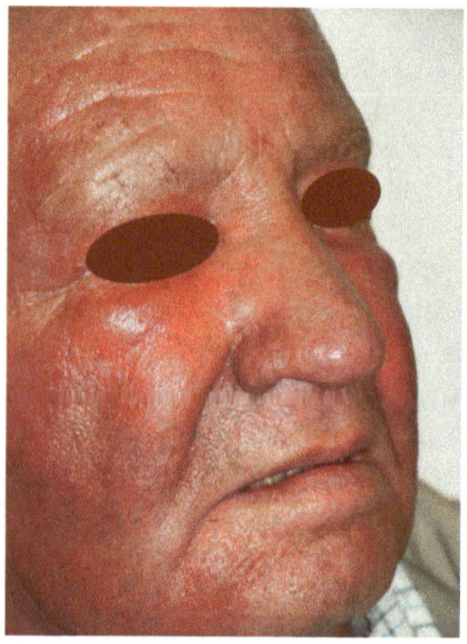

FIGURE 16.1 Dermatomyositis FST1. (Courtesy Prof. Ian Coulson, UK.)

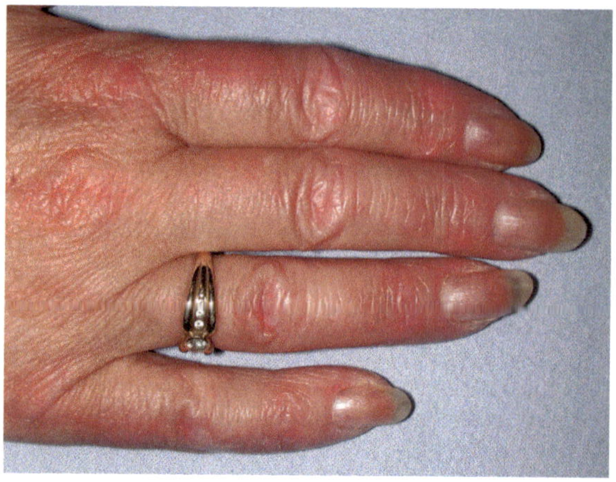

FIGURE 16.2 Dorsum of hand in dermatomyositis FST1. (Courtesy Prof. Ian Coulson, UK.)

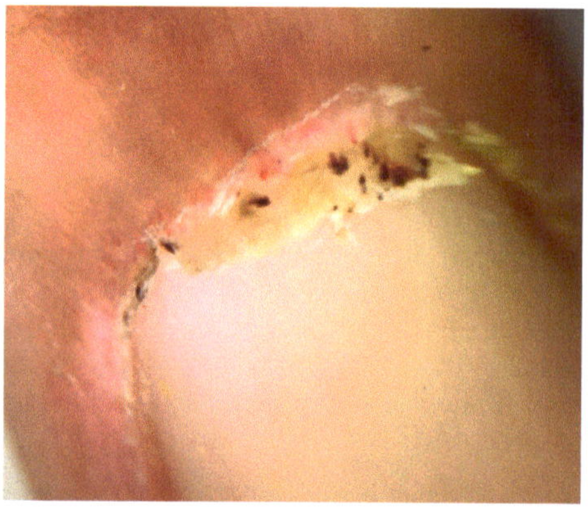

FIGURE 16.3 Capillaroscopy in dermatomyositis in FST2. The nail folds may show small hemorrhages and capillary changes that can be seen with the dermatoscope. (Courtesy Prof. Eckart Haneke & Prof. Osvaldo Correia, Germany.)

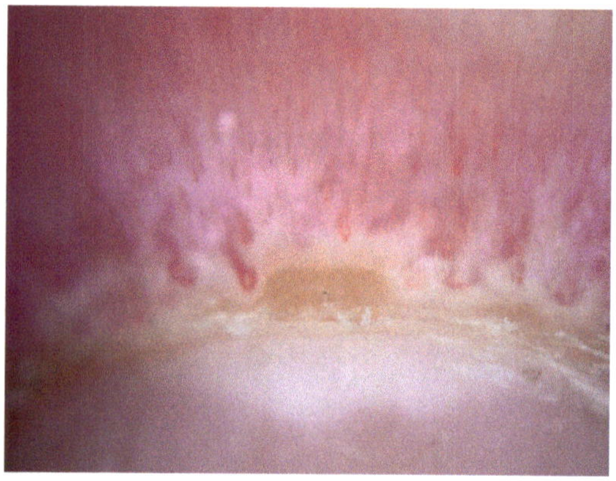

FIGURE 16.4 Capillaroscopy in dermatomyositis in FST2. (Courtesy Prof. Ian Coulson, UK.)

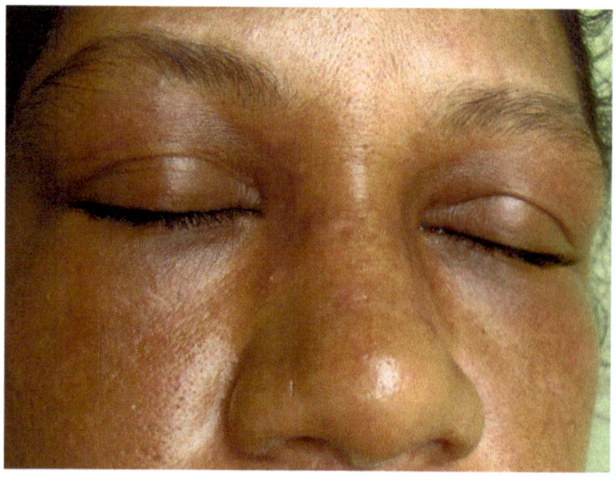

FIGURE 16.5 Edema of the eyelids and periorbital skin in a 45-year-old woman FST5 with proximal myopathy. Note even though the periorbital edema is marked, erythema or heliotropic rash is not a feature in dark skin.

17
DYSCHROMATOSIS

Introduction

Dyschromatosis universalis hereditaria (DUH) is a rare autosomal genodermatosis characterized by hyper- and hypopigmented macules distributed over the entire surface of the skin. The lesions usually appear in infancy or early childhood.

Epidemiology

This is a rare genodermatosis.

Associated diseases

DUH has been associated with neurological, ophthalmological, and hematological complications.

Clinical characteristics in light skin (Fitzpatrick skin types I–III)

DUH is a very rare genetic condition thought to be recessive; however, there are apparently different clinical types that are not clearly defined. Typically, the pigmentation is much more obvious in light-skinned persons and appears somewhat reticular, including the palms and soles (Figures 17.1 to 17.3). The differential diagnosis comprises a number of other rare genodermatoses such as poikiloderma congenitale, some types of xeroderma pigmentosum, pigmented xerodermoid, and many different forms of drug-induced hyperpigmentation, Dowling–Degos disease, etc. New melanocorticotropine agonists may lead to disfiguring generalized hyperpigmentation. Addison disease is usually associated with diffuse hyperpigmentation and pigmentation of the palmar creases. It usually has a later onset of the pigmentation.

Histopathology can exclude some of these diseases.

Clinical characteristics in dark skin (Fitzpatrick skin types IV–V)

Very rare skin condition. In dark skin, this color variation may be concealed and be hardly visible (Figures 17.4 and 17.5).

Investigations

This is diagnosed clinically.

Treatments

Assess for neurological, ophthalmological, and hematological complications and manage appropriately.

Further reading

Morice-Picard F, Taieb A (2024). Genetic Disorders of Pigmentation. In: Griffiths C, et al. (eds). *Rook's Textbook of Dermatology*, 10th ed. John Wiley & Sons Ltd., UK: 68.14.

Rajendiran P (2021). Hyperpigmentary Disorders. In: Ranawaka RR, et al. (eds). *Atlas of Dermatoses in Pigmented Skin*. Springer, Singapore; 869–871.

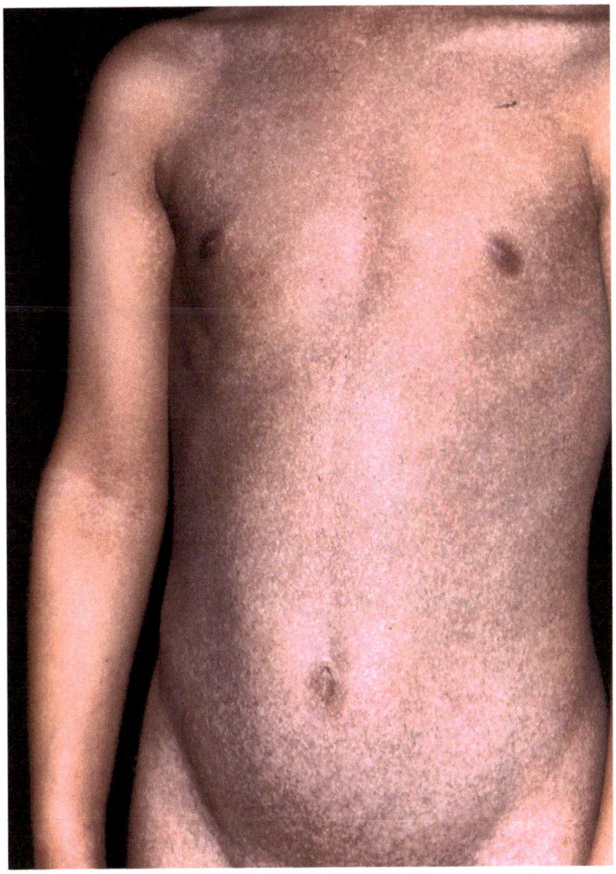

FIGURE 17.1 Dyschromatosis universalis in a young girl, aged 7, with this dirty-looking pigmentation. Both parents were of FST2. (Courtesy Prof. Eckart Haneke, Germany.)

DOI: 10.1201/9781003479512-17

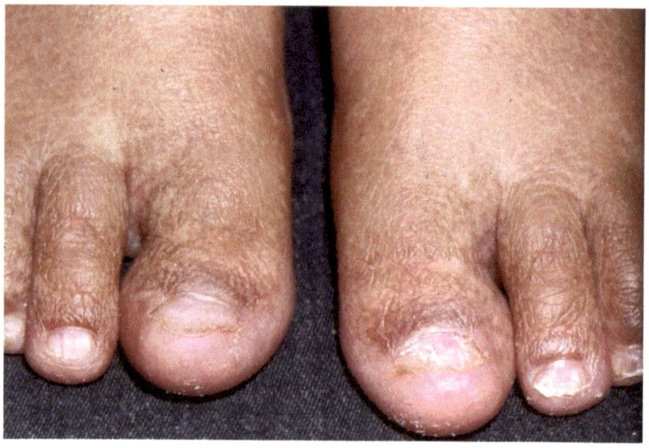

FIGURE 17.2 A 10 year old girl with dyschromatosis universalis, cousin of girl in previous photo. (Courtesy Prof. Eckart Haneke, Germany.)

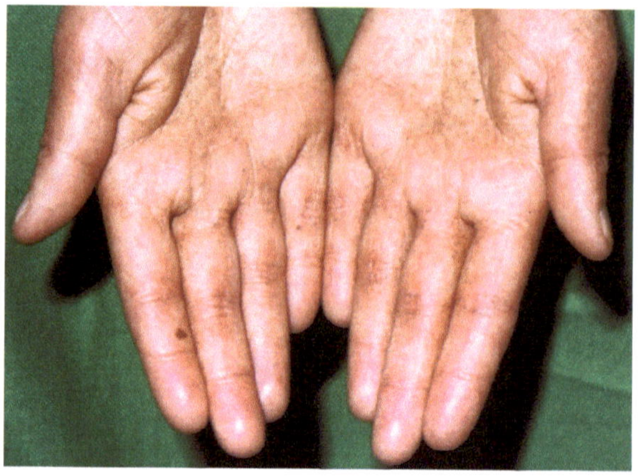

FIGURE 17.3 A 10-year-old girl with dyschromatosis universalis. (Courtesy Prof. Eckart Haneke, Germany.)

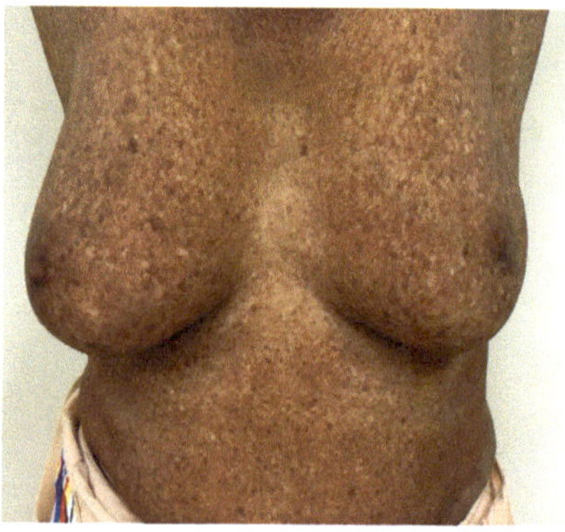

FIGURE 17.4 Dyschromatosis universalis hereditaria in a 45-year-old woman FST5. As this is familial and asymptomatic they tend to ignore this color variation in skin.

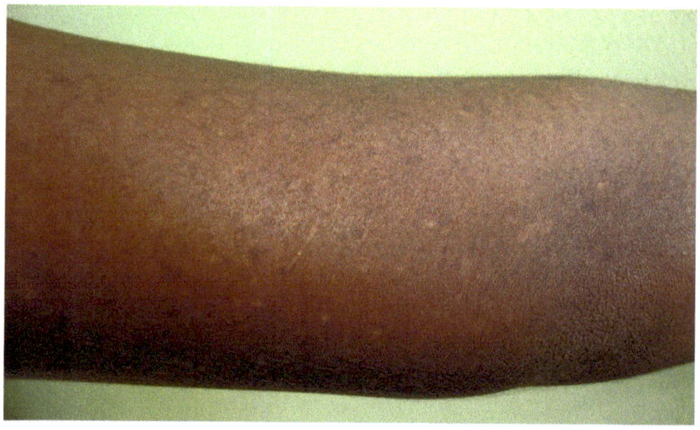

FIGURE 17.5 Dyschromatosis universalis hereditaria in a 16-year-old girl FST5. Note this dyschromatosis is hidden and barely visible in dark skin.

18
ECCHYMOSES, BRUISES

Introduction

Purpura and bruising are the main terms used to describe bleeding into the skin. Purpura is discoloration of the skin or mucous membranes due to extravasation of red blood cells. Petechiae are small, 1–2 mm, purpuric lesions. Ecchymoses (bruises) are larger extravasations of blood. The causes of petechiae and ecchymoses overlap. Thrombocytopenia usually causes petechiae, but more extensive bleeding may occur at lower levels of platelet count. Coagulation disorders cause ecchymoses rather than petechiae.

Extravasated blood is broken down into pigments derived from hemoglobin, usually within 2 or 3 weeks. Characteristic color changes include red, purple, and blue in the first 5 days, later turning green and yellow until the bruise slowly disappears.

(In the German and French literature, there is a clear distinction between bruises that are more or less deep-seated hematomas, ecchymoses that are more superficial and particularly Schamberg's disease which is [a group of] progressive lichenoid purpura.)

Epidemiology

This can affect all ages and both sexes.

Associated diseases

Associated with inherited or acquired platelet disorders (deficiencies or abnormal function), coagulation disorders (inherited, drug-induced, metabolic, disseminated intravascular coagulation (DIC), or secondary to systemic diseases), or hemorrhagic vasculitis.

Clinical characteristics in light skin (Fitzpatrick skin types I–III)

Bruises are common after direct blunt trauma, more often in women than in men. They are usually painful for some days depending on the intensity of the trauma (Figures 18.1 and 18.2).

Purpura is characterized by small non-palpable red spots due to extravasation of blood. They occur first on the lower legs, later on other dependent body parts, but may also occur around the eyes in certain situations. So-called stasis purpura is common in people with varicose veins, obesity, and on anticoagulants. All purpura forms on the lower legs will lead to brown discoloration due to degradation of the erythrocytes to compounds containing iron. Iron itself is brown but also stimulates melanocyte activity. The result is often a yellowish to dark brown color called purpura jaune d'ocre, which characteristically fades toward the knees.

Another condition is progressive pigmented purpura of Gourgerot–Blum or Schamberg's disease, consisting of tiny, often lichenoid-appearing papules that start with a point of blood and then slowly turn brown. It is more frequent in men. The buttocks may be involved and are more of a brownish-yellow color. Alcohol, drinks containing quinine, and a variety of drugs, probably also genetic factors, play an etiological role. A rare form is purpuric contact allergy to textile dyes.

Ecchymoses are frequently seen on the dorsa of the hands, lower arms, and lower legs of elderly people with chronic actinic elastosis and are also called actinic or senile purpura. They are an obligatory constituent of dermatoporosis. In addition, the skin is extremely fragile and tends to be abraded by the slightest trauma, leaving stellate pseudoscars that are white areas of superficial scarring.

Clinical characteristics in dark skin (Fitzpatrick skin types IV–V)

In dark skin, the erythematous early stage in purpura or ecchymoses may be unnoticeable (Figures 18.3 to 18.5). This would be apparent later when it turns to a bluish or purple color. This may lead to fatal consequences in inexperienced settings.

Investigations

This is diagnosed clinically.

Treatments

- Manage the causative factors.
- Reassure the patient that the skin lesion will resolve in 1–2 weeks.

Further reading

Braun-Falco O, Balda BR (1970). Sogenannte Pseudo-Cicatrices Stellaires Spontanées [So-called pseudo-cicatrices stellaires spontanées]. *Hautarzt*;21(11):509–513.

Ceilley RI (2017). Treatment of Actinic Purpura. *J Clin Aesthet Dermatol*;10(6):44–50.

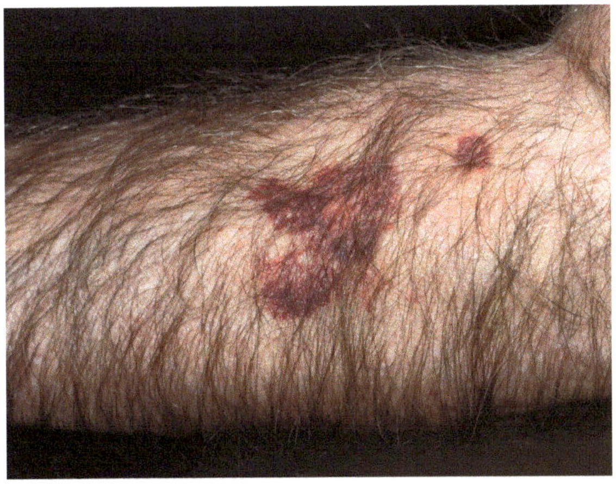

FIGURE 18.1 Ecchymoses following steroids FST1. (Courtesy Prof. Ian Coulson, UK.)

DOI: 10.1201/9781003479512-18

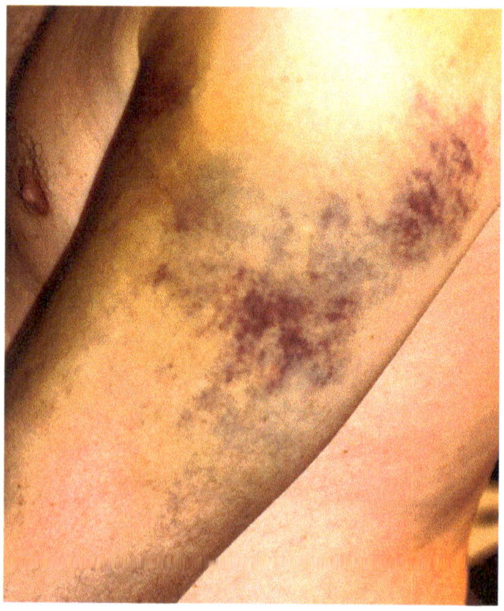

FIGURE 18.2 Bruises FST1. (Courtesy Dr. Richard Ashton, UK.)

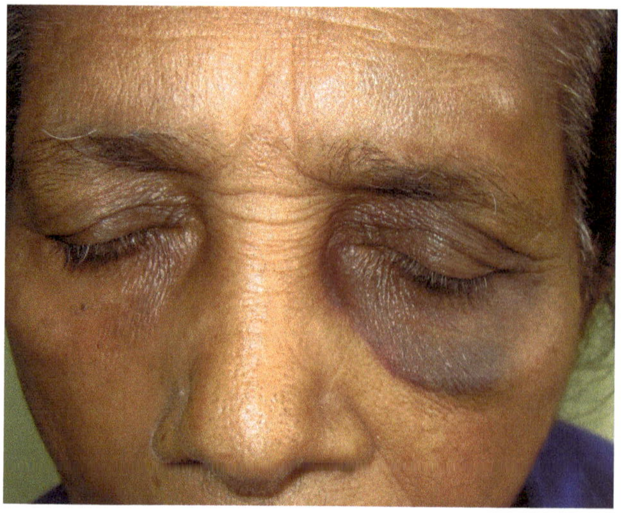

FIGURE 18.3 Ecchymoses around the left eye following a trauma FST5. Patient presented 2 days after the trauma when they noticed darkening.

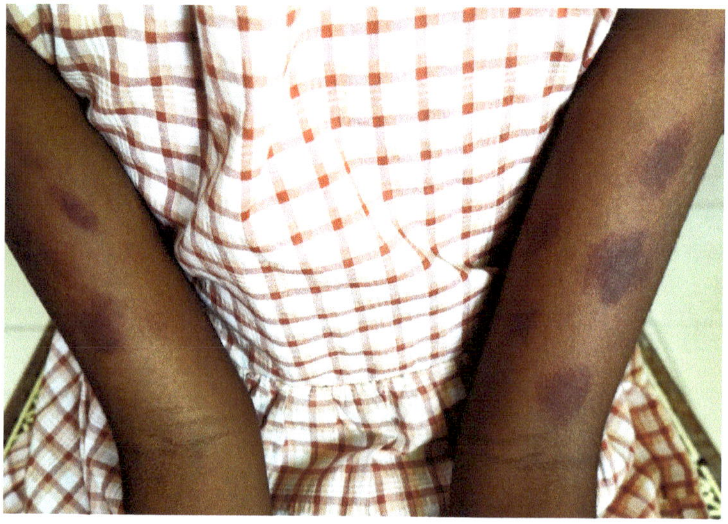

FIGURE 18.4 Self-induced ecchymoses and bruises in a 9-year-old girl FST5.

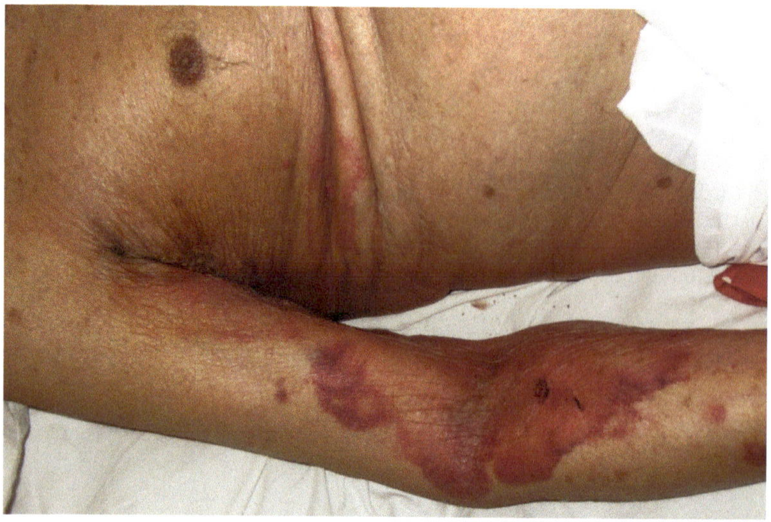

FIGURE 18.5 Echymoses and bruises in a 94-year-old hospitalized man FST4.

19

ASTEATOTIC ECZEMA (ECZEMA CRAQUELÉ, WINTER ECZEMA)

Introduction

Asteatotic eczema is eczema developing in very dry skin, commonly in the elderly. It usually affects the legs, arms, and hands of elderly people in the context of dry skin. A characteristic 'crazy paving' pattern is observed on the legs. It may flare during winter due to a reduction in humidity associated with central heating.

Epidemiology

Seen in the elderly, the prevalence increases with age, equally in men and women. It is more prevalent in the winter season.

Associated diseases

May associate or exacerbate with hypothyroidism. It can also be due to zinc deficiency, diuretics, and malnutrition. Extensive or generalized forms should raise the suspicion of internal malignancy: Lymphoma, angioimmunoblastic lymphadenopathy, gastric adenocarcinoma, and carcinoma of the breast.

Clinical characteristics in light skin (Fitzpatrick skin types I–III)

Eczema craquelé is a descriptive term as the skin looks like old porcelain with net-like cracks, or like mud that dried in the hot sun and breaks in a characteristic pattern (Figure 19.1).

Asteatotic means without fat (sebum), and this eczema type is therefore predominantly found where sebaceous glands are rare, such as the lower legs, and sometimes on the arms, thighs, rarely other skin regions. Inflammation is absent to mild but may exacerbate upon harsh treatment when the diagnosis is not made correctly. True eczematization may then occur with oozing and serous scabs, sometimes with the development of annular lesions as in microbial eczema. The condition is typically seen in the cold season but also in persons who shower frequently. Although urea is a good moisturizer, high concentrations may cause itching and should therefore not be used at the beginning of treatment.

Clinical characteristics in dark skin (Fitzpatrick skin types IV–V)

Even though seasonal variation is not marked in the tropics, this gets worse in colder months, from November to January. This is seen in elderly men and women who have very dry skin (Figure 19.2). The asteatotic skin is dry and slightly scaly. On the legs, the pattern of superficial markings is more marked and deeper ('crazy-paving' pattern or eczema craquelé). Frank eczematous changes finally develop.

Investigations

This is diagnosed clinically.

Treatments

- Restoration of skin hydration is key management using frequent moisturizers.
- Emollients, with or without urea, bath oil, and soap substitutes.
- Mild steroid with moisturizer such as Vaseline or emulsifying ointment in oozy eczemas.
- Pimecrolimus 1% cream.

Further reading

Chan CX, Zug KA (2021). Diagnosis and Management of Dermatitis, Including Atopic, Contact, and Hand Eczemas. *Med Clin North Am*;105(4):611–626.

Choudhary C, Kravvas G, Jones HT (2024). What You Need to Know about Common Skin Problems in Older Adults. *Br J Hosp Med*;85(4):1–8.

Mughal AA, Ingram JR (2024). Eczematous Disorders. In: Griffiths C, et al. (eds). *Rook's Textbook of Dermatology*, 10th ed. John Wiley & Sons Ltd., UK; 39.9.

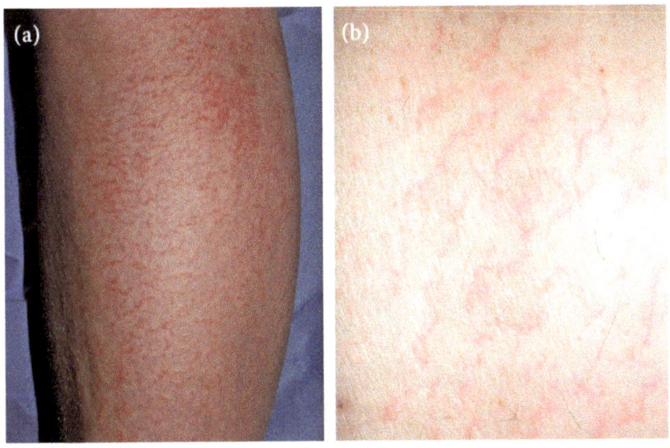

FIGURE 19.1 (a) Asteotoic eczema FST2, and (b) closer view. (Courtesy Prof. Ian Coulson, UK.)

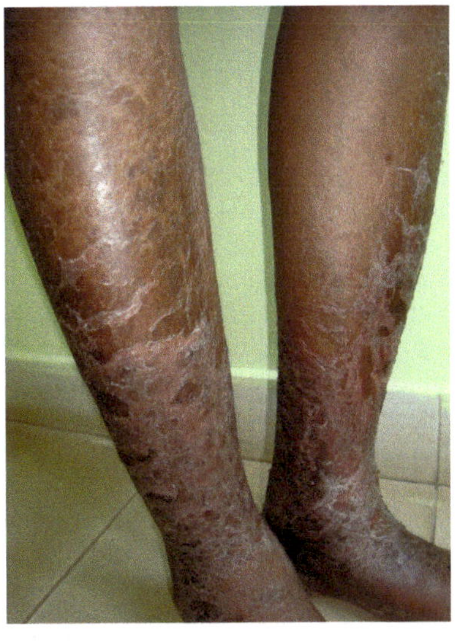

FIGURE 19.2 Asteotoic eczema in a 60-year-old woman FST5.

DOI: 10.1201/9781003479512-19

20
ATOPIC ECZEMA

Introduction

Atopic eczema (AE) is an itchy, chronic, or chronically relapsing inflammatory skin condition that often starts in early childhood. It is a difficult condition to define strongly because it lacks a diagnostic test and shows variable clinical features. The UK refinement of Hanifin and Rajka's diagnostic criteria for atopic dermatitis (eczema) allows for uniformity of diagnosis.

In the majority of cases, AE starts during infancy (usually less than 2 years of age). The pattern of the rash varies with age:

Infantile phase: The lesions most frequently start on the face. When the child begins to crawl, the exposed surfaces, as well as the extensor aspects of the knees and elbows, are affected.

Childhood phase: From 18 to 24 months onward, characteristically involved are the elbow and knee flexures. Note the atopic dirty neck in some.

Adult phase: The picture is similar to that in later childhood, with lichenification, especially of the flexures and hands.

There are numerous proposed scoring systems for assessing the severity of AE. The three that have been most appropriately tested and validated are (1) SCORing Atopic Dermatitis (SCORAD), (2) Eczema Area and Severity Index (EASI), and (3) Patient-Orientated Eczema Measure (POEM) – are predominantly used in research and clinical trials.

Epidemiology

AE occurs worldwide, equally prevalent in both affluent and low-income countries.

Associated diseases

The eruption is frequently associated with other atopic conditions (e.g., allergic rhinitis, hay fever, bronchial asthma) in the individual or other family members. AE patients have filaggrin mutation-associated clinical features such as ichthyosis vulgaris, keratosis pilaris, and hyper linear palms.

Clinical characteristics in light skin (Fitzpatrick skin types I–III)

AE is extremely common and very complex (Figures 20.1 to 20.5). Multiple volumes of books could be filled with the results of research and studies on AE; however, the problem is still not solved for the often extremely uncomfortable patients.

In babies, it may appear a few days after birth, though usually after 4–6 weeks, as so-called cradle cap, which might be difficult to differentiate from seborrheic dermatitis. Later, an oozing redness of the cheek may develop that bothers the parents more than the baby. Itching starts later with the involvement of other body areas such as the extremities and trunk. Further on, the skin lesions concentrate more on the flexural skin of the elbows and knees and also the trunk. The older the children get, the more they are usually disturbed by symptoms such as itching, lack of sleep, and attendance. Scratching may aggravate the skin. The children learn to rub with the backs of the fingertips rather than scratch with the free margins of the nails so that they get very shiny nails.

With time, the skin takes on a grayish hue around the acutely inflamed areas; the skin thickens and develops folds, a condition called lichenification. Furthermore, most atopic subjects have a reduced defense against staphylococci and secondary infection; thus, impetiginization is very common.

Later, the acute inflammation may subside and give way to dry, infiltrated skin.

There are many minor criteria for atopic eczema, such as the Dennie–Morgan folds (double lower lid fold), the anteriorly moved frontotemporal hair margin, the atopic palms with the characteristic increased number of palmar creases, the white dermographism after stroking on the skin of the trunk, the tendency to develop skin fissures on the fingertips called pulpitis sicca, a single deep rhagade extending from the nail fold of the thumb onto the pulp, the patchy pityriasiform lichenoid eczema often seen on the arm and also known as sandbox dermatitis, fissures on the soles of the feet after walking barefoot on sandy beaches, and the atopic winter feet. Umbilical jeans button eczema from the extremely frequent nickel allergy, wool intolerance, etc. Intolerance to some foods may occur and disappear without proof of a true alimentary allergy. The skin color is often gray to pale despite some inflammatory redness.

AE may last into adulthood or first occur after adolescence. It is a general observation that late-onset atopic dermatitis often lasts longer. It may then have different predominant localizations such as the lower eyelids in adult women. Neurogenic and psychogenic factors often aggravate the skin and increase the itch, hence the term neuroderm(at)itis.

Atopic subjects often have a positive family history for atopic diseases such as pollinosis, conjunctivitis, or asthma, and rarely also diarrhea. Curiously, whereas no allergy is normally found in AE except for nickel, allergic rhinitis may be due to well-defined pollen or animal epithelia.

Clinical characteristics in dark skin (Fitzpatrick skin types IV–V)

A mixture of erythema, crusting, excoriation, hyper- and hypopigmentation, and warty lichenification may be seen. Clinical features are the same as in above except for post-inflammatory hypo and hyperpigmentation are common in darker skin (Figures 20.6 to 20.12).

Investigations

This is diagnosed clinically.

Treatments

- Treatment should be tailored to an individual's needs, bearing in mind age, sex, social conditions, sites of involvement, and severity.
- Advice on the reduction of trigger factors (e.g., dry skin, food allergens, exposure to pets, bubble bath, skin infections, wool clothing, airborne allergens, sweating, excessive heat, winter chapping) is important.
- Use of frequent emollients is the mainstay of therapy:

DOI: 10.1201/9781003479512-20

- Use of bathing/showering with emollients.
- The regular use of emollients softens the skin and reduces itching. They make topical corticosteroids more effective and reduce the quantities required.

- Use of topical corticosteroids: Topical corticosteroids are the predominant treatment for the inflammation of AE. The strength and mode of application of the topical steroids depend on the severity of the dermatitis, the sites to be treated, and the age of the patient.
  - Short course of potent topical corticosteroids.
  - If lesions are exudative, topical corticosteroid creams or lotions may be required for a short time.
  - Bleach soaks are given in cases of infection.
  - Ointments are preferred, particularly when lichenification is prominent and suppression of inflammation is intended to induce remission.
- Oral sedating antihistamines and antibiotics may be added for short periods (when there is clinical evidence of infection). H1-receptor antagonists are used predominantly for their sedative effect.
- Topical calcineurin inhibitors (pimecrolimus and tacrolimus) to sensitive areas, wet wrap therapy, and phototherapy (adults) are second-line therapies in resistant cases.
- Systemic therapy is used in severe recalcitrant itching and for a short period; oral corticosteroids (short course), azathioprine, ciclosporin, methotrexate, and mycophenolate mofetil.

Further reading

Blauvelt A, Guttman-Yassky E, Lynde C, et al. (2024). Cendakimab in Patients with Moderate to Severe Atopic Dermatitis: A Randomized Clinical Trial. *JAMA Dermatol*;Aug 1;160(8):856–864:e242131.

Gammanpila RR, Kannangara AP (2024). Eczema, Dermatitis and Ichthyosis in Children with FST 5. In: *Paediatric Cases in Coloured Skin*. CRC Press/Taylor & Francis, UK; 59–80.

Ranawaka RR (2021). Eczematous Disorders. In: Ranawaka RR, et al. (eds). *Atlas of Dermatoses in Pigmented Skin*. Springer, Singapore; 107–122.

Zhao DJ, Li X, Lin HX, et al. (2024). Efficacy and Safety of Upadacitinib in the Treatment of Moderate-to-Severe Atopic Dermatitis: A Systematic Review. *PLoS One*;Jul 26;19(7):e0306463.

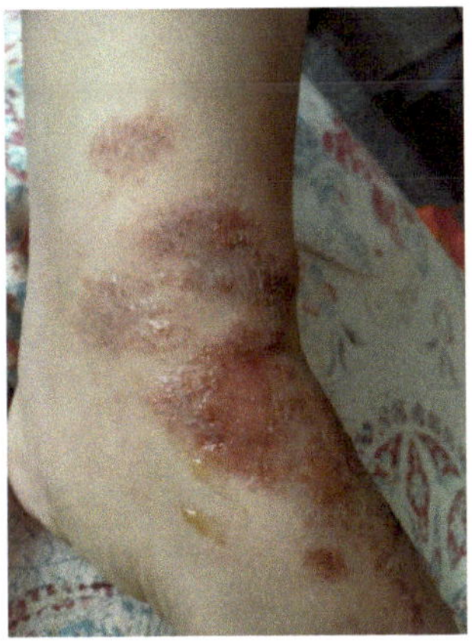

FIGURE 20.1 Acute eczema FST1. (Courtesy Prof. Eckart Haneke, Germany.)

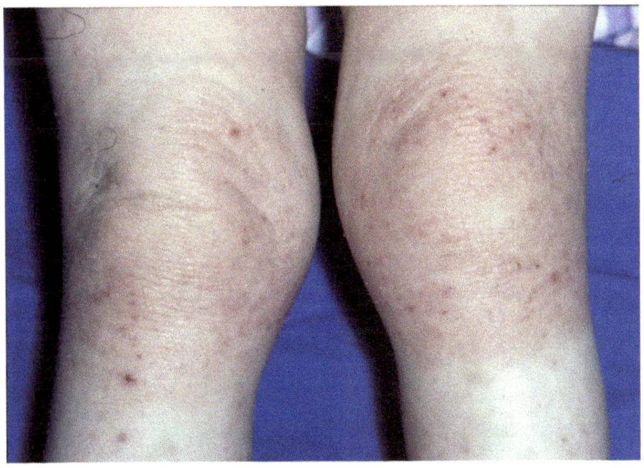

FIGURE 20.2 Atopic eczema reverse pattern on knees FST1. (Courtesy Prof. Ian Coulson, UK.)

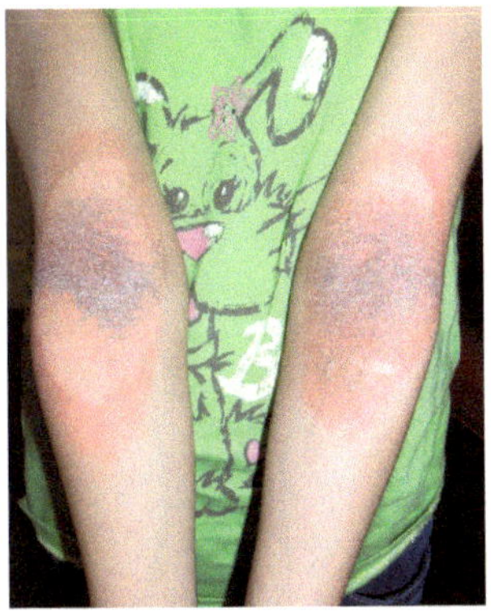

FIGURE 20.3 Atopic eczema in antecubital fossa FST1. (Courtesy Prof. Ian Coulson, UK.)

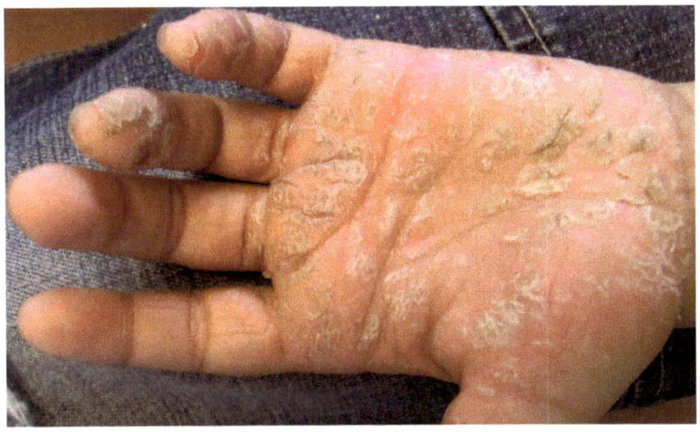

FIGURE 20.4 Hyperkeratotic palmar plantar eczema in FST2. (Courtesy Prof. Eckart Haneke, Germany.)

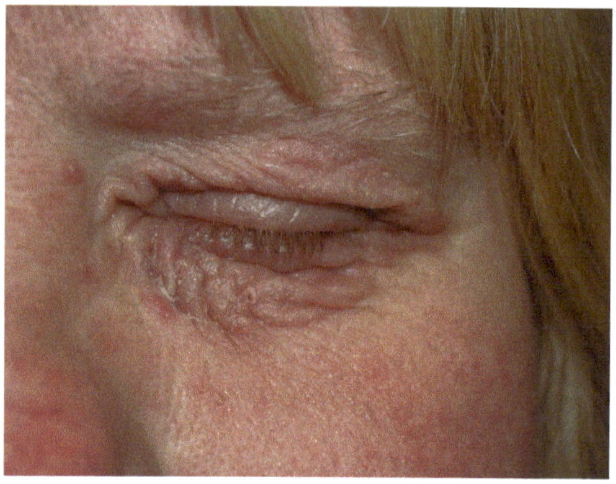

FIGURE 20.5 Atopic eye lid eczema FST1. (Courtesy Prof Ian Coulson, UK.)

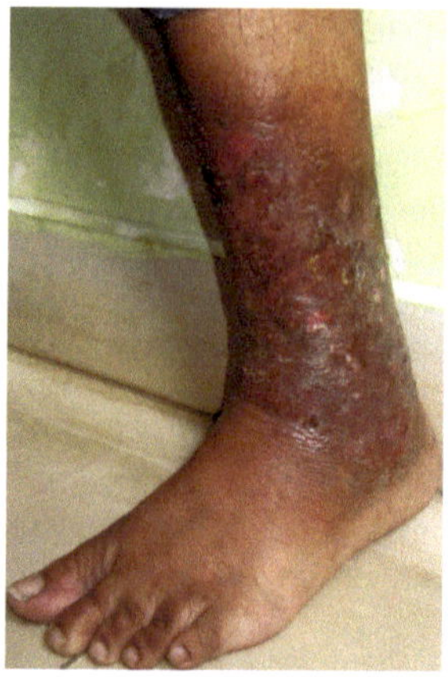

FIGURE 20.6 Acute infected eczema FST5. Note post-inflammatory hyperpigmentation on the affected area.

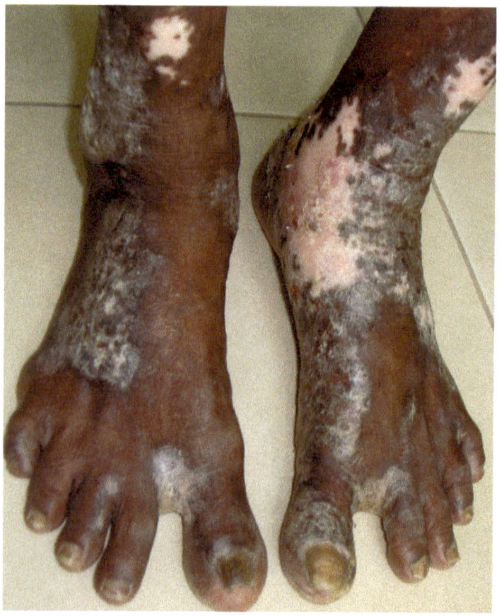

FIGURE 20.7 Chronic lichenified eczema FST5. Note both post-inflammatory hypo- and hyperpigmentation in the same person.

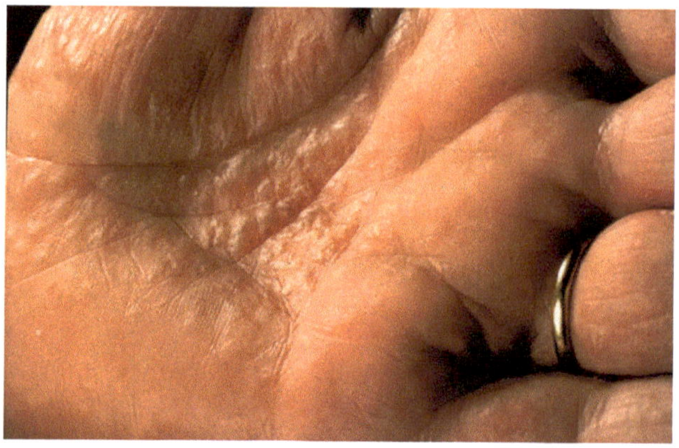

FIGURE 20.8 Pompholyx (dyshidrotic eczema) FST5.

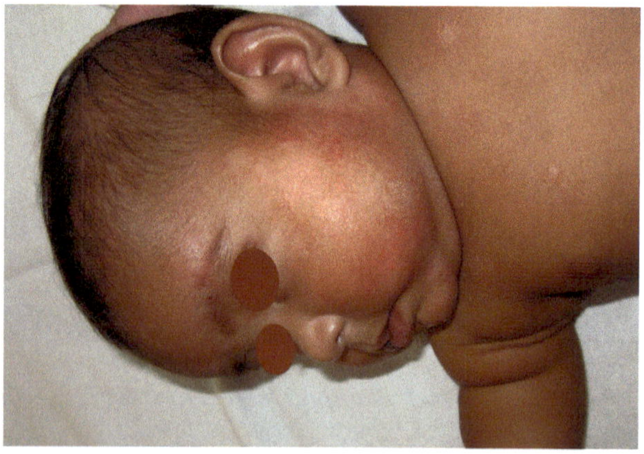

FIGURE 20.9 Infantile phase the atopic eczema most frequently starts on the face, cheeks FST5.

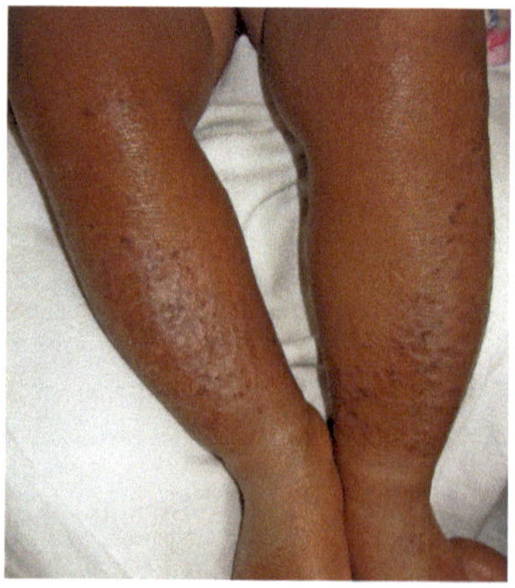

FIGURE 20.10 When the child begins to crawl, the exposed surfaces, extensor aspect of the knees and elbows are affected FST5.

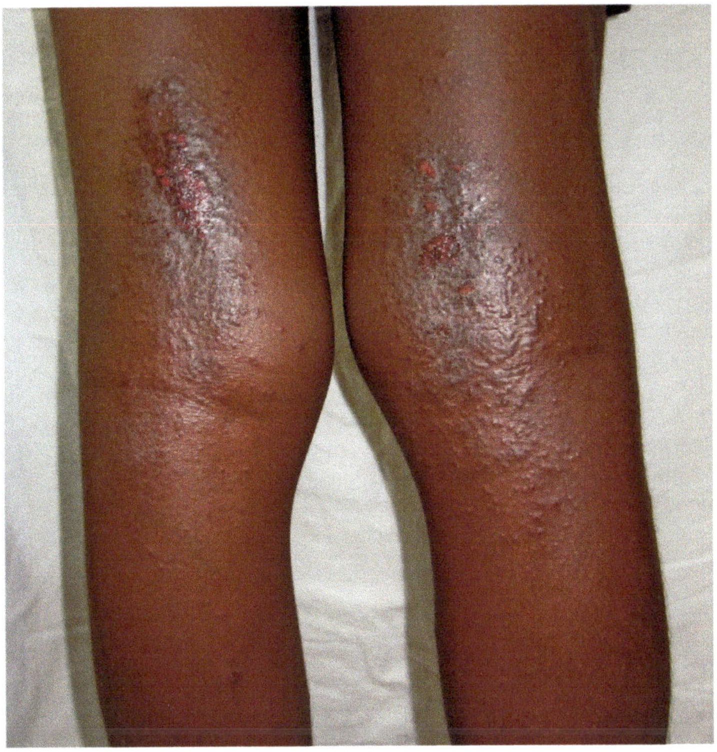

FIGURE 20.11 In children over 18 months and in adults atopic eczema characteristically involves elbow and knee flexures FST5.

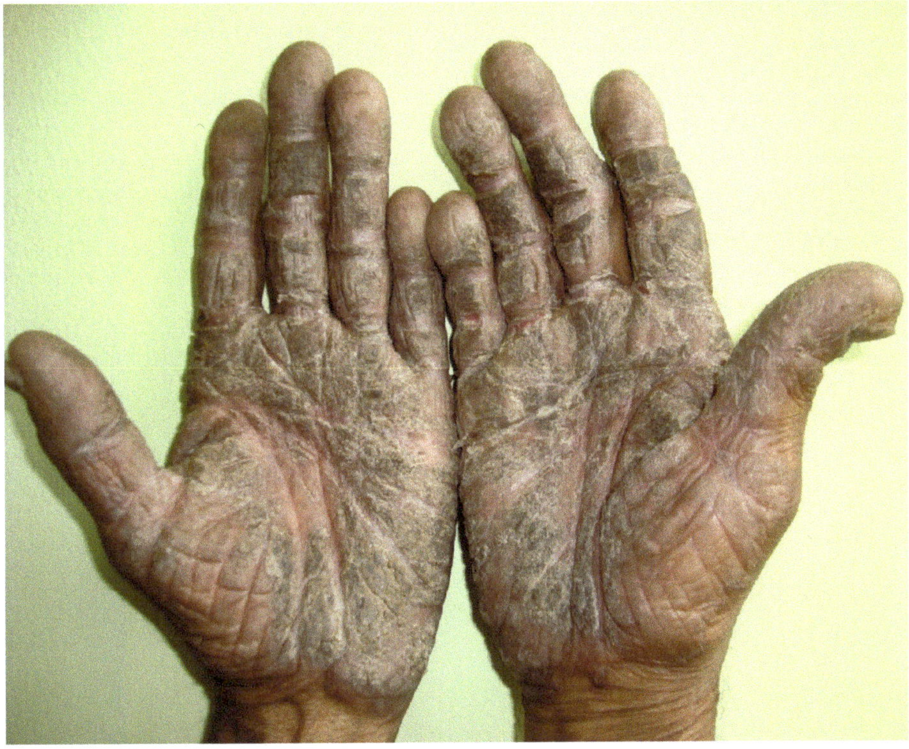

FIGURE 20.12 Hyperkeratotic palmar eczema in FST5.

21
ECZEMA HERPETICUM/KAPOSI VARICELLIFORM ERUPTION

Introduction

A widespread cutaneous infection with a virus (which normally causes localized or mild vesicular eruptions) occurs in a patient with pre-existing skin disease. The majority of cases are infections with HSV-1. However, HSV-2, VZV, coxsackie A6 and A16 (eczema coxsackium), and vaccinia (eczema vaccinatum) have all been associated with a similar eruption. Eczema herpeticum can result from primary or recurrent infection.

Atopic eczema is by far the most common predisposing condition, but is also reported with Darier disease, pemphigus foliaceus, benign familial pemphigus, exfoliative dermatitis, and widespread or erythrodermic psoriasis. If the skin disease is more localized, the varicelliform eruption may be limited to the affected skin.

Epidemiology

No seasonal variation. Seen in all ages and both sexes.

Clinical characteristics in light skin (Fitzpatrick skin types I–III)

Eczema herpeticum is a characteristic disease of atopic patients with recurrent herpes simplex, usually type 1, rarely type 2 (Figure 21.1). A patient with an acute flare of atopic eczema experiencing a first (rare!) or recurrent herpes simplex may get a widespread outbreak of herpetic lesions on the eczematous skin. The lesions are first vesicular with a yellow color and often oozing, which soon dry and become crusted. Untreated, it takes about 10 to 14 days for the scabs to fall off. They often leave very shallow scars, hence the old term of Kaposi's varicelliform eruption.

At the time when vaccinia vaccination was obligatory, eczema vaccinatum was a feared complication in atopics.

In severe cases, hundreds of Mollusca contagiosa may appear on atopic eczema skin.

A varicelliform eruption may also be seen after full-face abrasion (mechanical dermabrasion, laser skin resurfacing).

Clinical characteristics in dark skin (Fitzpatrick skin types IV–V)

In our setting, this is more common in elderly men with exfoliative dermatitis (Figure 21.2). Existing skin disease suddenly becomes worse with the appearance of vesicles, which rapidly become pustular and erupt in massive crops. Typical vesicles or subsequent erosions, generally confined to eczematous or inflamed areas, should cause the suspicion of eczema herpeticum. The patient becomes ill with fever, painful skin, generalized erythema, and regional lymphadenopathy. Punched-out tiny ulcers of 1–2 mm diameter are typical of HSV infection.

Investigations

High suspicion is essential for a clinical diagnosis.

Blister fluid or a surface swab may be analyzed for HSV and multinucleated epidermal giant cells.

Treatments

- Patents with atopic eczema or Darier disease should avoid close contact with relatives and friends with active herpes simplex.
- Antiviral treatment is recommended for all ages and should be started as soon as possible after diagnosis.

Less ill patients respond well to oral aciclovir, valaciclovir, or famciclovir.

- Severe cases should receive intravenous acyclovir as early as possible.
- Frequently recurrent disease may benefit from low-dose prophylactic aciclovir or valaciclovir.
- Bacterial infection and the underlying eczema or other dermatoses should be treated in the usual way. However, avoid the use of steroid therapy until the viral lesions have healed.

Further reading

Harwood CA, Sterling JC (2024). Viral Infections. In: Griffiths C, et al. (eds). *Rook's Textbook of Dermatology*, 10th ed. John Wiley & Sons Ltd., UK; 25.43.

DOI: 10.1201/9781003479512-21

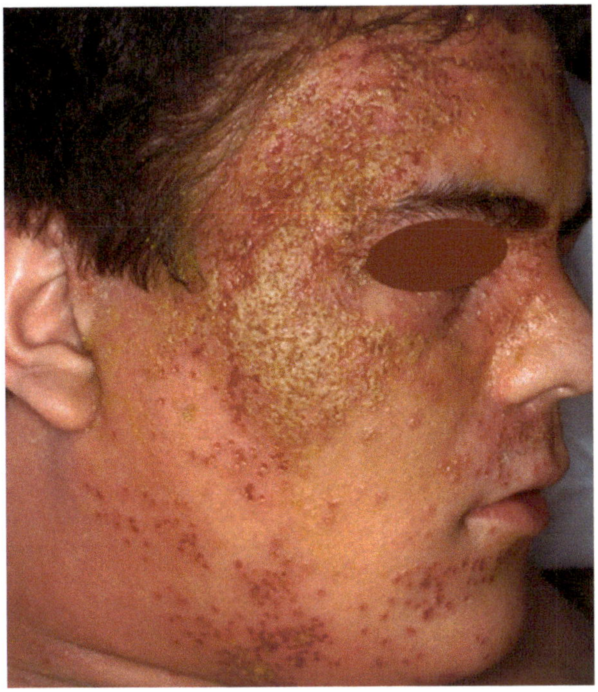

FIGURE 21.1 Eczema herpeticum FST2. (Courtesy Prof. Ian Coulson, UK.)

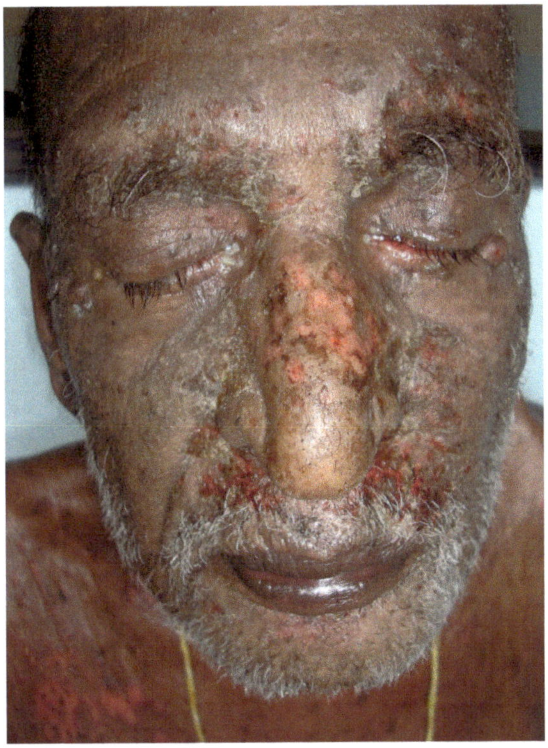

FIGURE 21.2 Eczema herpeticum in a 76-year-old man FST5 with generalized eczema. His eczema suddenly became worse with oozing, pus discharge, fever, and general ill health. Careful examination revealed punched-out ulcers on the trunk and face.

22
NIPPLE ECZEMA

Introduction

This is eczema arising on the nipple. It can be unilateral or bilateral. When it is bilateral, irritant contact dermatitis to undergarments should be considered. Eczema lacks the sharp, raised, and rounded margin and the superficial induration that differentiates it from Paget disease of the breast (Chapter 74). In doubtful cases, a biopsy should be conducted.

Epidemiology

Common in nulliparous and breastfeeding young women.

Associated diseases

Unilateral nipple eczema in elderly women should raise the possibility of Paget's disease of the breast.

Clinical characteristics in light skin (Fitzpatrick skin types I–III)

Nipple eczema is mainly seen in young women (Figure 22.1). Usually, both mamillae are red, develop tiny papules and minute vesicles, the roofs of which break off, and oozing starts. Contact allergy to diverse products is common; also, mechanical irritation may elicit eczema, particularly in atopics.

Unilateral nipple eczema raises the suspicion of Paget's disease. Other differential diagnoses are nipple psoriasis, nipple candidiasis, and scabies.

Clinical characteristics in dark skin (Fitzpatrick skin types IV–V)

We see this condition more frequently in mothers who continue to breastfeed older children (Figure 22.2). The saliva of older children aged 2 years and above may be an irritating factor in some. Oozing eczematous lesions on the nipple having a more fluctuating course, improving in response to local treatment, and spreading rapidly when irritated, are features of nipple eczema.

Investigations

This is a clinical diagnosis.

Biopsy is performed if Paget's disease of the breast is suspected.

Treatments

- Treatment of nipple eczema must effectively control the signs and symptoms of the disease, as it can have a negative effect on quality of life and can lead to premature cessation of breastfeeding.
- The key treatment step is starting with topical corticosteroids or calcineurin inhibitors, both of which are considered safe during lactation.
- Provoking factors, such as repetitive friction, chemical agents, or allergens, have to be avoided. Nipple protection devices can be proposed for nursing women, and sometimes adjustment of latch/suck positioning during breastfeeding is recommended.
- Patients are advised to intensively moisturize the nipple and to switch to emollient wash products. Warm water and black tea compresses or commercially available tannin-containing topicals can provide comfort.
- Treat as eczema with mild to moderate topical steroids with or without topical or oral antibiotics.
- When acute eczema is settled, regular emollients.

Further reading

Ranawaka RR, Madarasinghe NP, Kannangara AP, et al. (2020). Cutaneous Disorders of Breast. In: Smoller B, et al. (eds). *Atlas of Dermatology, Dermatopathology and Venereology*, Springer, Cham; 991–1038.

Reynaert V, Gutermuth J, Wollenberg A (2023). Nipple Eczema: A Systematic Review and Practical Recommendations. *J Eur Acad Dermatol Venereol*;37(6):1149–1159.

Wu C, Jia QN, Fang K, et al. (2023). Skin Diseases of the Nipple and Areola Complex: A Case Series Study from China. *Front Med*;10:1136482.

Zengin HB, Tan PH, Liu R, et al. (2024). 'Eczematous' Dermatitis of the Nipple: Clinical and Histopathological Differential Diagnosis of Paget Disease. *Pathology*;S0031-3025(24)00002–3.

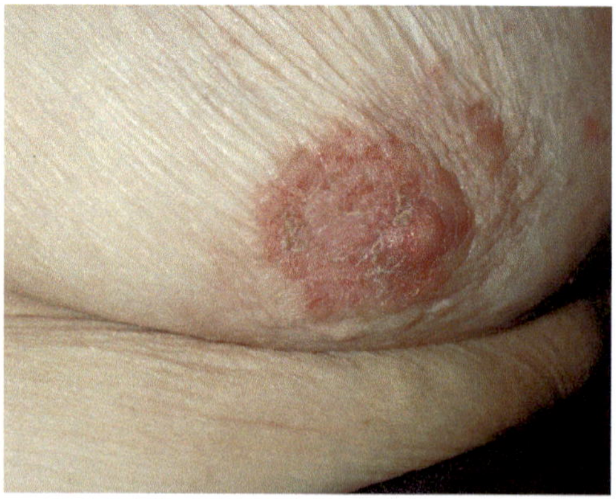

FIGURE 22.1 Nipple eczema in a 77-year-old woman FST1. (Courtesy Prof. Ian Coulson, UK.)

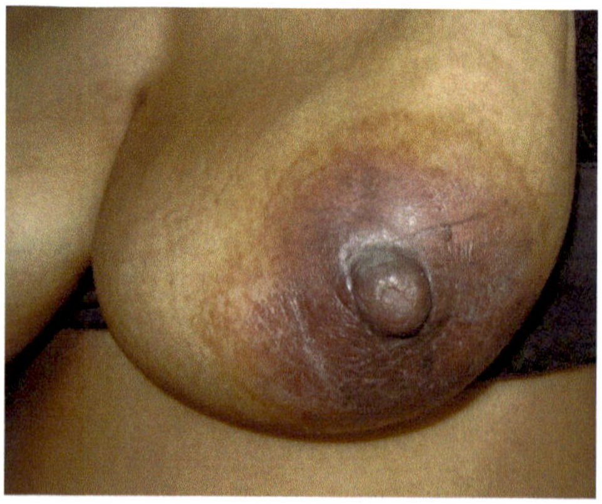

FIGURE 22.2 Unilateral nipple eczema in a 27-year-old breastfeeding mother FST5.

DOI: 10.1201/9781003479512-22

23
NUMMULAR ECZEMA OR DISCOID ECZEMA

Introduction

This is a non-specific morphological feature, namely circular or oval plaques of eczema with a clearly demarcated edge. This is a chronic problem, undergoing relapses and remissions.

There are a number of variants:

- Nummular dermatitis: Exudative type
- Nummular dermatitis: Dry type
- Nummular dermatitis of the hands
- Exudative discoid and lichenoid chronic dermatosis

Epidemiology

Common in children and the elderly.

Clinical characteristics in light skin (Fitzpatrick skin types I–III)

Nummular eczema is also called microbial eczema. Characteristically, a small round papule develops that enlarges to a diameter of 3–10 mm, before more well-demarcated round erythematous infiltrated plaques develop (Figures 23.1 and 23.2). They exhibit tiny papules that tend to erode and finally form a round plaque of five or more centimeters in diameter covered with a sero-sanguinolent scab. There may be one single plaque, but in most cases, several to many and sometimes symmetrical lesions are found. The lower legs are predominantly affected, followed by the forearms and later the lower trunk.

Although bacteria, particularly staphylococci, may colonize the oozing surface this is not an infection; the etiology of nummular eczema is not clear; however, some authors speculate that an allergic reaction to microbial agents may play a role. In our experience, most middle-aged men are heavy smokers and consume considerable amounts of alcohol. The course is chronic or chronic relapsing.

Histopathology is relatively characteristic, with exocytosis and a tiny serous crust on top.

The differential diagnosis comprises a number of different dermatoses: Single lesions may resemble tinea corporis. In children and adolescents, atopic eczema may be nummular. Asteatotic eczema on the distal extremities may develop inflammatory round plaques. Allergic contact dermatitis may be nummular, particularly the jeans-button eczema due to nickel or lesions on the dorsa of the hands and feet due to various topical skin care products, as well as nickel and cobalt.

Clinical characteristics in dark skin (Fitzpatrick skin types IV–V)

Oval or coin-shaped, well-defined, discrete eczema is commonly seen in children (Figure 23.3).

Investigations

This is diagnosed clinically.

Treatments

- Lifestyle changes such as stopping tobacco use and alcohol intake.
- Emollient and topical corticosteroid with or without topical or oral antibiotics.
- Topical calcineurin inhibitors are second-line therapies.
- Phototherapy (narrow-band UVB/PUVA), oral immunosuppressants including methotrexate, or oral steroids in resistant, troublesome lesions.

Further reading

Gammanpila RR, Kannangara AP (2024). Eczema, Dermatitis and Ichthyosis in Children with FST 5. In: *Paediatric Cases in Coloured Skin*. CRC Press, UK; 59–80.

Ranawaka RR (2021). Eczematous Disorders. In: Ranawaka RR, et al. (eds). *Atlas of Dermatoses in Pigmented Skin*. Springer, Singapore; 107–122.

DOI: 10.1201/9781003479512-23

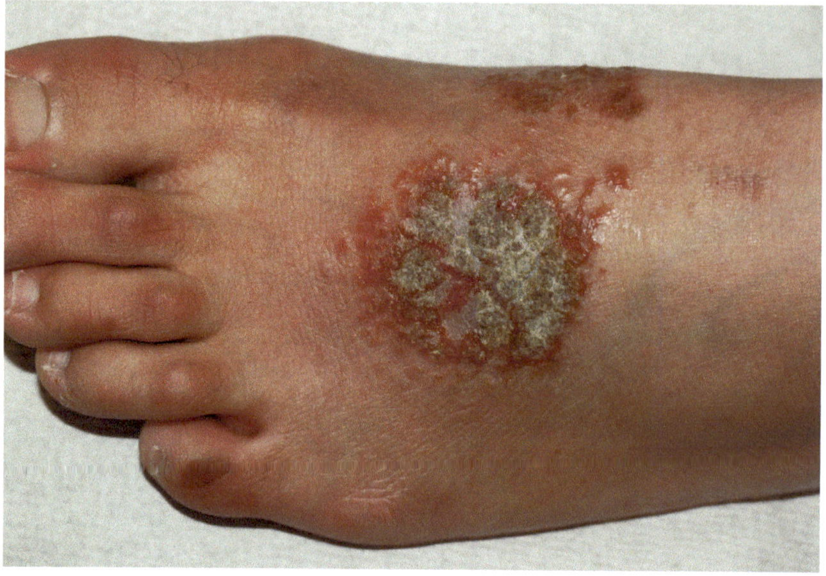

FIGURE 23.1 Nummular eczema FST2. (Courtesy Prof. Ian Coulson, UK.)

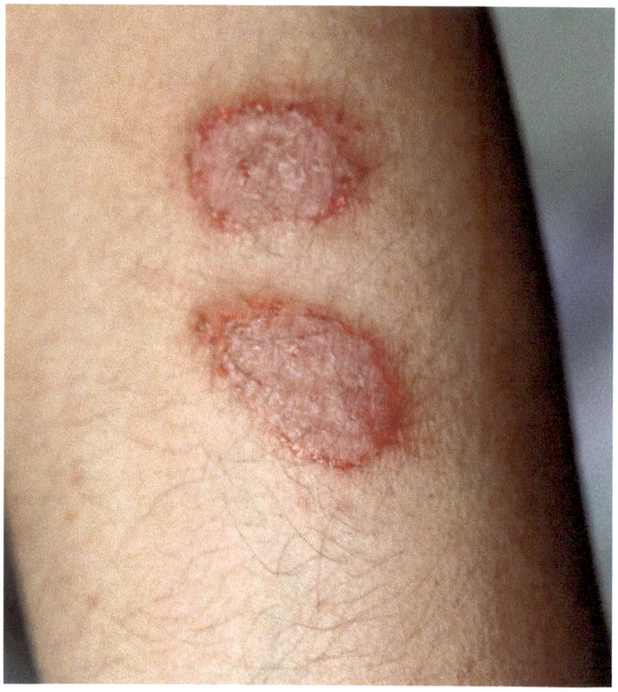

FIGURE 23.2 Discoid eczema FST1. (Courtesy Dr. Richard Ashton, UK.)

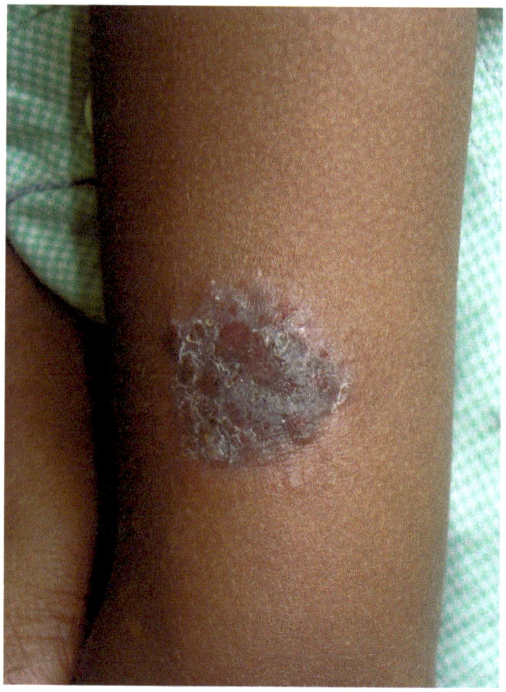

FIGURE 23.3 Nummular eczema in a 3-year-old girl FST5.

24
ERYSIPELAS AND CELLULITIS

Introduction

Erysipelas is a bacterial infection of the dermis and upper subcutaneous tissue; its hallmark is a well-defined raised edge reflecting the more superficial (dermal) involvement. Erysipelas is a form of cellulitis rather than a distinct entity, so that the definition of cellulitis would include inflammation of dermal as well as subcutaneous tissue. In patients with normal immunity, this is predominantly a streptococcal disease; *Staphylococcus aureus* and *Haemophilus influenzae* type b (in facial cellulitis in children) are also occasionally implicated. *S. pneumoniae*, *Pseudomonas aeruginosa*, and *Campylobacter jejuni* have been reported in the immunocompromised.

Epidemiology

Common disease in all ages and both sexes, although more prevalent in elderly diabetics.

Associated diseases

May be associated with fasciitis, myositis, subcutaneous abscesses, septicemia, and, in some, post-streptococcal nephritis.

Clinical characteristics in light skin (Fitzpatrick skin types I–III)

Erysipelas is a rather common infection of the skin by streptococci, usually group A, less frequently group G. It is seen in all age groups, although more frequently in adults (Figures 24.1 to 24.3). The disease starts with chills, fever, and a diffuse erythema of the skin that progresses and often has a flame-like extension proximally. Small skin fissures, for instance from interdigital tinea pedum or from chronic rhagades around the nares or at the earlobes, are the portal of entry for this bacterial infection. Regional lymph node swelling often occurs. In severe cases, the erythema may be hemorrhagic, become bullous and finally necrotic, particularly in immunocompromised and diabetic patients. A phlegmonous form is the most serious one, with extremely rapid necrosis of the deep dermis, fascia, and muscle, called necrotizing fasciitis; this requires intensive care and immediate surgical intervention. The diagnosis is made clinically and confirmed by the characteristic symptomatology such as high fever, chills, elevated erythrocyte sedimentation rate, and leucocytosis.

Treatment is with high-dose penicillin. Recurrences are common as the patients do not develop infection immunity. Chronic lymphedema may result (elephantiasis nostras). Frequently recurring erysipelas is treated with long-term antibiotic prophylaxis.

Differential diagnosis is acute toxic contact dermatitis, which always presents without fever. On the face, an early herpes zoster has to be considered. On the hands, erysipeloid caused by *Erysipelothrix rusiopathiae*, is an acute infection usually due to inoculation of the pathogen through a minor skin laceration, often acquired during work (fishmongers, butchers). The onset is less acute and the color of the skin is livid red.

Clinical characteristics in dark skin (Fitzpatrick skin types IV–V)

Since erythema is obscured in darker skin, late diagnosis, underestimation of severity, and delayed management may lead to higher morbidity in dark-skinned patients (Figures 24.4 and 24.5). Other features of inflammation such as swelling and tenderness are important signs and symptoms in these instances.

Investigations

This is diagnosed clinically.

Swab cultures, blood, and tissue cultures would help to identify the offending organisms and antibiotic sensitivity (ABST).

Treatments

Identify the organisms and systemic antibiotics according to ABST.

Further reading

Wootton C, Elliott I (2024). Bacterial Infections. In: Griffiths C, et al. (eds). *Rook's Textbook of Dermatology*, 10th ed. John Wiley & Sons Ltd., UK; 26.17.

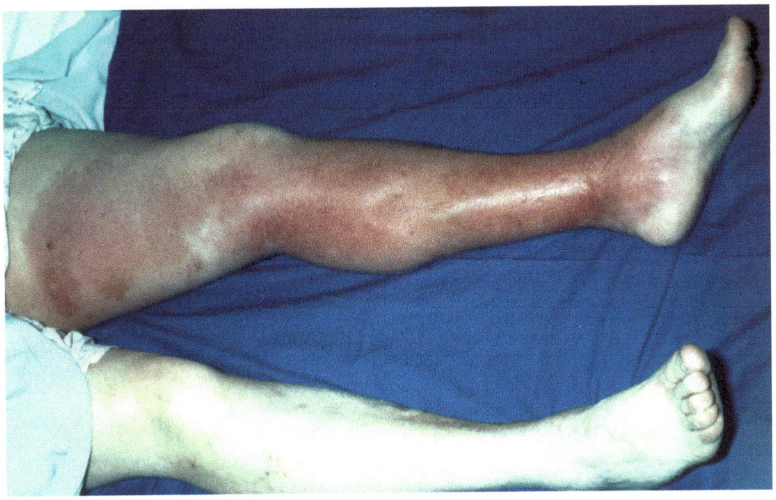

FIGURE 24.1 Cellulitis in an obese diabetic woman FST1. (Courtesy Prof. Ian Coulson, UK.)

DOI: 10.1201/9781003479512-24

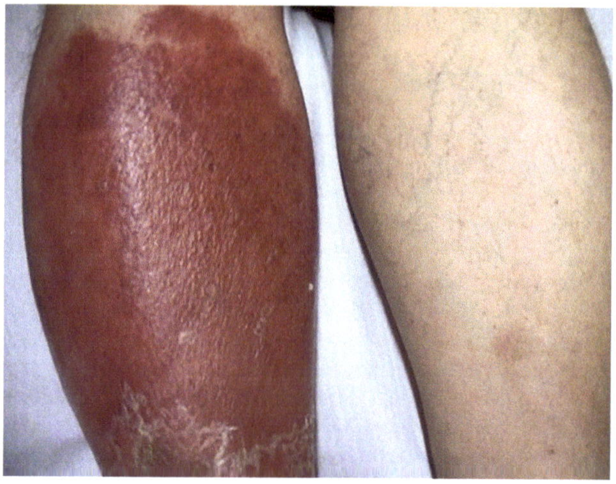

FIGURE 24.2 Erysipelas in a patient with FST2. (Courtesy Prof. Osvaldo Correia, Portugal.)

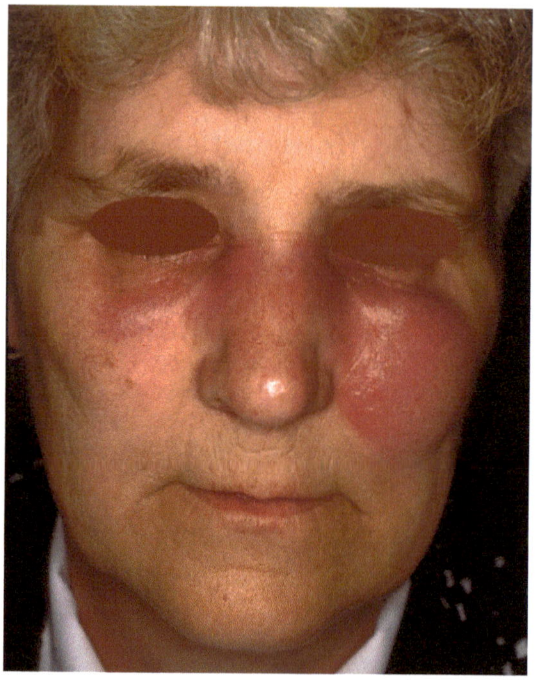

FIGURE 24.3 Erysipelas on the face FST2. (Courtesy Prof. Ian Coulson, UK.)

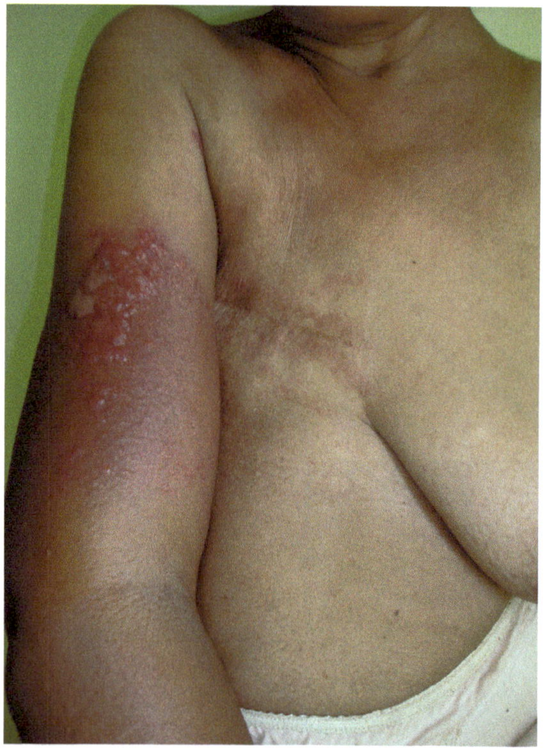

FIGURE 24.4 Cellulitis on lymphedematous right arm in a woman with mastectomy FST5.

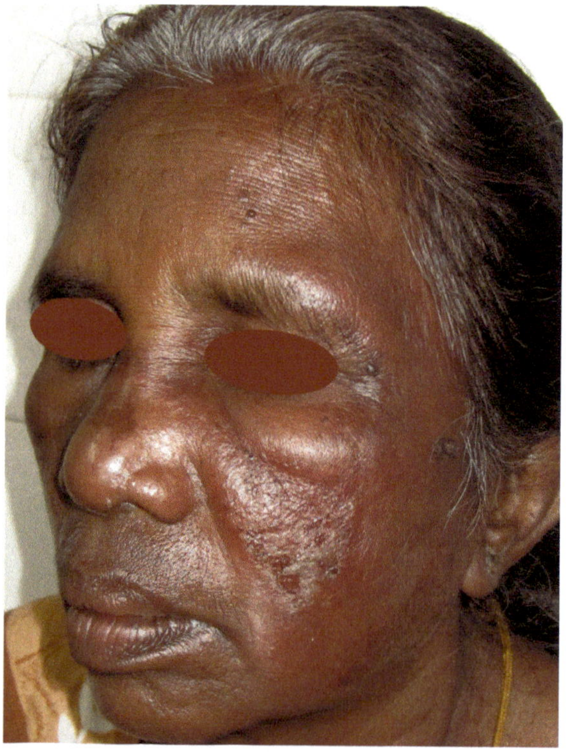

FIGURE 24.5 Erysipelas on the face in a very dark-skinned woman FST5. Note severity of erythema is obscured in dark skin.

25
ERYTHEMA ANNULARE CENTRIFUGUM

Introduction

Erythema annulare centrifugum (EAC) is a gyrate erythema that is typically characterized by annular, polycyclic, erythematous plaques with scaling behind the advancing edge. It slowly enlarges to form a ring as the central area flattens and fades. EAC is a reactive process that may be precipitated by infections, drugs, or malignancy. Concurrent infection is the most common underlying association, which include viral (Epstein–Barr virus), bacterial (streptococcal infections, *Escherichia coli*), mycobacterial, fungal (dermatophytes in 48%), or parasitic. However, in the majority of cases, no underlying cause is identified.

This may be superficial (pruritic, scaling) or deep (non-pruritic, non-scaling) type. EAC may last days to decades in spite of treatments.

Epidemiology

EAC can occur at any age. There is no sex predilection.

Associated diseases

Infections, thyroid disease, liver disease, and malignancy (lymphoma, leukemia, thyroid, gastric, breast, ovarian, prostate carcinomas).

Clinical characteristics in light skin (Fitzpatrick skin types I–III)

This is a peculiar, clinically well-characterized, etiologically unclear condition, which is thought by some authors to be an allergic reaction (Figure 25.1); however, a pathogenic allergen has rarely, if ever been found. Infections, infestations, malignant tumors, autoimmune diseases, drugs, and food allergens were considered. It is seen mainly in middle-aged adults of either gender. Mainly on the trunk and proximal extremities, asymmetrically distributed urticarial erythemas develop that soon form annular or serpiginous lesions with gradual central clearing. The disease may disappear spontaneously or recur in irregular periods. Itching is common in the newly forming lesions, otherwise it is not pronounced.

Histopathology shows superficial or deep lymphocytic perivascular infiltrates under a normal epidermis and papillary dermis. This is characteristic of all so-called figurate erythemas.

The differential diagnosis is wide and spans from annular urticaria to erythema multiforme, dermatitis herpetiformis, bullous pemphigoid, annular psoriasis, tinea corporis, erythema gyratum repens, erythema gyratum perstans, erythema chronicum migrans, and necrolytic migratory erythema, in addition to some other dermatoses that can occasionally be annular.

Clinical characteristics in dark skin (Fitzpatrick skin types IV–V)

EAC is not frequently identified in our setting.

Figure 25.2 shows a 58-year-old woman who complained of these itchy annular erythematous lesions that have been expanding by up to 2–3 mm per day with central clearing for more than 6 months. As fungal infections are the most common cause, she was treated with oral terbinafine 250 mg daily for one month, which led to the disappearance of the lesions.

Investigations

This is diagnosed clinically.

- Skin biopsy for histopathology: A spectrum of non-specific histological findings is seen in EAC, and it is critical to have clinicopathological correlation. The characteristic histological feature in EAC is a perivascular 'sleeve-like' lymphohistiocytic infiltrate, which may be mainly superficial, mainly deep, or mixed.
- As fungal infections are the most common, fungal cultures are performed from suspected lesions (skin, nail).
- Full blood count, liver and thyroid function tests, abdominal ultrasound and chest X-ray, antinuclear antibody profile, serum angiotensin-converting enzyme (ACE), and HIV serology
- If a malignancy is suspected, appropriate investigations should be conducted.

Treatments

- Identify and treat any underlying conditions.
- Moderately potent or potent topical corticosteroids or topical calcipotriol should be used after infection is ruled out.
- Topical tacrolimus and phototherapy are second-line therapies.
- Oral chloroquine, hydroxychloroquine, or systemic steroids in resistant cases.

Further reading

Erduran F (2024). Evaluation of Clinicopathological Features and Associated Conditions in Erythema Annulare Centrifugum: A Retrospective Observational Analysis of 63 Patients. *Dermatol Pract Concept*;Jan 1;14(1):e2024039.

Mu EW, Sanchez M, Mir A, et al. (2015). Paraneoplastic Erythema Annulare Centrifugum Eruption (PEACE). *Dermatol Online J*;Dec 16;21(12):13030/qt6053h29n.

Murphy R (2024). Reactive Inflammatory Erythemas. In: Griffiths C, et al. (eds). *Rook's Textbook of Dermatology*, 10th ed. John Wiley & Sons Ltd., UK; 47.6.

DOI: 10.1201/9781003479512-25

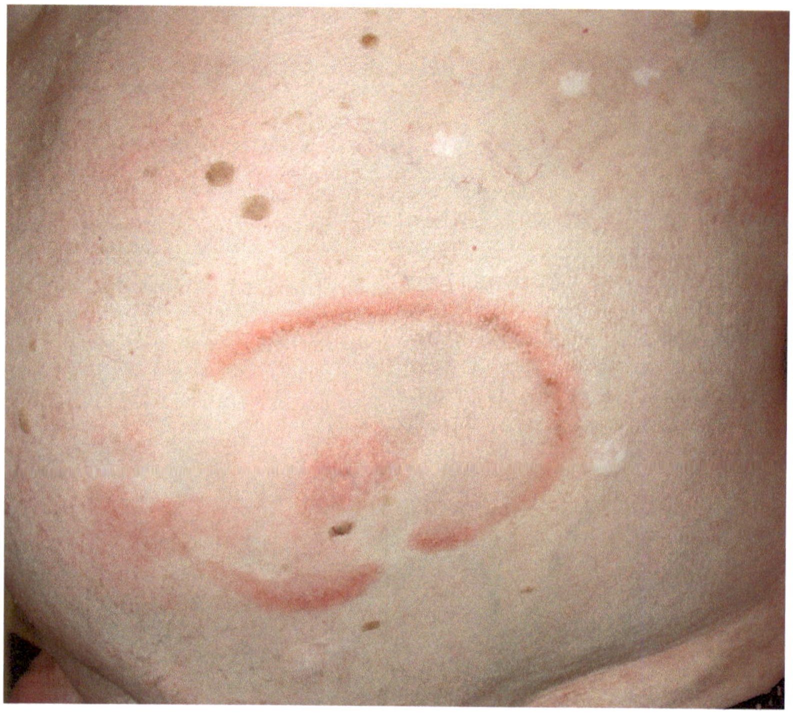

FIGURE 25.1 Erythema annulare centrifugum FST1. (Courtesy Prof. Ian Coulson, UK.)

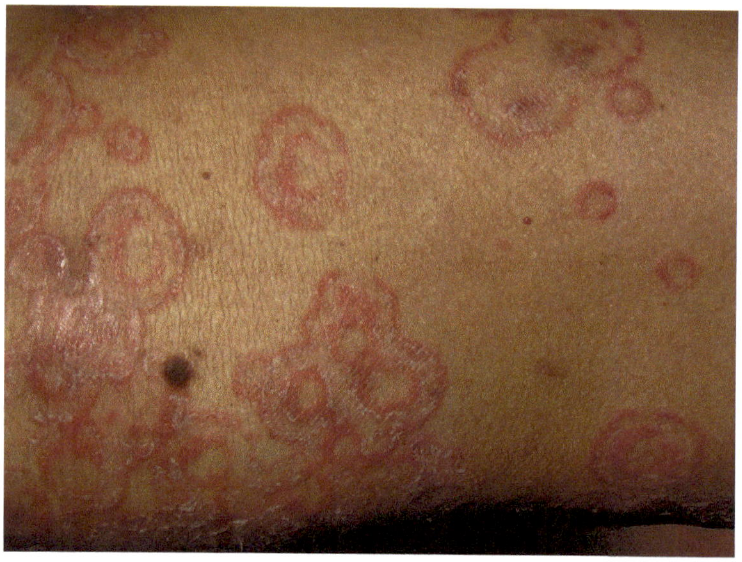

FIGURE 25.2 Erythema annulare centrifugum in a 58-year-old woman FST5 who presented with these itchy lesions lasting for more than 6 months in spite of varied treatments by family physicians.

26
ERYTHEMA MULTIFORME

Introduction

Erythema multiforme (EM) is described in a group of conditions called reactive erythemas that do not necessarily lead to a specific underlying diagnosis. EM is a self-limiting cytotoxic dermatitis resulting from cell-mediated hypersensitivity to drugs or infections (especially with herpes virus). This is now considered EM minor and EM major as part of one spectrum. It presents clinically with macular, papular, or urticarial lesions, as well as the classic 'target lesions.' Lesions may involve the palms, trunk, oral, and genital mucosal membranes.

Epidemiology

EM can occur at any age, including in neonates or young children. There is no sex predilection.

Associated diseases

EM may be triggered by viral (herpes simplex virus, *Mycoplasma* infections are the most common), bacterial and fungal infections, malignancy (carcinoma, lymphoma, leukemia), lupus erythematosus (Rowell syndrome), polyarteritis nodosa, and sarcoidosis.

Clinical characteristics in light skin (Fitzpatrick skin types I–III)

Erythema multiforme, a cutaneous and mucosal hypersensitivity, is a relatively common condition in light-skinned people (Figures 26.1 and 26.2). With or without a recognizable trigger, round red papules and plaques arise anywhere on the skin, particularly the extremities and mucosae that may soon develop a central bulla and then resemble a target lesion. In most cases, between 10 and 20 such lesions appear; however, in severe cases, many more lesions can develop, and the patients feel severely ill. The roof of the bullae is necrotic and sloughs off, leaving a red raw surface. This may develop a hemorrhagic crust that tends to crack when located in areas of movement, such as the lips and corners of the mouth. In the mouth, typical bullae are not seen; instead, fibrin-covered shallow ulcerations develop, rendering eating and chewing very painful. Genital lesions cause dyspareunia. The lesions take 2 to 3 weeks to heal.

Whereas EM was thought to be a drug reaction in most cases some decades ago, post-herpetic EM appears to outnumber other causes even when there is no visible herpes simplex outbreak, as asymptomatic virus shedding as a sign of herpes virus activation is frequent. Herpes-induced EMs also tend to recur frequently and often present with oral mucosal lesions. Other causes are streptococcal and mycoplasma infections as well as COVID-19 infection and vaccination. Drugs associated with EM include antipyretics and antibiotics like penicillins, cephalosporins, macrolides, sulfonamides, tuberculostatic agents, and many others. In some patients, contact with heavy metals, herbal agents, topical therapies, and poison ivy can trigger EM. Some lesions are photosensitive.

Treatment is topical with mild steroids and antibiotics to prevent secondary infection, and mouthwashes for oral mucosal lesions. Even if herpes simplex is not seen, recurrent oral EM warrants a trial with long-term acyclovir.

EM may be differentiated into erythema multiforme minor, essentially involving the skin with typical lesions and symmetrical acral distribution with rare mucosal lesions, often affecting the mouth, and into EM major with more extensive skin lesions but not exceeding 10% of the body surface area. Typical target lesions are present. Mucosal involvement is severe and affects at least two different mucosal sites; the oral mucosa is typically affected as well as, often, the genital and conjunctival mucosae.

EM major takes 4–6 weeks to heal.

Clinical characteristics in dark skin (Fitzpatrick skin types IV–V)

Erythematous macular, papular, urticarial lesions, or target lesions may be inconspicuous in darker skin leading to delayed diagnosis, and therefore increased complications and morbidity (Figure 26.3).

Investigations

This is diagnosed clinically.

Investigations are performed depending on the underlying disease.

Treatments

- Treat the underlying problem.
- Symptomatic treatments.
- Recurrent EM without overt herpes infection can be treated with prophylactic acyclovir.
- Thalidomide has been used in a few cases to prevent relapses of recurrent EM.

Further reading

Murphy R (2024). Reactive Inflammatory Erythemas. In: Griffiths C, et al. (eds). *Rook's Textbook of Dermatology*, 10th ed. John Wiley & Sons Ltd., UK; 47.1.

Saleh W, Alharbi H, Cha S (2024). Increased Prevalence of Erythema Multiforme in Patients with COVID-19 Infection or Vaccination. *Sci Rep*;Feb 2;14(1):2801.

DOI: 10.1201/9781003479512-26

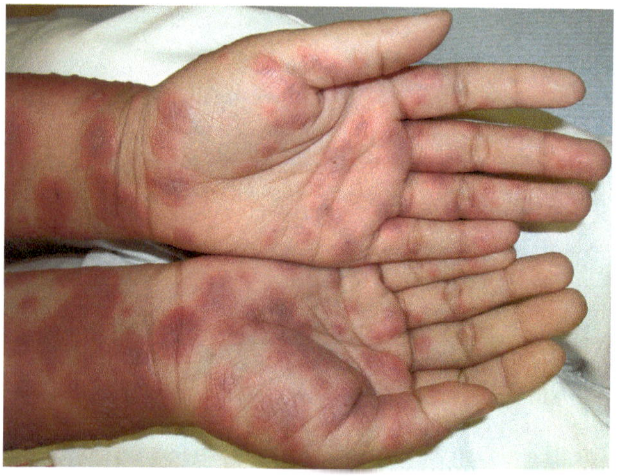

FIGURE 26.1 Erythema multiforme FST1. (Courtesy Prof. Ian Coulson, UK.)

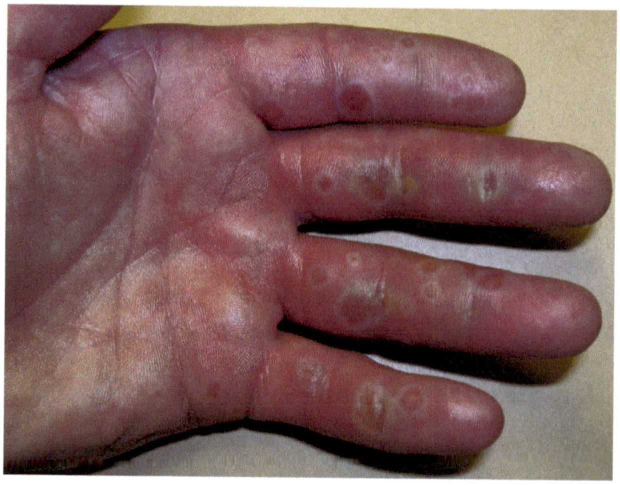

FIGURE 26.2 Erythema multiforme, post-herpes simplex FST2. (Courtesy Prof. Ian Coulson, UK.)

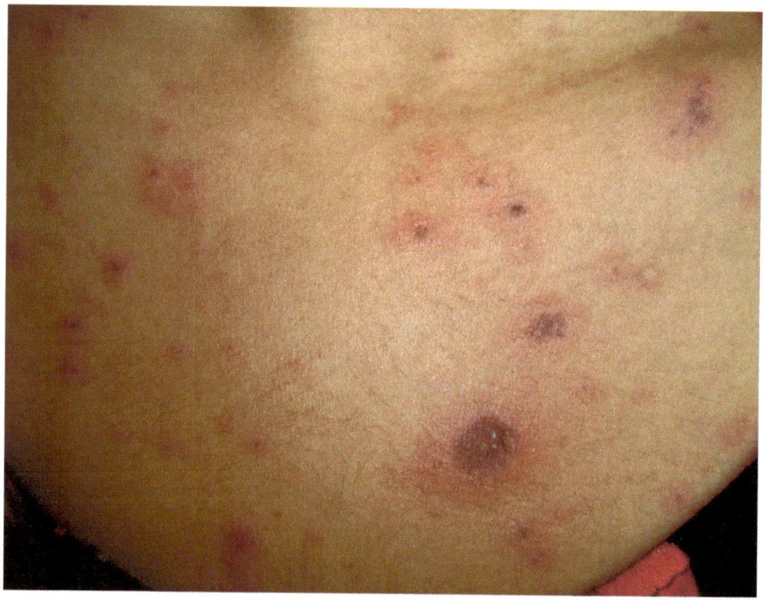

FIGURE 26.3 Erythema multiforme; target lesions in a 24-year-old woman FST5 with gingival herpes infection.

27
ERYTHEMA NODOSUM

Introduction

Erythema nodosum (EN) is the most common panniculitis that shows an acute onset and self-limited course. It is clinically characterized by the sudden eruption of several erythematous, tender, non-ulcerating nodules and plaques, typically located on the shins. It resolves spontaneously without ulceration, scarring, or atrophy. The most common triggers are bacterial infections, sarcoidosis, and inflammatory bowel disease (not ulcerative colitis).

Epidemiology

EN occurs at any age; most cases appear between the second and fourth decades of life, with the peak between 20 and 30 years of age, and it is six times more frequent in women.

Associated diseases

Etiological factors show considerable geographical variation related to specific endemic infections. In Europe, streptococcal infections (2–3 weeks after a throat infection), sarcoidosis, and Crohn's disease are the most common associations. Tuberculosis is a common cause of erythema nodosum in Asia and Africa.

Clinical characteristics in light skin (Fitzpatrick skin types I–III)

EN is a well-known disease of the cutaneous fat that almost exclusively occurs over the shin and rarely over the extensor surface of the lower arms (Figure 27.1). Sudden onset of warm, red, tender-to-painful nodes is characteristic. Sometimes they may take on a bluish hue due to a mild hemorrhagic component. Most patients report a previous streptococcal infection, particularly streptococcal angina, some weeks before the onset of the lesions. Other causes include other infections, malignancies, inflammatory diseases, autoimmune diseases, pregnancy, and medications. No specific treatment is needed in uncomplicated cases; however, recurrent EN should prompt a search for its etiology and adequate therapy. This may be the case in sarcoidosis (Löfgren syndrome with acute sarcoidosis and arthritis) and Crohn's disease (found by Mendelian randomization).

EN has to be differentiated from EN leprosum, which is a completely different disease concerning its clinical and immunological characteristics.

Clinical characteristics in dark skin (Fitzpatrick skin types IV–V)

The patients present with tender, painful subcutaneous nodules on the shins (Figure 27.2). They are mostly skin-colored and are detected by palpation rather than visualization. Erythema, if present, may be obscured by darker skin color. Tuberculosis, pulmonary or extra-pulmonary, is a common cause in our setting.

Investigations

This is diagnosed clinically.

Investigate to identify the possible etiological factors. Initial laboratory investigations should include a complete blood count, erythrocyte sedimentation rate, ASO titre, urinalysis, throat culture, intradermal tuberculin test and/or chest X-ray.

Treatments

Treat the underlying disease.

Further reading

Requena L, Cerroni L (2024). Panniculitis. In: Griffiths C, et al. (eds). *Rook's Textbook of Dermatology*, 10th ed. John Wiley & Sons Ltd., UK; 97.18.

Zhu H, Jiang Y, Ma G, et al. (2024). Causal Relationship between Inflammatory Bowel Disease and Erythema Nodosum: A Two-Sample Bidirectional Mendelian Randomization Study. *Skin Res Technol*;30(2):e13600.

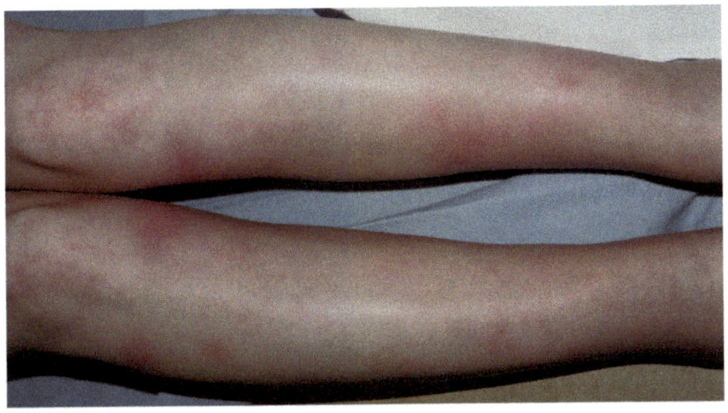

FIGURE 27.1 Erythema nodosum FST1. (Courtesy Prof. Ian Coulson, UK.)

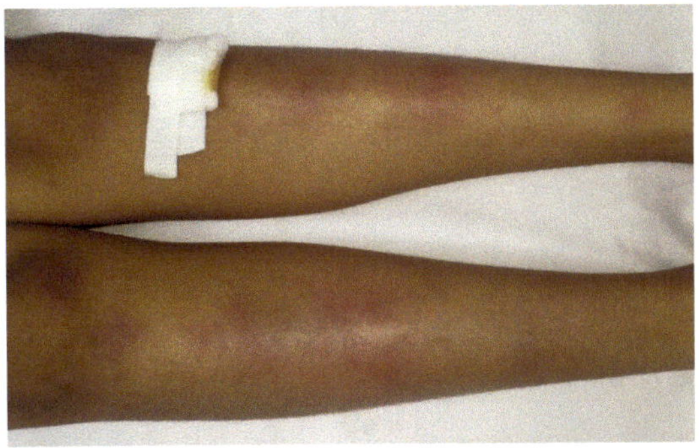

FIGURE 27.2 Erythema nodosum in an 8-year-old boy FST5.

DOI: 10.1201/9781003479512-27

28
ERYTHRASMA

Introduction

Localized superficial infection of the skin caused by aerobic coryneform bacteria, usually known as *Corynebacterium minutissimum*. It is a common disease in warm, humid climates, affecting the axillae, groin, and toe webs. This is mostly asymptomatic but may mildly itch in warm, hot, sweaty climate.

Epidemiology

Occurs at any age but is more common among adults than in children.

Associated diseases

Erythrasma may be the presenting feature in diabetics.

Clinical characteristics in light skin (Fitzpatrick skin types I–III)

Erythrasma is a fairly common condition occurring in the big folds of persons living in warm climates or sweating a lot. The skin is discolored with a slightly reddish-brown tinge (Figure 28.1). The lesions are usually sharply demarcated. A Wood's lamp shows a coral red fluorescence.

Symptoms are rare and mild; itching occurs occasionally. Treatment is by aeration of the diseased skin folds and antibacterial topicals such as erythromycin; azole antifungals are also active.

Clinical characteristics in dark skin (Fitzpatrick skin types IV–V)

Erythrasma is a common skin infection in hot, humid climates. Irregularly shaped, sharply marginated, slightly scaly asymptomatic dark brown or blackish patches in the axillae are the most common presentation (Figure 28.2). They are never red or erythematous in dark skin. Patients are worried about the cosmetically unacceptable appearance. Hyperpigmented pityriasis versicolor is a common association.

Toe cleft infection, if present, may go unnoticed in dark skin due to its brown color and asymptomatic nature. Extensive erythrasma involving axillae, groin, and submammary areas has been observed in middle-aged obese diabetic women.

Investigations

This is diagnosed clinically.

Coral-red fluorescence under a Wood's lamp is diagnostic and helps to differentiate from hyperpigmented pityriasis versicolor.

Smartphone applications that simulate UV light are helpful when a Wood's lamp is unavailable (Zagales and Korman 2024).

Treatments

Without treatment, the bacteria tend to grow slowly, spreading the disease that persists indefinitely.

- Topical azole antifungal, such as clotrimazole, miconazole, econazole, oxiconazole, or ketoconazole for 2–4 weeks, until complete clearance.
- Topical azole creams can be alternated with topical fucidic acid cream or mupirocin ointment for a faster cure.
- For more extensive lesions, oral erythromycin or oral tetracycline is prescribed for 2 weeks. A single dose of 1 g clarithromycin is also effective (Khan 2020).
- Relapse is a problem in some patients. In these cases, long-term antiseptics, such as povidone–iodine, and drying agents, such as powders, should be applied in the affected areas.

Further reading

Forouzan P, Cohen PR (2020). Erythrasma Revisited: Diagnosis, Differential Diagnoses, and Comprehensive Review of Treatment. *Cureus*;12(9):e10733.

Khan MJ (2020). Interdigital Pedal Erythrasma Treated with One-Time Dose of Oral Clarithromycin 1 g: Two Case Reports. *Clin Case Rep*;8(4):672–674.

Wootton C, Elliott I (2024). Bacterial Infections. In: Griffiths C, et al. (eds). *Rook's Textbook of Dermatology*, 10th ed. John Wiley & Sons Ltd., UK; 26.38.

Zagales R, Korman AM (2024). Need a Wood Lamp Alternative? Grab Your Smartphone. *Cutis*;113(6):271–272.

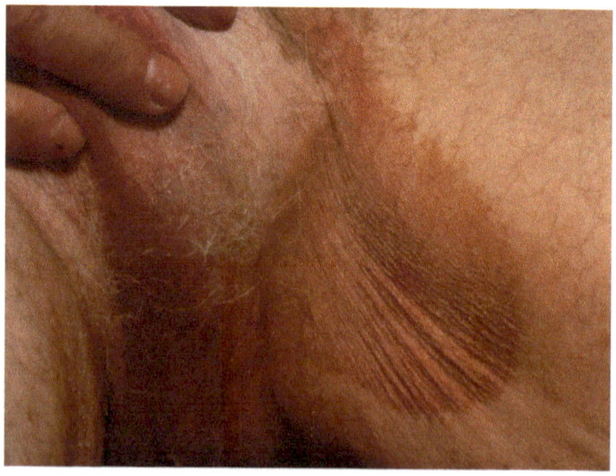

FIGURE 28.1 Erythrasma FST2. (Courtesy Prof. Ian Coulson, UK.)

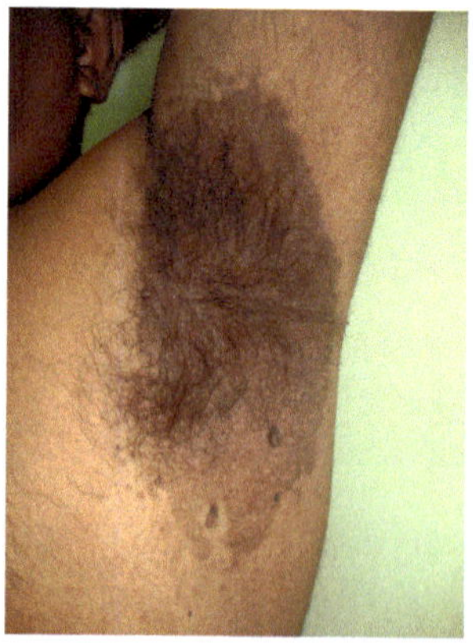

FIGURE 28.2 Erythrasma in a 32-year-old man FST5. Note multiple skin tags on axilla.

DOI: 10.1201/9781003479512-28

29
ERYTHRODERMA

Introduction

Erythroderma is the term applied to any inflammatory skin disease that affects more than 90% of the body surface. Eczema (40%), psoriasis (25%), lymphoma and leukemias (15%), and drugs in 10% (including phenylbutazone, phenytoin, carbamazepine, gold salts, lithium, cimetidine) are the most common causes of erythroderma. Ichthyosiform erythroderma and pityriasis rubra pilaris, even though less than 1% of cases reported, are important causes of erythroderma.

Erythema may obscure in dark skin, giving false security and causing management delay. Impaired thermoregulation (hypo- and hyperthermia), high-output cardiac failure, high fluid loss by transpiration, systemic infections, and hypoalbuminemia are well-known complications. Erythroderma is a potentially fatal condition, particularly in elderly people.

Epidemiology

Common in males of 45–50 years of age.

Associated diseases

Eczema and psoriasis are the diseases frequently encountered with erythroderma. Cutaneous T-cell lymphoma is the most common malignancy to cause erythroderma, followed by Hodgkin disease.

Clinical characteristics in light skin (Fitzpatrick skin types I–III)

Erythroderma is a chronic skin condition involving more than 90% of the body surface. Due to its enormous extension, many functions of the skin can no longer be maintained and the disease may run a fatal course.

The more acute form is characterized by generalized erythema with scaling (Figure 29.1). The patients shiver as thermoregulation no longer functions. They lose electrolytes, structural and serum proteins, and fluids resulting in hypoalbuminemia, hypovolemia with cardiac and circulatory insufficiency, edema, hypoglycemia, and generalized lymph node enlargement. If this is not treated like a burn patient, the patient will not survive.

Another type is erythroderma with insidious onset and chronic course; this is usually less severe as the general symptoms are less pronounced. This condition is seen in atopics and also in secondarily erythrodermic mycosis fungoides, whereas in relatively acute Sézary syndrome, it may be as dramatic as in the more acute onset forms.

Often, the underlying primary dermatosis can no longer be diagnosed, not even by histopathology.

Clinical characteristics in dark skin (Fitzpatrick skin types IV–V)

Patients with erythroderma present with generalized erythema, edema, and bran-like scaling (Figure 29.2). They are unwell with fever, shivering, and malaise. Erythema may obscure in dark skin, giving false security and causing management delay. Blanching pressure on the surface makes erythema more apparent in dark skin.

Investigations

This is diagnosed clinically.

Histopathology can help identify the cause of erythroderma in up to 50% of cases, particularly if multiple and repeated skin biopsies are examined.

Treatments

- Consider hospital or day unit admission in acute phase.
- Withdraw or switch medications that may be implicated as a cause.
- Protein and electrolyte balance, circulatory status, and body temperature require close monitoring.
- Appropriate fluid intake.
- Treat any secondary infection.
- Frequent application of greasy emollients is necessary to restore skin barrier function.
- Systemic therapy is dependent on the underlying cause.

Further reading

Mughal AA, Ingram JR (2024). Eczematous Disorders. In: Griffiths C, et al. (eds). *Rook's Textbook of Dermatology*, 10th ed. John Wiley & Sons Ltd., UK; 39.31.

DOI: 10.1201/9781003479512-29

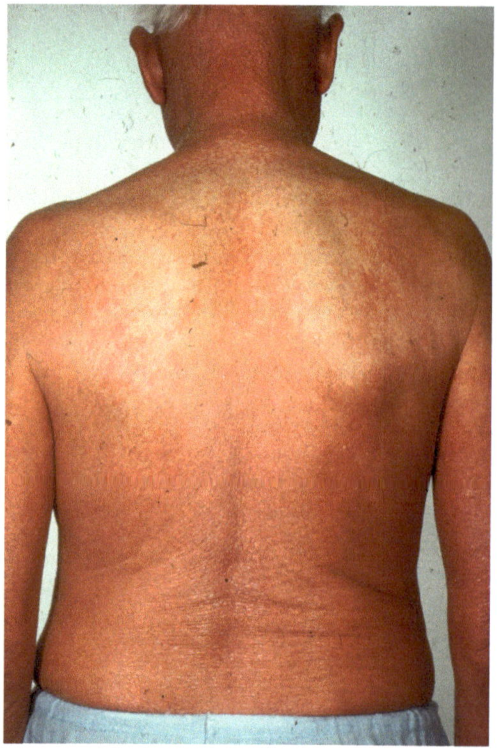

FIGURE 29.1 Erythroderma FST1. (Courtesy Dr. Richard Ashton, UK.)

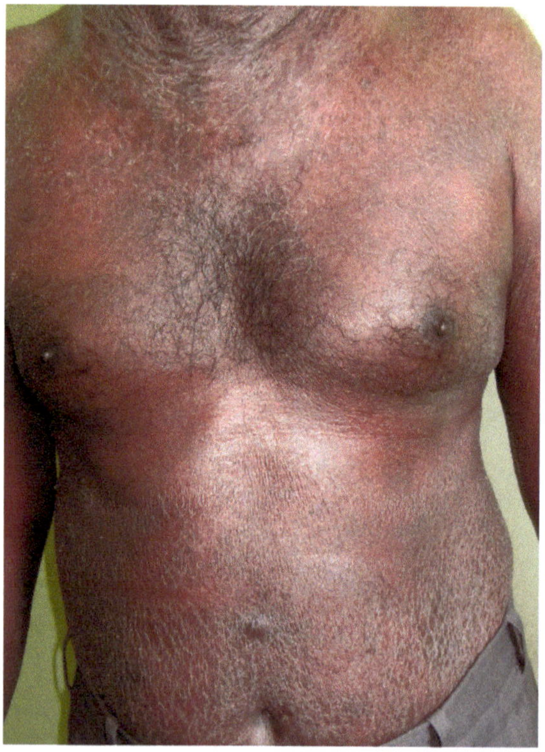

FIGURE 29.2 Erythroderma in a 56-year-old man. Note erythema is concealed in dark skin.

30
EXFOLIATIVE DERMATITIS

Introduction

Exfoliative dermatitis and erythroderma are synonymously used in Western books. However, they are not clinically the same in our settings, even though the causative factors, epidemiology, and associated diseases are somewhat similar in both conditions. Exfoliative dermatitis is the term applied to any inflammatory skin disease that affects more than 90% of the body surface. Eczema, psoriasis, lymphomas, contact allergy, photoallergy, and drugs are the most common causes. Even after extensive searches, predisposing factors are not clearly identified in most of our patients, leading to a chronic and is recurrent nature of the disease.

Erythema is not a feature in dark-skinned patients with exfoliative dermatitis. Impaired thermoregulation (hypo- and hyperthermia), high-output cardiac failure, high fluid loss by transpiration, systemic infections, and hypoalbuminemia are well-known complications in both conditions. Exfoliative dermatitis, even extensive is not fatal, but chronic and recurrent in most patients, and lasts for many years.

Epidemiology

Common in males of 45–50 years of age. However, this continues and is recurrent throughout their lives.

Associated diseases

Eczema, psoriasis, contact allergy, photoallergy, and drug allergy are the diseases frequently encountered with exfoliative dermatitis. Mycosis fungoides may present as exfoliative dermatitis.

Clinical characteristics in light skin (Fitzpatrick skin types I–III)

Dermatitis exfoliativa, as understood in the Anglo-American dermatological literature, is a descriptive term for sub-erythroderma of different causes, whereas *dermatitis exfoliativa neonatorum* is the staphylococcal scalded syndrome of newborns and infants in the German dermatological language.

Exfoliative dermatitis is characterized by a near-generalized erythema with scaling (Figure 30.1). The patients are in a reduced general condition. Dermopathic lymph node swelling is common. The hair thins, the nails become dystrophic, brittle, and tend to split. Itching is variable from moderate to intolerable.

The underlying skin disease is often not clear; even histopathology may be non-specific.

Clinical characteristics in dark skin (Fitzpatrick skin types IV–V)

Exfoliative dermatitis is very common among middle-aged to elderly men in our settings (Figure 30.2). They present with a generalized eczematous rash, edema, bran-like scaling, and generalized lymphadenopathy. The skin is darker than their original color, possibly due to persistent post-inflammatory hyperpigmentation. In chronic patients, the skin is shiny, with loss of body and scalp hair, and lichenified palms and soles are common. In the acute stage they are unwell with fever, shivering, and malaise with oozing eczematous skin. Itching is a predominant feature which is exceedingly troublesome and their main complaint.

Investigations

This is diagnosed clinically.

Histopathology can help identify the cause of exfoliative dermatitis in up to 50% of cases, particularly if multiple and repeated skin biopsies are examined.

Treatments

- Consider hospital or day unit admission in acute phase.
- Withdraw or switch medications that may be implicated as a cause.
- Protein and electrolyte balance, circulatory status, and body temperature require close monitoring. Appropriate fluid intake.
- Treat any secondary infections.
- Diluted topical corticosteroids help to resolve their symptoms, combined with the frequent application of greasy emollients, in order to restore skin barrier function.
- Systemic therapy is dependent on the underlying cause.
- If the underlying cause is not identified, a short course of oral steroids helps to regain near-normal skin, and a low dose of 7.5–10 mg daily is continued long-term as maintenance therapy if permitted by other coexisting medical conditions.

Further reading

Mughal AA, Ingram JR (2024). Eczematous Disorders. In: Griffiths C, et al. (eds). *Rook's Textbook of Dermatology*, 10th ed. John Wiley & Sons Ltd., UK; 39.31.

DOI: 10.1201/9781003479512-30

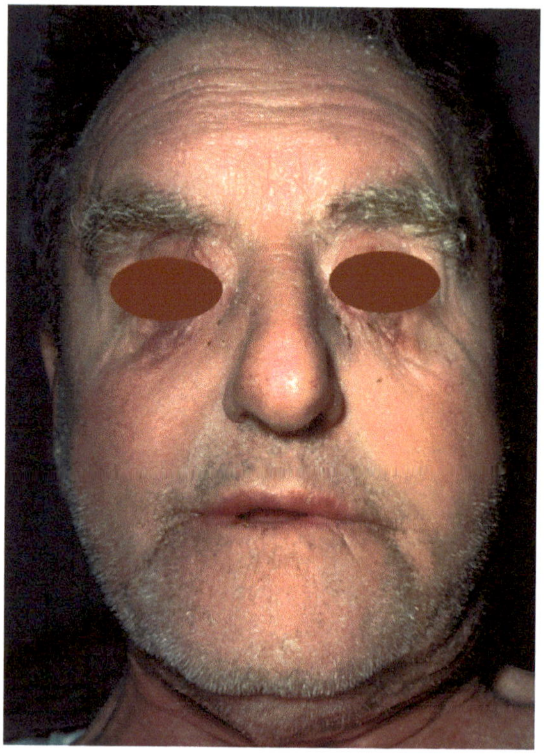

FIGURE 30.1 Exfoliative dermatitis FST1. (Courtesy Prof. Ian Coulson, UK.)

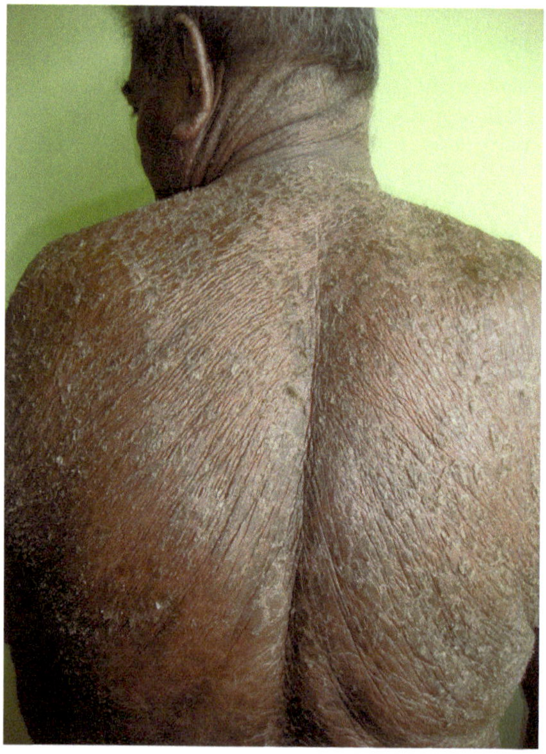

FIGURE 30.2 Exfoliative dermatitis in a 45-year-old man FST5. Note erythema is not a feature in this condition and generalized post-inflammatory hyperpigmentation leads to darken skin color. This is very chronic and recurrent, with frequent exacerbations and therefore frequent hospital admissions are common.

31
FIXED DRUG ERUPTION

Introduction

Fixed drug eruption (FDE) is an adverse reaction to drugs, foods, food additives, and herbal medicines. The most frequently reported drugs include tetracyclines, non-steroidal anti-inflammatory drugs (NSAIDs), sulfonamides, co-trimoxazole, paracetamol, omeprazole, and sedatives. Lesions appear on the skin or mucosa 30 minutes to 8 hours post-exposure. It is characterized by solitary or multiple lesions. FDE first appears as a sharply defined, round or oval erythematous and bullous lesion, which is followed by well-circumscribed areas of hyperpigmentation. The lesions increase in size and/or number with the continuation of the causative drug, leaving deeper residual pigmentation. Generalized bullous FDE (GBFDE) is a form of extensive FDE that may be misdiagnosed as toxic epidermal necrolysis (TEN).

Epidemiology

Reported in all ages and both sexes.

Clinical characteristics in light skin (Fitzpatrick skin types I–III)

FDE is a fairly common condition (Figures 31.1 and 31.2). It is characterized by recurrent episodes of a single round red spot that soon turns bullous. The roof of the blister is gray as it is necrotic epidermis. This may slough off and leave a raw surface that may crust. Healing takes roughly 2 weeks and is followed by a brown spot.

The causative drugs are already mentioned, but it has to be kept in mind that some foods and over-the-counter medicines may also be the culprit. We have seen a young woman who got an FDE each time she menstruated, even though she did not take any remedy.

Histopathology is characteristic of extensive epidermal necrosis and little inflammation.

Clinical characteristics in dark skin (Fitzpatrick skin types IV–V)

FDE first appears as erythematous or bullous lesions which turn into blackish round or oval patches (Figures 31.3 and 31.4). The erythematous stage is transient and may go unnoticed. Most of our patients present with asymptomatic or mildly itchy blackish well-demarcated oval patches.

Investigations

This is diagnosed clinically.

Treatments

- It has a good prognosis; after drug discontinuation, lesions resolve spontaneously.
- Treatment options include antihistamines and mild to moderate topical corticosteroids.

Further reading

Ardern-Jones MR (2024). Benign Cutaneous Adverse Reactions to Drugs. In: Griffiths C, et al. (eds). *Rook's Textbook of Dermatology*, 10th ed. John Wiley & Sons Ltd., UK; 117.4.

Wijenayake BKS (2021). Cutaneous Adverse Reactions to Drugs. In: Ranawaka RR, et al. (eds). *Atlas of Dermatoses in Pigmented Skin*. Springer, Singapore; 1034–1037.

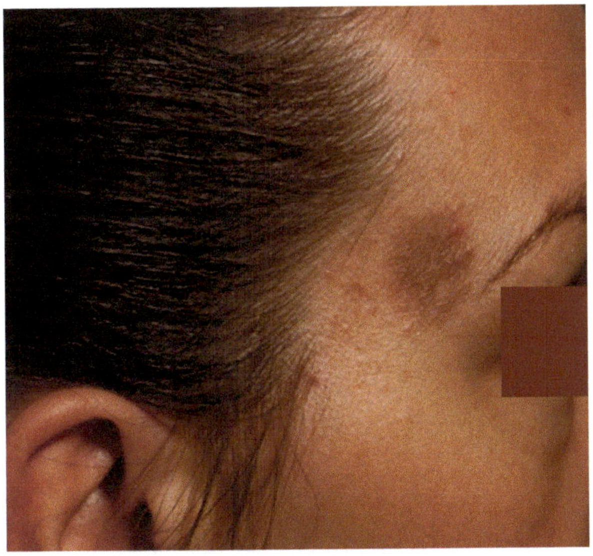

FIGURE 31.1 Fixed drug eruption FST3. (Courtesy Prof. Ian Coulson, UK.)

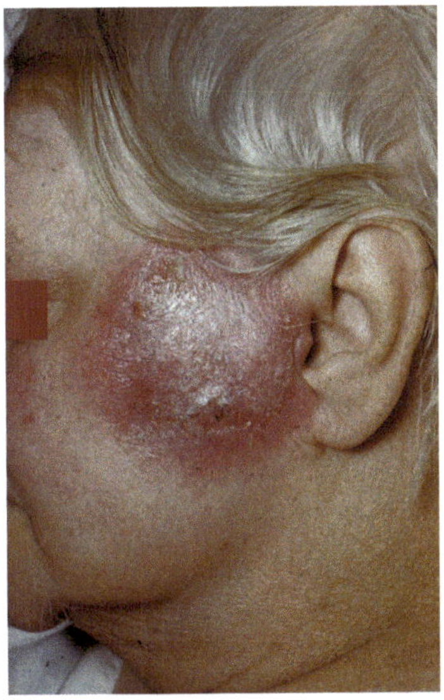

FIGURE 31.2 Fixed drug eruption in acute stage FST1. (Courtesy Prof. Ian Coulson, UK.)

DOI: 10.1201/9781003479512-31

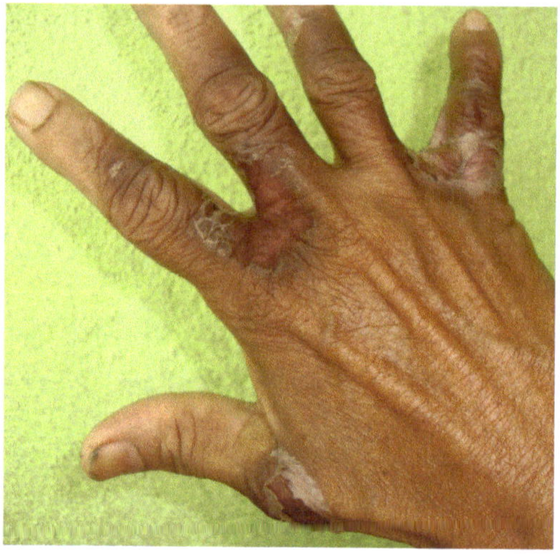

FIGURE 31.3 Fixed drug eruption in acute stage with ruptured bullae in a 66-year-old woman FST5.

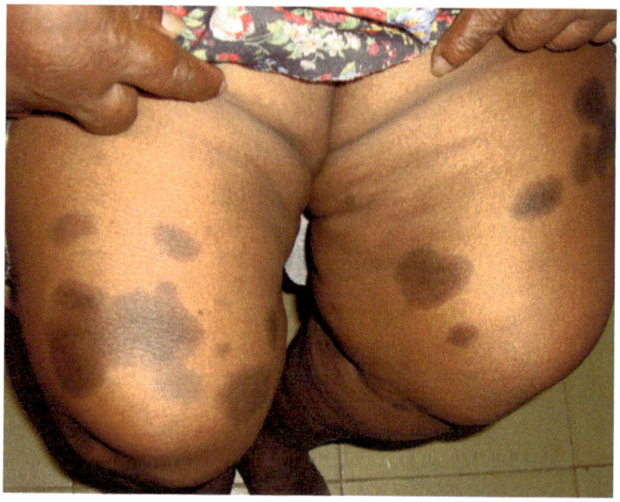

FIGURE 31.4 Multiple fixed drug eruptions in a 64-year-old woman FST5 due to repeated exposure to the offending drug.

32
FRECKLES/EPHELIDES

Introduction

Freckles, or ephelides are very common on the light-exposed skin of fair-skinned individuals, FST1 to FST3. They first appear at about the age of 5 years as light-brown pigmented macules on the light-exposed skin. This is uncommon in darker skin.

Epidemiology

Very common in individuals from FST1 to FST, red or blond hair, fair skin, and blue eyes.

Associated diseases

Freckles are a feature of a number of inherited and acquired disorders; xeroderma pigmentosum, neurofibromatosis, hereditary symmetrical dyschromatosis, and progeria. In neurofibromatosis I, freckling occurs frequently in the axillae, where it is virtually pathognomonic (Crowe's sign). It is present in about 70% of affected subjects and appears a little later than the café-au-lait spots.

Clinical characteristics in light skin (Fitzpatrick skin types I–III)

Freckles are autosomal dominant and very common in light-skinned persons, particularly in persons with blond to red hair and blue to green eyes (Figures 32.1 and 32.2). Often beginning over the bridge of the nose, they develop under the influence of sunlight in spring and summer, extend over large portions of the face, and may spread to all sun-exposed skin areas. The lesions are yellow to brown with bizarre delimitation. They become more intense in childhood and adolescence and have a tendency to regress in later life.

The differential diagnosis comprises a number of syndromes with multiple lentigines; however, these do not show regression in wintertime. Many persons with ephelides try to get a suntan and often develop larger pigment spots on their shoulders; these are so-called sunburn spots.

Freckling around the axillae is typical for neurofibromatosis I. Small labial and mucosal lentiginous pigment spots are seen in Laugier–Hunziker syndrome; if they are associated with longitudinal melanonychia, it is called Laugier–Hunziker–Baran syndrome. Periorificial lentigines of Peutz–Jeghers are associated with intestinal polyposis. LEOPARD syndrome is an acronym for diffuse **l**entiginosis, **e**lectrocardiographic abnormalities, **o**cular symptoms and hypertelorism, **p**ulmonary stenosis, **a**bnormal genital organ development, growth **r**etardation, and **d**eafness.

Clinical characteristics in dark skin (Fitzpatrick skin types IV–V)

Freckles are rare in dark skin (Figure 32.3). Once freckles appear, they are persistent and without seasonal variation in color or severity. Since sunlight exposure is constant and unavoidable in a tropical country, they gradually darken and increase in number over time.

Investigations

This is diagnosed clinically.

Treatments

Ephelides (freckles) and actinic (solar) lentigines respond well to treatment with the Q-switched KTP laser (532 nm). Unlike the Q-switched ruby (694 nm) and Q-switched alexandrite lasers, this laser may cause bruising. Each lesion has to be treated individually, a sometimes tedious exercise in photodamaged patients.

Further reading

Haneke E (1991). Laugier-Hunziker-Baran Syndrom [Laugier-Hunziker-Baran syndrome]. *Hautarzt*;42:512–515.

Van Geel N, Speeckaert R (2024). Acquired Pigmentary Disorders. In: Griffiths C, et al. (eds). *Rook's Textbook of Dermatology*, 10th ed. John Wiley & Sons Ltd., UK; 86.15.

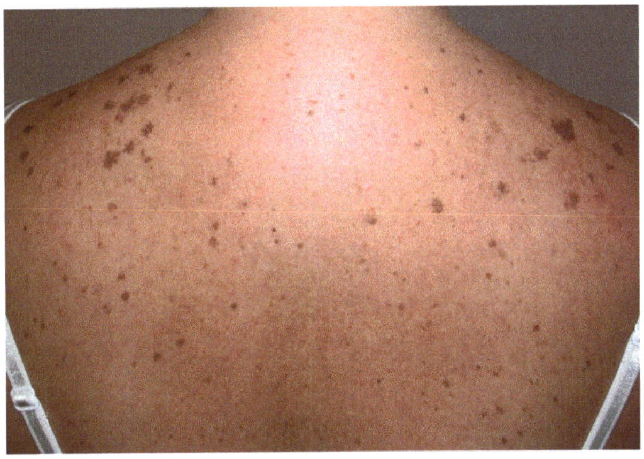

FIGURE 32.1 Freckles following sunburn FST3. (Courtesy Prof. Ian Coulson, UK.)

DOI: 10.1201/9781003479512-32

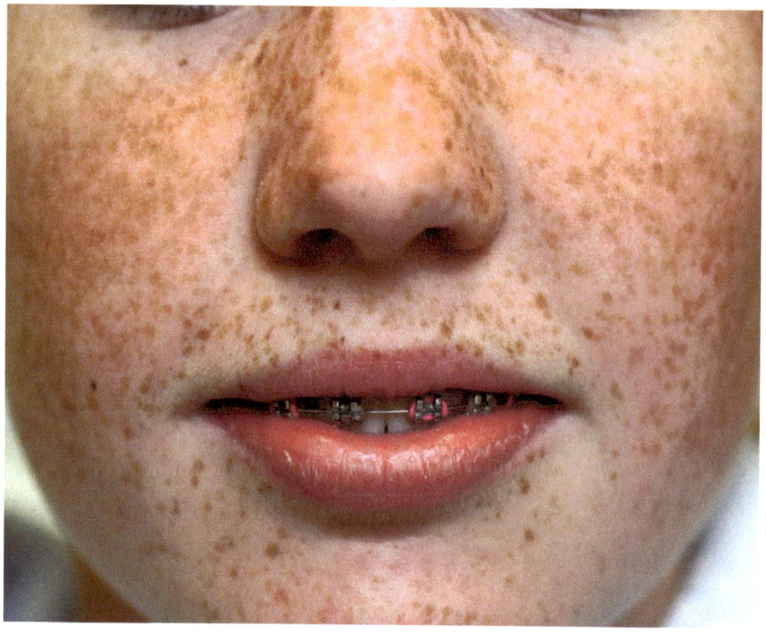

FIGURE 32.2 Freckles FST1. (Courtesy Dr. Richard Ashton, UK.)

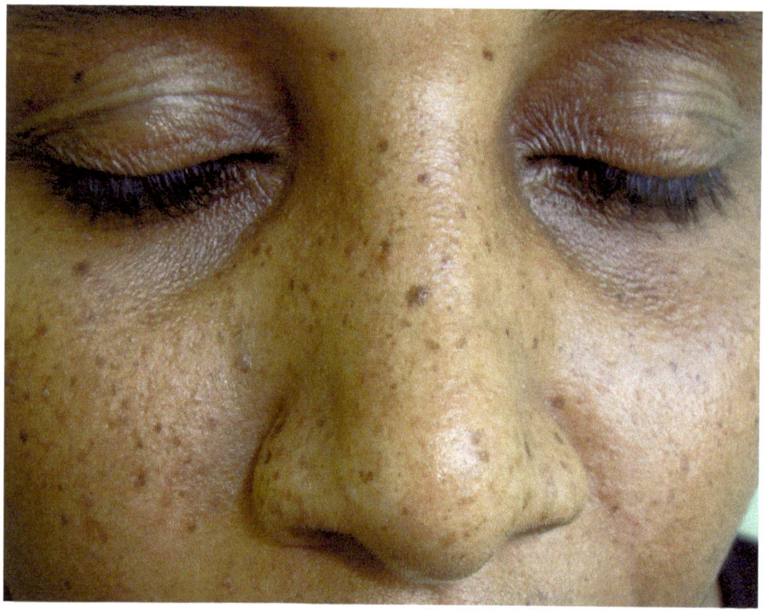

FIGURE 32.3 Freckles in a 32-year-old woman FST5. Freckles are uncommon in dark skin.

33
INFANTILE HEMANGIOMA

Introduction

Infantile hemangiomas (strawberry nevus, capillary hemangioma) are the most common benign vascular tumors encountered in infancy, occurring in up to 10% of infants, more commonly in girls than boys.

The natural history is of proliferation in the first few months of life and spontaneous involution over 3–7 years. Most infantile hemangiomas reach 80% of their final size by 3 months of age. If untreated, involution is complete at a median age of 3 years. The main complications of infantile hemangiomas are ulceration, disfigurement, and functional impairment.

Epidemiology

Appear at birth, and are more common in girls.

Associated diseases

Hemangiomas overlying the spine may be associated with spinal defects.

Clinical characteristics in light skin (Fitzpatrick skin types I–III)

Hemangiomas are very common capillary proliferations (Figures 33.1 and 33.2); they begin at birth or shortly thereafter, grow rapidly within a few weeks, remain at this size for a few months, and take another few years to involute spontaneously. They are raised purple-red lesions, often compressible, non-tender. If located in close proximity to the eyes, mouth, nose, genital, or anal region, follow-up of the baby is warranted to initiate early treatment in order to avoid functional impairment.

Clinical characteristics in dark skin (Fitzpatrick skin types IV–V)

In dark-skinned individuals, hemangiomas may appear very dark (Figures 33.3 to 33.6).

Investigations

This is diagnosed clinically.

Occasionally, ultrasound may be required:

- To distinguish infantile hemangiomas from other soft tissue masses or vascular malformations.
- For plaque-type infantile hemangiomas on the face and lower trunk and before treatment with β-blockers.

Treatments

Treatment will depend on the location, morphology, and stage of evolution, impact on function, risk of disfigurement, and co-morbidities.

- Propranolol is now the first-line treatment. Propranolol has been shown to induce a better and faster response than systemic steroids, and is associated with fewer and less concerning adverse effects.
- Pulsed dye laser (PDL) can be helpful for the treatment of ulcerations, telangiectases, and erythema post-involution.
- Surgery may very occasionally be required in the proliferative phase if functional impairment or ulceration cannot be managed medically. Surgical reconstruction, if indicated, may be best undertaken after 3.5 years, as further aesthetically beneficial spontaneous improvement is unlikely to occur.
- Embolization may have a role for life-threatening hemangiomas, particularly those leading to congestive cardiac failure that have not responded to medical therapy.

Further reading

Ling LCT, Aan MKJ (2024). Beta-Blockers for the Treatment of Infantile Haemangiomas in Premature Infants. *Australas J Dermatol*;Nov;65(7):e194–e197.

Ranawaka RR (2021). Vascular Tumours and Malformations. In: Ranawaka RR, et al. (eds). *Atlas of Dermatoses in Pigmented Skin*. Springer, Singapore; 65–80.

Sharma A, Gupta M, Mahajan R (2024). Infantile Hemangiomas: A Dermatologist's Perspective. *Eur J Pediatr*;Oct;183(10): 4159–4168.

Sharma A, Venkatesan V, Sharma A, et al. (2024). Association of Attention Deficit Hyperactivity Disorder with the Use of Oral Propranolol in Infantile Haemangiomas: An Ambispective Comparative Study. *Indian J Dermatol*;69(2):171–173.

Solman L, Glover MT (2024). Haemangiomas and Other Non-Malignant Tumours of Infancy. In: Griffiths C, et al. (eds). *Rook's Textbook of Dermatology*, 10th ed. John Wiley & Sons Ltd., UK; 116.1.

DOI: 10.1201/9781003479512-33

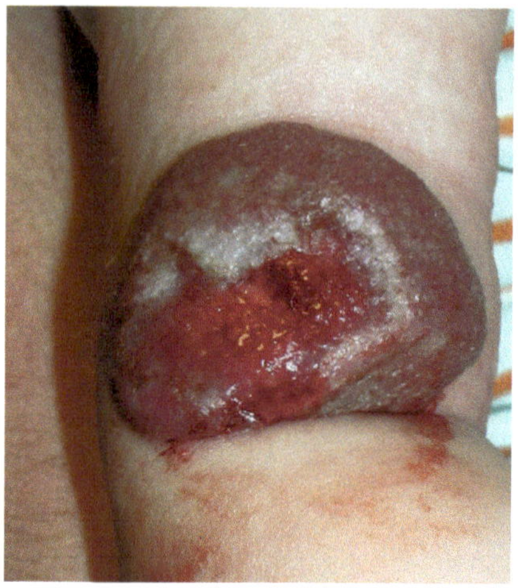

FIGURE 33.1 Ulcerated infantile hemangioma FST1. (Courtesy Prof. Ian Coulson, UK.)

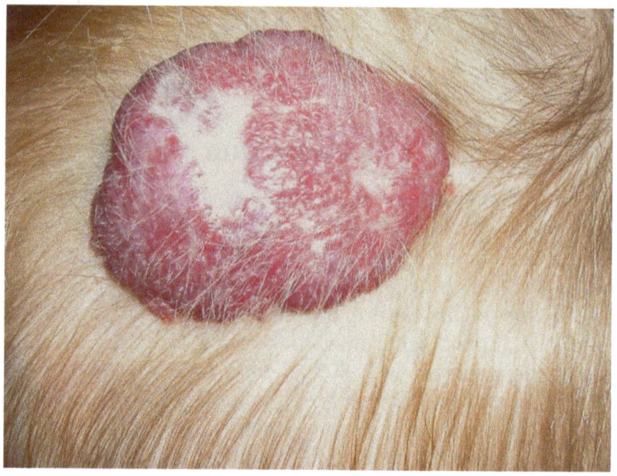

FIGURE 33.2 Infantile hemangioma on the anterior fontanelle FST1. (Courtesy Prof. Ian Coulson, UK.)

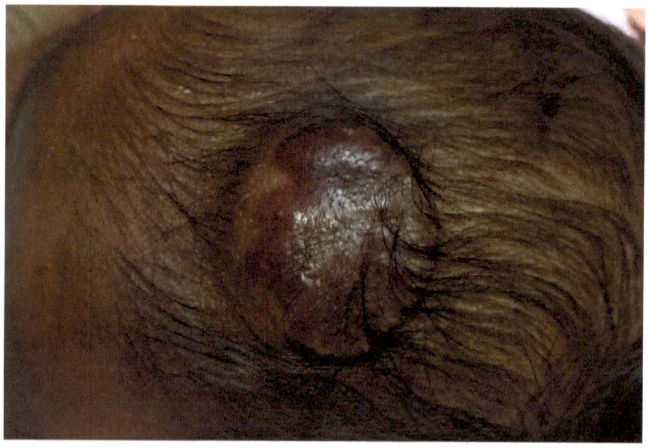

FIGURE 33.3 Infantile hemangioma on the anterior fontanelle FST5. In dark-skinned babies hemangiomas may appear dark as in this 6-week-old baby.

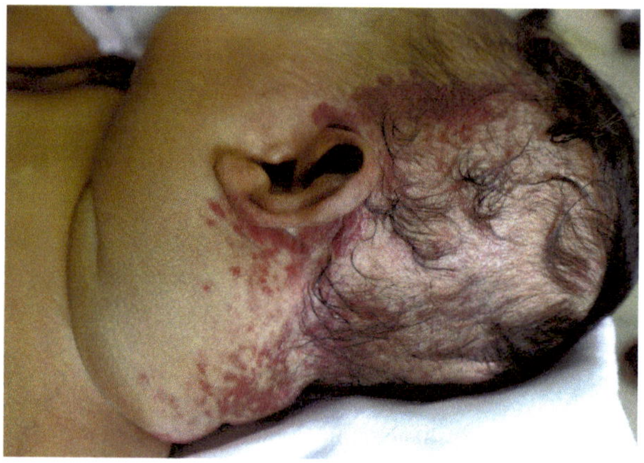

FIGURE 33.4 Large hemangioma compressing the aorta, deviating the trachea, and extending to the thoracic cavity FST5.

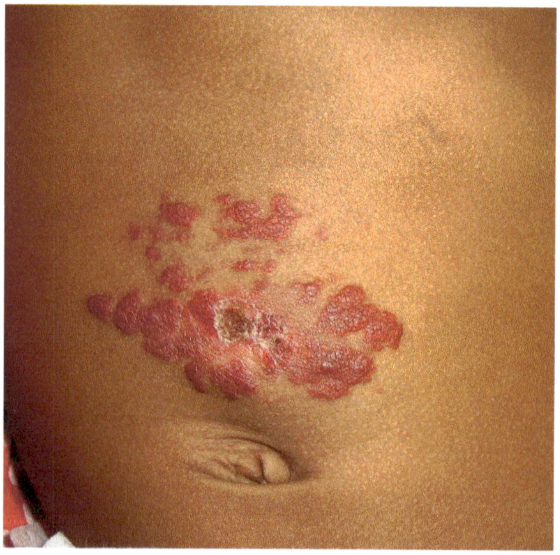

FIGURE 33.5 Ulcerated infantile hemangioma in a 7-month-old baby FST5.

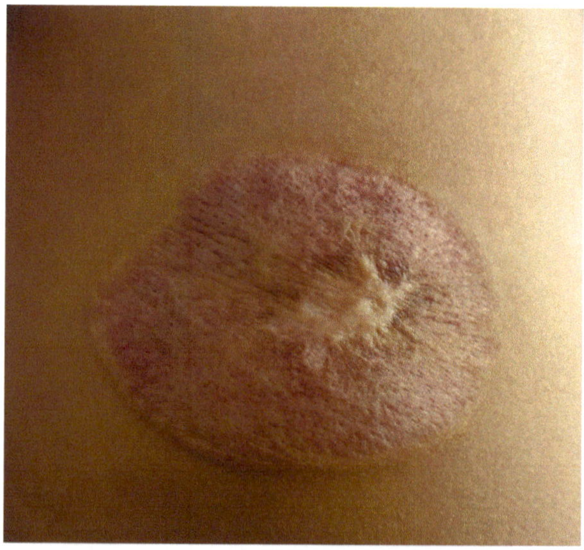

FIGURE 33.6 Residual textural change and central scarring after involution of ulcerated infantile hemangioma in a 5-year-old child FHT5.

34
HALO NEVUS

Introduction

Development of a halo of hypomelanosis around a central cutaneous tumor. This tumor is usually a benign melanocytic nevus, rarely primary or secondary malignant melanoma. The nevus tends to flatten and may disappear completely over time. The depigmented areas often persist but may pigment after many years.

Epidemiology

Seen in all ages, but common in the young.

Associated diseases

Rarely, primary or secondary malignant melanoma may present with a hypomelanotic halo.

Vitiligo can be present in the personal or family history.

Clinical characteristics in light skin (Fitzpatrick skin types I–III)

Halo nevus is not a rare event in light-skinned children and adolescents (Figures 34.1 and 34.2). One or more acquired, very rarely congenital, nevi suddenly develop a white halo. There may be a slight redness in the immediate surroundings of the nevus. Sometimes, classical vitiligo develops after some time.

In the author's experience, complete excision is recommended as this may prevent the development of independent vitiligo.

Clinical characteristics in dark skin (Fitzpatrick skin types IV–V)

Vitiliginous halo surrounding an existing nevus is not uncommon in our patients. They present early as this is striking in dark skin, and they fear vitiligo (Figure 34.3).

Investigations

This is diagnosed clinically.

Treatments

Reassurance.

Further reading

Cohen PR, Gutierrez N, Erickson CP, et al. (2023). Halo Phenomenon in Lobular Capillary Hemangioma: A Case Report of a Pyogenic Granuloma with Surrounding Cutaneous Hypopigmentation and Review of Tumors with Halo Phenomenon. *Cureus*;15(8): e43228.

van Geel N, Speeckaert R (2024). Acquired Pigmentary Disorders. In: Griffiths C, et al. (eds). *Rook's Textbook of Dermatology*, 10th ed. John Wiley & Sons Ltd., UK; 86.40.

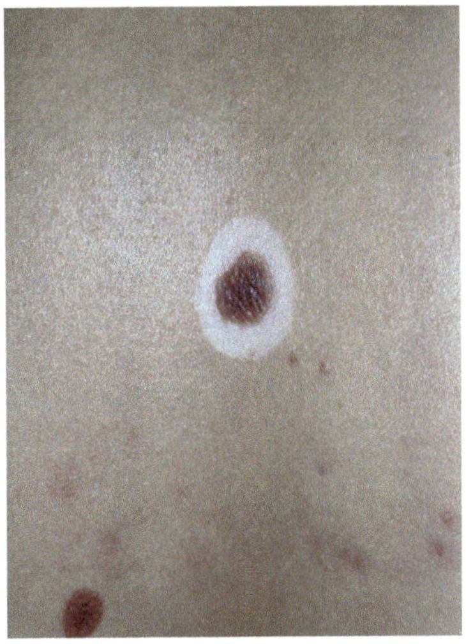

FIGURE 34.1 Halo nevus FST2. (Courtesy Prof. Ian Coulson, UK.)

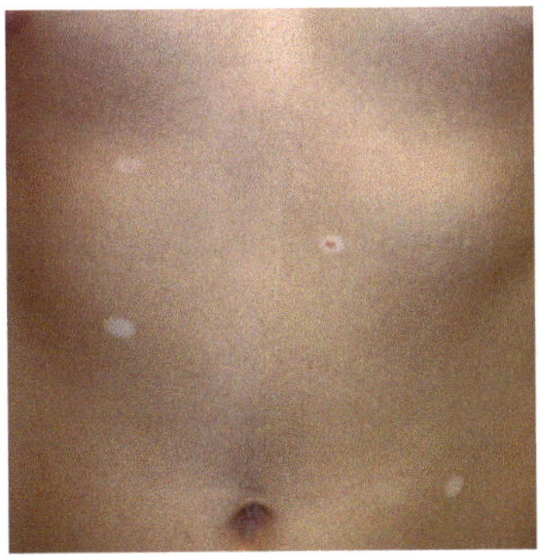

FIGURE 34.2 Vitiligo and halo nevus more marked in tanned skin FST3. (Courtesy Prof. Ian Coulson, UK.)

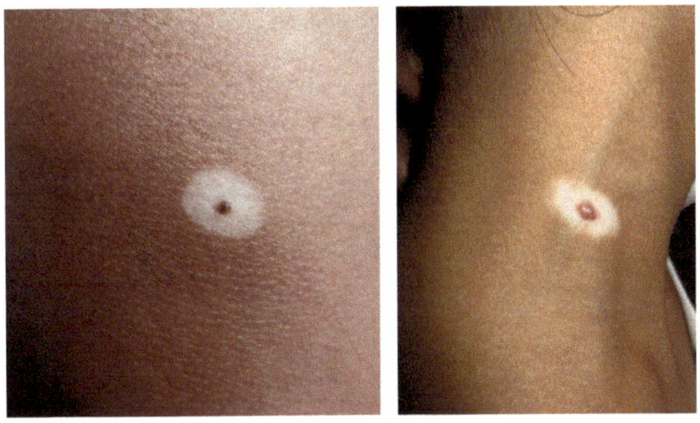

FIGURE 34.3 Halo nevus FST5.

DOI: 10.1201/9781003479512-34

35
HERPES SIMPLEX INFECTION

Introduction

Herpes simplex (HS) infections are caused by HSV, or human herpesvirus 1 and 2 (HHV-1, HHV-2). There are two major antigenic types: Type 1, which typically causes facial infections; and type 2, which is typically genital, though overlap of infection is common. After the initial infection, the virus becomes latent and may reactivate in later life. Genital herpes is a sexually transmitted infection (STI).

Epidemiology

The most common viral infections of humans throughout the world.

Associated diseases

HSV infection can lead to eczema herpeticum. Disseminated or systemic infection may occur in the immunodeficient and in neonates.

Clinical characteristics in light skin (Fitzpatrick skin types I–III)

The first contact with HS virus may go unnoticed, cause slight general symptoms like a minor common cold, or cause a serious and widespread infection, in most cases as a gingivostomatitis herpetica. This takes some time to heal and the child usually remains free from HSV infection for years.

For an unknown reason, groups of tiny clear vesicles may appear at the lip margin that turn yellow after a few days, break off and crust (Figure 35.1). These may fall off after some more days and leave a circumscribed redness. Depending on individual immunity, this event may recur at regular or irregular intervals as the virus DNA remains in the sensory ganglia after the primary infection. Many patients know their precipitating events; young women may get recurrent HS labialis with each menstruation, and young men with particular stress situations.

Herpes simplex genitalis is usually observed with the beginning of sexual activity. When observed in childhood, sexual abuse has to be considered. Tiny groups of vesicles appear on the prepuce, glans, or penis shaft, on the labia majora, labia minora, in the perineum. Particularly, those on the penis shaft and labia minora are very painful, whereas those in the vaginal tract run an almost asymptomatic course and are rarely diagnosed but may be the source of infection for the partner.

There are many special situations in which HS may be atypical: Eczema herpeticum in atopic eczema, herpes gladiatorum in wrestlers, continually appearing recurrences in the sacro-gluteal region. Ulcerative HS may be seen in immunosuppressed subjects. Vegetating lesions are seen in leukemia patients.

Clinical characteristics in dark skin (Fitzpatrick skin types IV–V)

HSV gingivostomatitis is commonly seen in young adults (Figure 35.2) and rare in children in our setting. It presents with a recurrent vesicular eruption around the mouth at the same site that resolves spontaneously even if untreated. Constitutional symptoms are mild; however, rarely, some may complicate with fever, malaise, secondary bacterial infection, ulcers, and regional lymphadenopathy.

HSV genitalis is very common among adults (Figure 35.3), but not seen in children. They present with very painful and sore punched-out ulcers on the genitalia and perineum, frequently associated with secondary bacterial infection, edema, ulcers, and general ill health. Pain and dysuria are common in women. Genital lesions can last for 2–3 weeks if untreated.

Investigations

This is diagnosed clinically.

Treatments

- Educate the patient on the recurrence and prevention of the spread of the disease.
- Oral acyclovir, valacyclovir, or famciclovir. Oral acyclovir 400 mg three times daily for one week.
- Intravenous aciclovir or cidofovir for extensive or systemic infection.
- Frequently recurring HS may deserve long-term antiviral prophylaxis.

Further reading

Harwood CA, Sterling JC (2024). Viral Infections. In: Griffiths C, et al. (eds). *Rook's Textbook of Dermatology*, 10th ed. John Wiley & Sons Ltd., UK; 25.20.

Rajendiran P (2021). Viral Infections. In: Ranawaka RR, et al. (eds). *Atlas of Dermatoses in Pigmented Skin*. Springer, Singapore; 297–318.

DOI: 10.1201/9781003479512-35

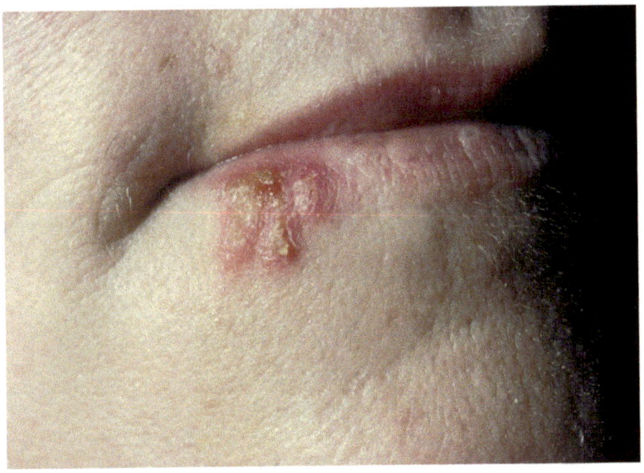

FIGURE 35.1 Herpes simplex labialis. (Courtesy Dr. Richard Ashton, UK.)

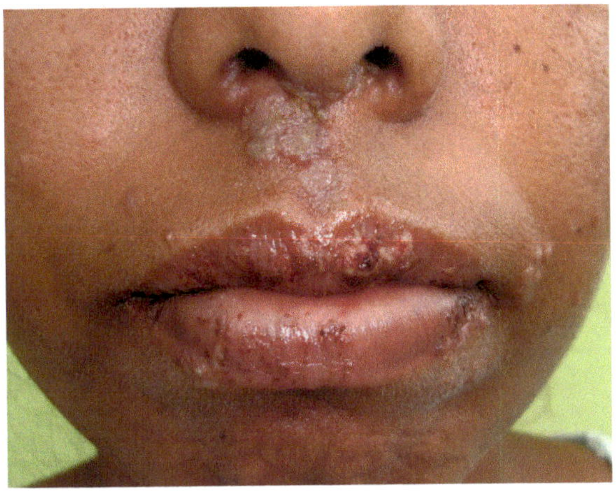

FIGURE 35.2 Extensive Herpes simplex labialis.

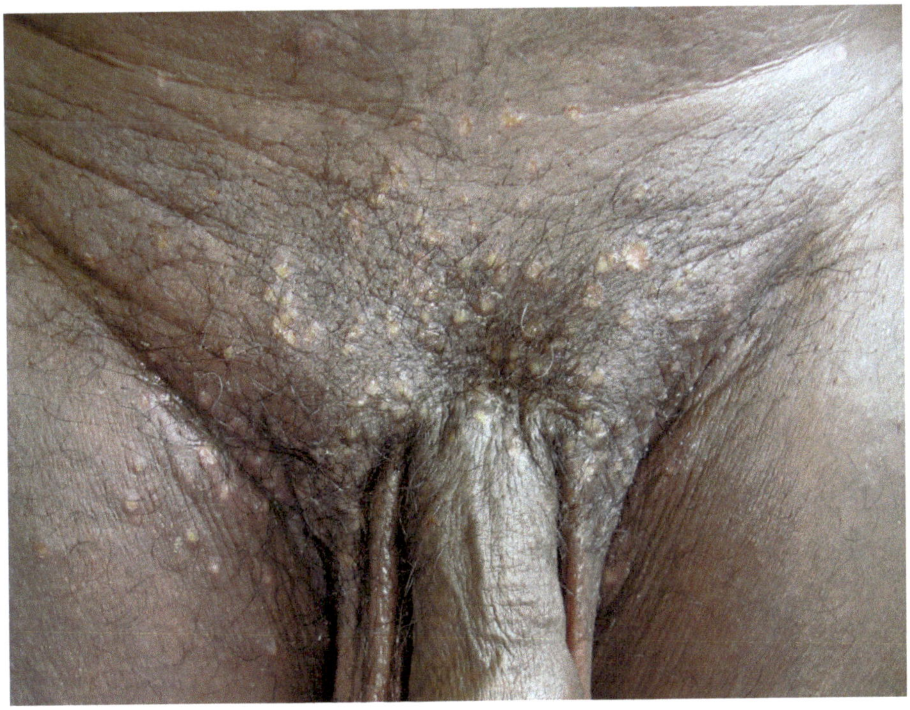

FIGURE 35.3 Herpes genitalis in a 76-year-old man FST5. Note the punched-out ulcers.

36
IDIOPATHIC GUTTATE HYPOMELANOSIS

Introduction

Idiopathic guttate hypomelanosis (IGH) is an acquired leukoderma with discrete round to oval porcelain-white macules approximately 2–5 mm in diameter. The borders are sharply defined, often angular and irregular. The number increases with age, and there is no spontaneous re-pigmentation.

Epidemiology

Common in the elderly, more reported by women.

Associated diseases

Some suggest that IGH reflects the normal aging or photo aging process.

Clinical characteristics in light skin (Fitzpatrick skin types I–III)

This is a common type of hypopigmentation mostly seen on the lower legs of women, but also in men and on both entire legs and arms with a history of extensive sun exposure (Figures 36.1 to 36.4). It was recently hypothesized to be due to melanocyte exhaustion.

Clinical characteristics in dark skin (Fitzpatrick skin types IV–V)

A very common skin condition in middle-aged to elderly men and women (Figure 36.5). Women seek reassurance more than men for fear of vitiligo. These appear more frequently on sun-exposed areas of the body, commonly on the pretibial side of the legs and the forearms; however, it is not uncommon to see them on unexposed areas too.

Investigations

This is diagnosed clinically.

Treatments

- Reassurance.
- 5-Fluorouracil tattooing helps in worried patients (Arbache and Hirata 2023, Rambhia and Rambhia 2020).

Further reading

Arbache S, Hirata SH (2023). Efficacy and Safety of 5-Fluorouracil Tattooing to Repigment Idiopathic Guttate Hypomelanosis: A Split-Body Randomized Trial. *Dermatol Surg*;49(6):603–608.

Rambhia SH, Rambhia KD (2020). Treatment of Idiopathic Guttate Hypomelanosis with 5-Fluorouracil Tattooing Using a Handheld Needle. *JAAD Int*;1(2):200–201.

Ranawaka RR (2021). Hypopigmentory Disorders. In: Ranawaka RR, et al. (eds). *Atlas of Dermatoses in Pigmented Skin*. Springer, Singapore; 107–122.

van Geel N, Speeckaert R (2024). Acquired Pigmentary Disorders. In: Griffiths C, et al. (eds). *Rook's Textbook of Dermatology*, 10th ed. John Wiley & Sons Ltd., UK; 86.45.

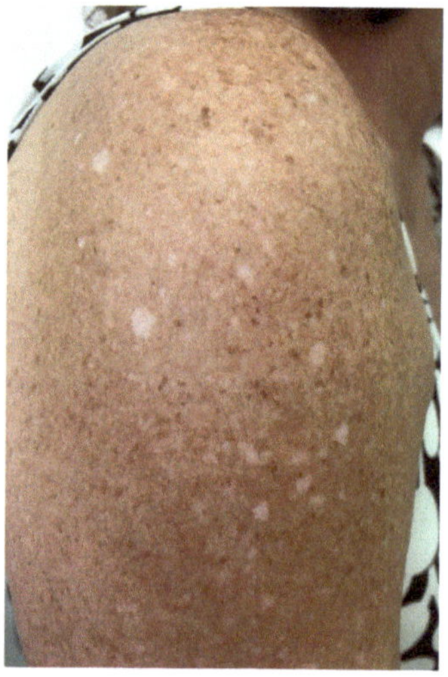

FIGURE 36.1 Idiopathic guttate hypomelanosis FST2. (Courtesy Dr. Richard Ashton, UK.)

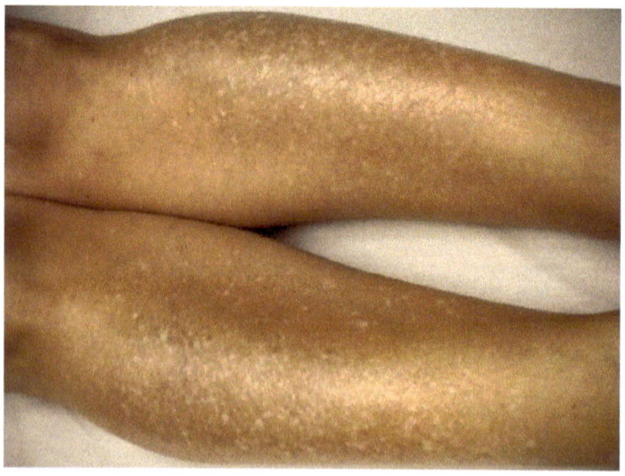

FIGURE 36.2 Hypomelanosis guttata idiopathica in a sun-tanned woman with FST2. (Courtesy Prof. Osvaldo Correia, Portugal.)

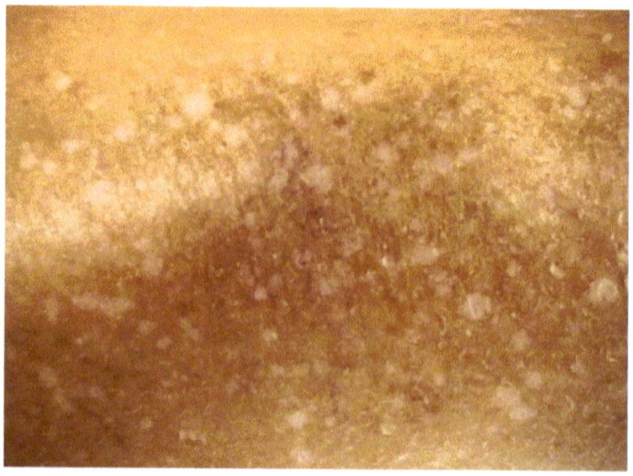

FIGURE 36.3 Hypomelanosis guttata idiopathica in a sun-tanned woman with FST2. (Courtesy Prof. Osvaldo Correia, Portugal.)

DOI: 10.1201/9781003479512-36

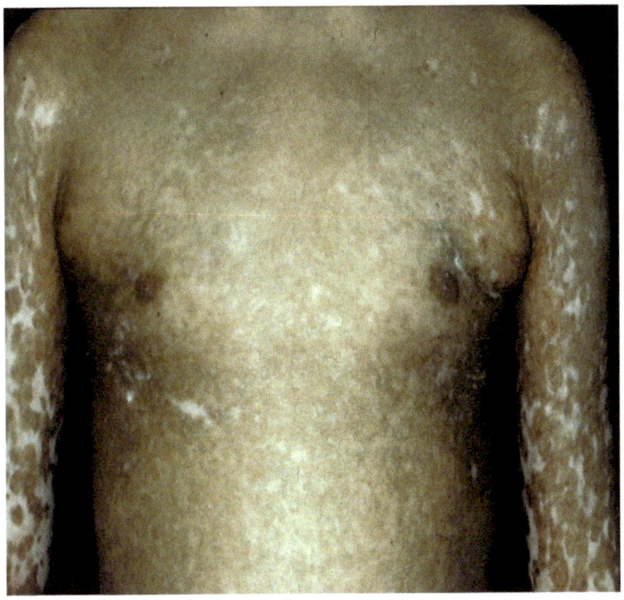

FIGURE 36.4 Guttate hypopigmentation like white spots in a SFT2 patient with chronic graft-versus-host reaction. (Courtesy Prof. Osvaldo Correia, Portugal.)

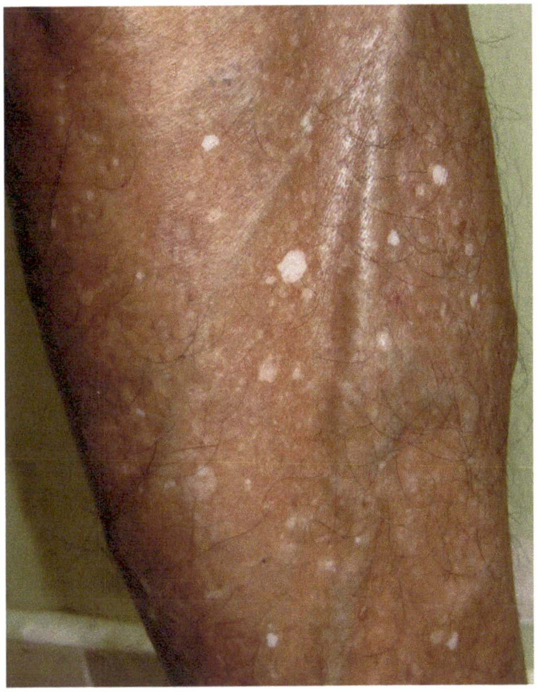

FIGURE 36.5 Idiopathic guttate hypomelanosis in a 75-year-old man FST5.

37
INTERTRIGO

Introduction

Intertrigo, also known as intertriginous dermatitis, is one of the four conditions that fall under the umbrella term of moisture-associated skin damage (MASD). MASD is strongly associated with obesity. MASD is caused by prolonged exposure to various sources of moisture, including urine, stool, perspiration, wound exudate, mucus, saliva, and their contents. Four of the most common forms of MASD are incontinence-associated dermatitis, intertriginous dermatitis, periwound moisture-associated dermatitis, and peristomal moisture-associated dermatitis.

Common causes of genito-crural intertrigo are irritant contact dermatitis, seborrheic dermatitis, psoriasis (inverse pattern/flexural), erythrasma, candidosis, tinea, trichosporosis (in India), and pseudoacanthosis nigricans. In pseudoacanthosis nigricans, the associated obesity is almost always responsible for intertrigo and skin tags.

Candida intertrigo is the most common of all. It is cutaneous candidosis occurring in the skin folds where occlusion from clothing, medical dressings, or obesity that produces abnormally moist conditions. It also occurs in skin folds close to the orifices, and in finger and toe webs. Typically, erythema and a little moist exudation start deep in the fold. As the condition develops, it spreads beyond the area of contact, usually developing the typical features of candidosis with a fringed, irregular edge and subcorneal pustules rupturing to give tiny erosions. Soreness and itching are usual.

Intertrigo of the groin is a frequent problem in the heavily muscled athlete. 'Judo jogger's itch' occurs while jogging following vigorous judo but may be a manifestation of dry skin subjected to abnormal physical and climatic trauma.

Epidemiology

Intertrigo is common in obese subjects irrespective of sex or age.

Associated diseases

Candida intertrigo is associated with poorly controlled diabetes.

Clinical characteristics in light skin (Fitzpatrick skin types I–III)

Intertrigo is very common. (Figure 37.1) Most, but by far not all, patients are obese. It develops where skin lies on skin, and moisture and warmth create a humid climate plus friction that causes superficial abrasion of the horny layer. Depending on the subject, it may go unnoticed or cause burning and itching.

The skin of the flexures – nape of the neck, axillae, submammary folds, lower abdominal folds, groin, genito-anal region – is red and often denuded with a glistening moist surface. In the rima ani, groin, and abdominal and submammary folds, rhagades appear. With time, the erythematous skin may become more pigmented.

Intertrigo may also develop from prolonged sitting, particularly on plastic-covered chairs, after long marches in hot weather, and similar situations.

Psoriasis inversa is particularly prone to developing intertrigo. Intertriginous candidosis may be primary or secondary. Bacterial colonization is common, but not the cause.

Clinical characteristics in dark skin (Fitzpatrick skin types IV–V)

Erythema and moist exudation at deep skin folds, which is itchy and sore, are the most common presentation (Figures 37.2 and 37.3). In darker skin, erythema is obscured by intertriginous hyperpigmentation and/or cloudy exudate.

Investigations

This is diagnosed clinically.

Treatments

- Keeping the skin fold dry is the mainstay of prevention and therapy. Potassium permanganate soaks are effective for this purpose. Wash mitts containing octenidine (Octenisan wash mitts®) are recommended for body decontamination.
- *Candida* intertrigo requires specific topical therapy (azole or polyene antifungal creams), usually continued for about 2 weeks, but treatment may be required for longer periods and is likely to fail if attention is not given to drying the affected area. Antifungal powders may help to prevent re-growth of *Candida* and may keep the skin folds dry.
- Antibiotic creams if bacterial intertrigo is suspected. Potassium permanganate or bleach soaks have antibacterial properties, too.

Further reading

Dissemond J, Assenheimer B, Gerber V, et al. (2021). Moisture-Associated Skin Damage (MASD): A Best Practice Recommendation from Wund-D.A.CH. *J Dtsch Dermatol Ges*;19(6):815–825.

Gray M, Black JM, Baharestani MM, et al. (2011). Moisture-Associated Skin Damage: Overview and Pathophysiology. *J Wound Ostomy Continence Nurs*;38(3):233–241.

Voegeli D (2020). Intertrigo: Causes, Prevention and Management. *Br J Nurs*;29(12):S16–S22.

DOI: 10.1201/9781003479512-37

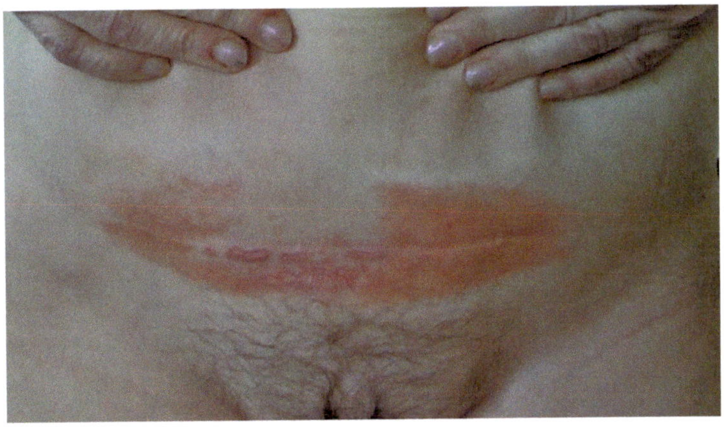

FIGURE 37.1 Intertrigo in FST1 woman. (Courtesy Prof. Uwe Wollina, Germany.)

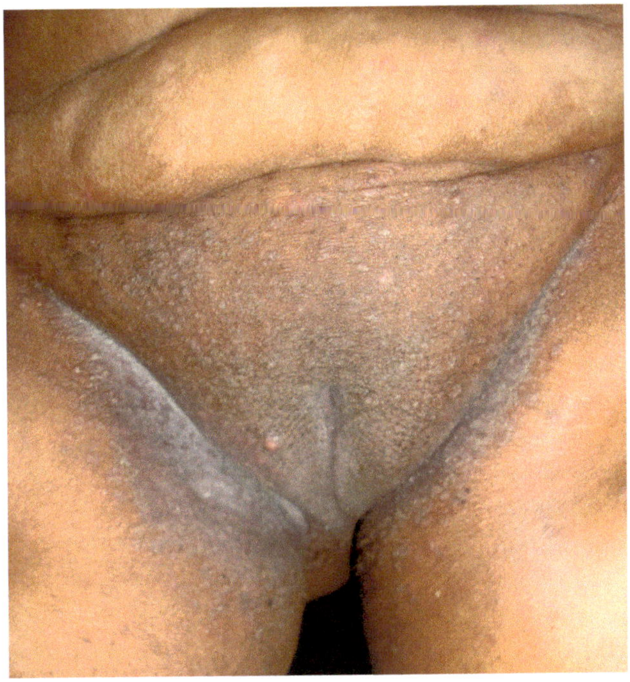

FIGURE 37.2 Intertrigo (intertriginous dermatitis) due to candida infection in a 57-year-old obese diabetic woman FST5.

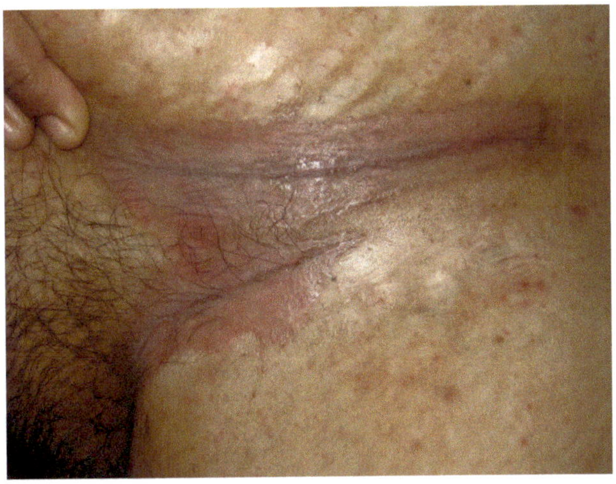

FIGURE 37.3 Intertrigo FST5.

38
KERATODERMA

Introduction

Palmoplantar keratodermas (PPKs) are hereditary or acquired disorders defined by excessive epidermal thickening of the palms and soles. This is observed as an isolated symptom or as part of a syndrome. There are several clinical patterns: Diffuse, focal/areate, striate, punctate, cicatrizing (mutilating), and pseudo-ainhum (constricting bands appear around digits). Water retention by an abnormally keratotic and porous stratum corneum contributes to maceration and microbial overgrowth.

Associated diseases

Associated hyperhidrosis, dermatophyte infections, and pitted keratolysis are common.

Clinical characteristics in light skin (Fitzpatrick skin types I–III)

Keratosis palmaris et plantaris comprises both genetic and acquired diseases characterized by the enormous thickening of the horny layer of the palms and soles (Figures 38.1 and 38.2). The genetic types may be autosomal dominant or recessive, occur without other skin symptoms or be associated with other skin and internal organ manifestations. They may be diffuse or punctate/papular/nodular/striate, be strictly confined to the palms and soles, or be transgredient. Many hyperkeratotic palms and soles are acquired in the course of another disease. The epidermis may look more or less normal under the hyperkeratosis or show granular degeneration (epidermolytic hyperkeratosis). They may remain asymptomatic or cause pain, such as in Richner–Hanhart syndrome and different pachyonychia congenita syndromes.

Generally, the palms and soles are diffusely hyperkeratotic and may show a red margin in Unna–Thost KPP. In the so-called epidermolytic KPP, larger sheets of the keratin may shed and leave a raw surface. In particular, the papular forms are often painful.

In tyrosinemia II of Richner–Hanhart, the tylomas are excessively painful and may prevent the patient from walking. This is also a common feature of pachyonychia congenita.

Clinical characteristics in dark skin (Fitzpatrick skin types IV–V)

Evenly yellow hyperkeratosis of the palms and sole is apparent, but red border is never observed in dark skin types (Figures 38.3 to 38.5).

Investigations

This is diagnosed clinically.

Subtyping may require molecular testing.

Treatments

- Keratolytic therapy, such as 5–10% salicylic acid in white soft paraffin, or a gel of 5–6% salicylic acid in 70% propylene glycol.
- Low-dose systemic acitretin (0.2–0.5 mg/kg) may be tried, especially in patients with functional impairment.
- Fungal superinfection and bacterial overgrowth should be treated.
- Biologics (brodalumab) and JAK inhibitors (topical tofacitinib) have been found effective in refractory severe keratoderma (Buononato et al. 2024, Maitiyaer et al. 2024).

Further reading

Buononato D, Giorgio CMR, Carraturo E, et al. (2024). Palmoplantar Psoriasis or Palmoplantar Keratoderma? Successful Treatment with Brodalumab. *Int J Dermatol*;63(9):1272–1273.

Karagaiah P, Gowda VM (2021). Inherited Disorders of Keratinization. In: Ranawaka RR, et al. (eds). *Atlas of Dermatoses in Pigmented Skin*. Springer, Singapore; 123–150.

Maitiyaer M, Liu Y, Keyimu N, et al. (2024). A Novel Approach with Tofacitinib for the Management of Keratoderma Blennorrhagicum in Reactive Arthritis: A Case Report. *Front Immunol*;15:1399249.

Oji V, SV, her K, Metze D, et al. (2024). Inherited Disorders of Cornification. In: Griffiths C, et al. (eds). *Rook's Textbook of Dermatology*, 10th ed. John Wiley & Sons Ltd., UK; 63.50.

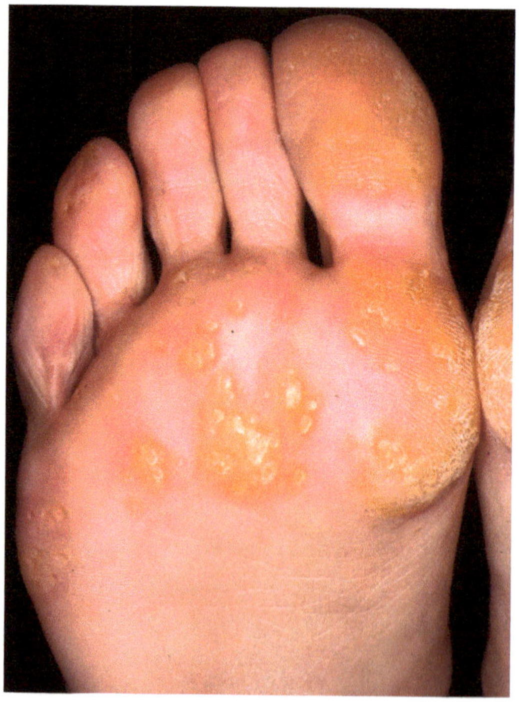

FIGURE 38.1 Punctate keratoderma FST2. (Courtesy Prof. Ian Coulson, UK.)

DOI: 10.1201/9781003479512-38

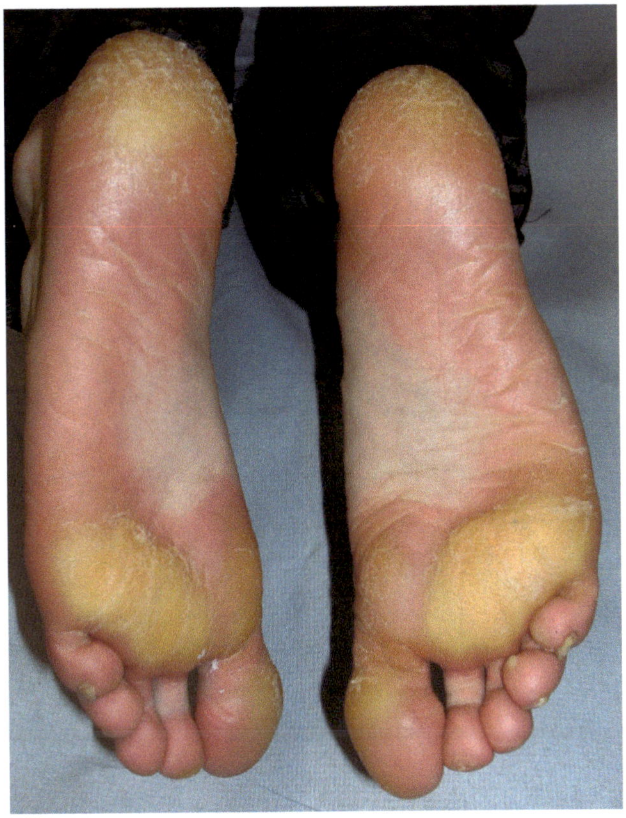

FIGURE 38.2 Focal plantar keratoderma FST2. (Courtesy Prof. Ian Coulson, UK.)

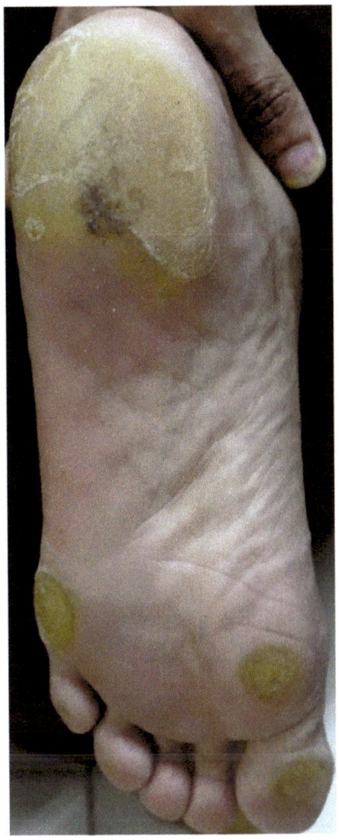

FIGURE 38.3 Focal plantar keratoderma FST5.

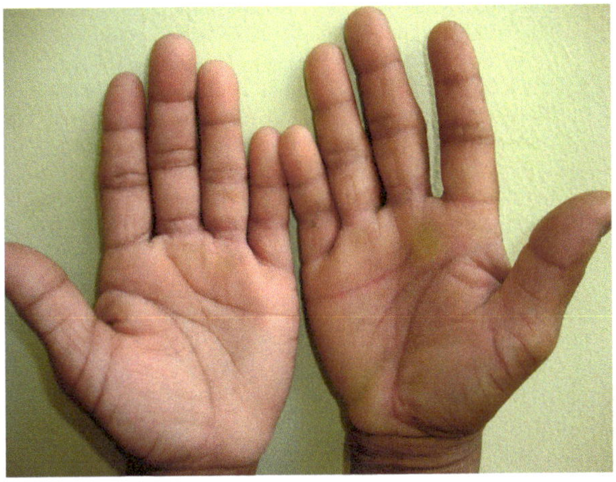

FIGURE 38.4 Punctate keratoderma in a 50-year-old farmer FST5 showing the areas of palmar skin under most pressure is disproportionately thickened. Note red border is never observed in dark skin.

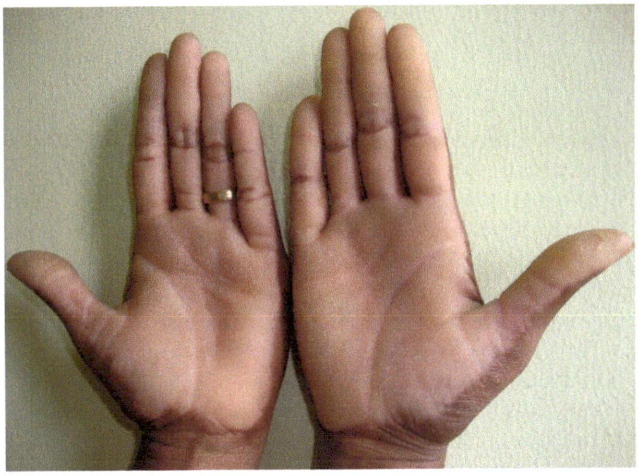

FIGURE 38.5 Diffuse keratoderma in a 32-year-old woman FST5 showing the whole of the palmar or plantar epidermis, including the centripalmar skin and the instep, is uniformly thickened. Evenly yellow hyperkeratosis of the palms and soles are apparent but a red border is never observed in dark skin.

39
KERATOSIS PILARIS/KERATOSIS FOLLICULARIS

Introduction

Keratosis pilaris (KP) is an inherited abnormality of keratinization affecting the follicular orifices. KP is a very common skin condition, characterized by follicular keratotic papules and perifollicular erythema. KP is inherited as an autosomal dominant trait with variable penetrance. KP generally starts in children, most commonly on the extensor surfaces of the upper arms and thighs, and can worsen around puberty. The buttocks and the lumbar areas are also frequently affected. These areas acquire a 'goose-bump' appearance and rough texture.

Please note that 'pilus' is the hair, but what is abnormally keratinized is the follicular opening; thus, the correct term has to be keratosis follicularis (not keratosis pilaris). However, it may then be confused with dyskeratosis follicularis Darier – this is a dilemma.

Epidemiology

KP affects 50–80% of adolescents and about 40% of adults. It appears in children around 9–10 years and may worsen around puberty, then it improves with age. Children and females present for treatment.

Associated diseases

KP may be associated with atopic dermatitis, ichthyosis vulgaris, obesity, diabetes mellitus, and malnutrition, but can also present in conjunction with syndromes such as Down syndrome and Noonan syndrome.

Clinical characteristics in light skin (Fitzpatrick skin types I–III)

KP is extremely common (Figures 39.1 and 39.2). It is seen in children, adolescents, and adults of both genders.

Often starting on the dorso-lateral aspect of the upper arm, the outer aspect of the proximal thighs and buttocks, and often in the lateral aspect of the face, tiny hard papules are seen in follicular distribution. The skin is dry and often a bit scaly. KP often improves over time.

Particularly in the face, the keratotic papules may be in erythematous skin, which tends to become atrophic, a condition called keratosis follicularis rubra atrophicans. A localized variant of this condition is found in the eyebrow region, leading to loss of eyebrow hair, this is called ulerythema ophryogenes (meaning scarring eyebrow erythema).

Most patients do not seek treatment once they are informed about the nature of this inborn anomaly. If therapy is wanted, consistent use of emollients is recommended. Regular vitamin A acid cream, as used for acne vulgaris treatment, is diluted 1:10 and applied daily. Over the course of months, the skin insidiously becomes smoother.

Clinical characteristics in dark skin (Fitzpatrick skin types IV–V)

Very common skin condition (Figure 39.3). Most of our patients are young adolescents who are worried about a 'goose-bump' appearance and rough texture. KP in dark skin is either skin colored or hyperpigmented, and erythema is not prominent. Clinical variants of KP, such as erythromelanosis follicularis faciei et colli or KP atrophicans, are not identified in our setting, possibly due to concealment in dark skin.

Investigations

This is diagnosed clinically.

Treatments

- KP is a cosmetic problem that improves with age. Reassurance and education are adequate in most cases.
- Keratolytics, such as salicylic acid, lactic acid, glycolic acid, and 20% urea preparations, reduce roughness of the skin.
- Topical retinoids may reduce hyperkeratosis and can be very successful when combined with 10% urea-containing moisturizers.
- In severe KP, oral isotretinoin has been successful.
- Pulsed dye laser in patients with severe fixed erythema from KP atrophicans faciei.
- 1064-nm Nd:YAG laser has proved to significantly and safely reduce skin roughness.

Further reading

Maitriwong P, Tangkijngamvong N, Asawanonda P (2020). Innovative 1064-nm Nd:YAG Laser Significantly Improves Keratosis Pilaris, A Randomized, Double-Blind, Sham-Irradiation-Controlled Trial. *Lasers Surg Med*;52(6):509–514.

McCormick E, Nussbaum D, Friedman A, et al. (2024). Evaluation of a Moisturizing Cream with 20% Urea for Keratosis Pilaris. *J Drugs Dermatol*;23(1):1274–1277.

Scorer MJ, Johnston GA (2024). Acquired Disorders of Epidermal Keratinization. In: Griffiths C, et al. (eds). *Rook's Textbook of Dermatology*, 10th ed. John Wiley & Sons Ltd., UK; 85.9.

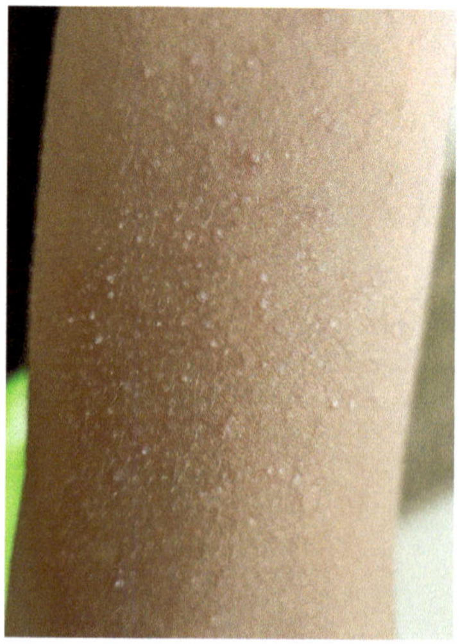

FIGURE 39.1 Keratosis pilaris FST1. (Courtesy Prof. Nooshin Bagherani, Iran.)

DOI: 10.1201/9781003479512-39

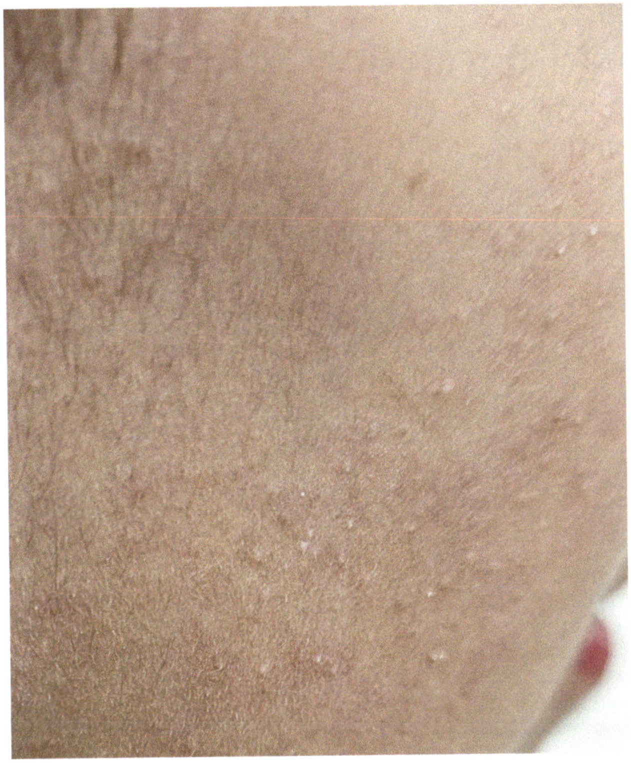

FIGURE 39.2 Keratosis pilaris FST1. (Courtesy Prof. Nooshin Bagherani, Iran.)

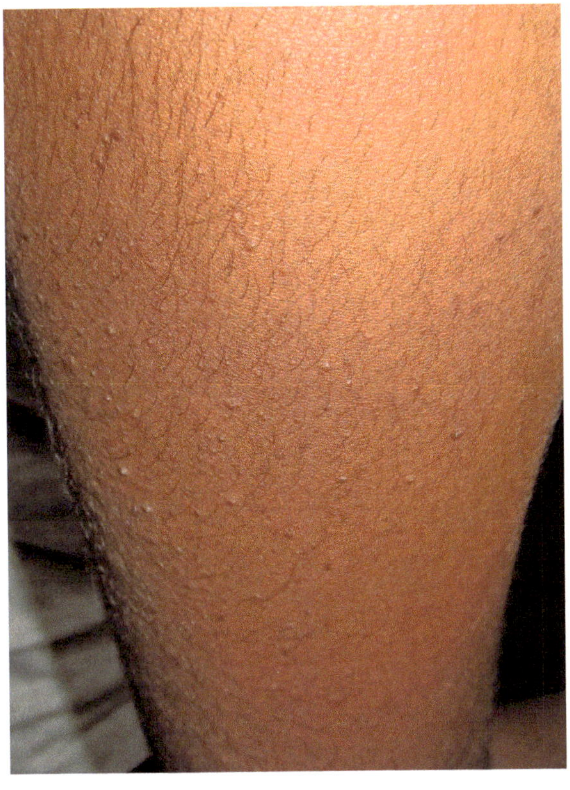

FIGURE 39.3 Keratosis pilaris FST5.

40
KERATOSIS SPINULOSA OR LICHEN SPINULOSUS

Introduction

Lichen spinulosus (LS) is an idiopathic condition that appears as hyperkeratotic follicular papules arranged into large plaques. They appear rapidly, and individual lesions measure 1–2 mm in size and are distributed symmetrically on the extensor surfaces of the limbs, elbows, knees, or on the trunk and neck. On the surface of the papule, there is a pointed keratotic spine that gives a spiky feeling to touch. They form plaques of 2–5 cm in diameter. LS is considered a variant of keratosis pilaris: The conditions share the same features on histology; hair follicles are dilated by a thick keratinous plug and surrounded by a mild to moderate chronic inflammatory infiltrate. LS can persist for many years, but in most patients, it resolves spontaneously within 1–2 years.

Epidemiology

This is not rare as reported earlier. It is underreported due to the benign asymptomatic nature. LS is a disease of children and young adults, with no sex predilection.

Associated diseases

None reported.

Clinical characteristics in light skin (Fitzpatrick skin types I–III)

LS is seen as a variant of keratosis follicularis. It predominantly occurs in adolescents (Figure 40.1). It is usually localized and associated with KF. The single lesion looks like a minute digitate hyperkeratosis; however, it should be differentiated from this condition called multiple minute digitate hyperkeratoses. Histopathologically, mucinosis follicularis was associated in one case.

Clinical characteristics in dark skin (Fitzpatrick skin types IV–V)

Keratosis spinulosa is common in our setting (Figure 40.2). It mostly appears in children aged 7–10 years, and is skin-colored and asymptomatic. The sudden appearance and spiky feeling worry the patients and parents. Even though the progression of the disease has not been studied, since this is not identified among adults, we may conclude that LS may resolve spontaneously with time.

Investigations

This is diagnosed clinically.

Treatments

- Treatment of LS is purely to improve the cosmetic appearance.
- Keratolytic agents including lactic acid (5–12%), salicylic acid (3–5%), and urea (10–20%) can be used.
- Topical retinoids have been successful.

Further reading

Correia O, Rocha N, Haneke E (2014). Multiple Minute Digitate Hyperkeratosis Affecting the Face and Folds: Clinical, Dermoscopic, and Histological Report of a Familial Case. *Acta Dermatovenerol Alp Pannonica Adriat*;23(4):79–80.

Gallo JC, de Wet J, Visser WI, et al. (2023). Generalized Lichen Spinulosus and Secondary Follicular Mucinosis. *JAAD Case Rep*;33:101–104.

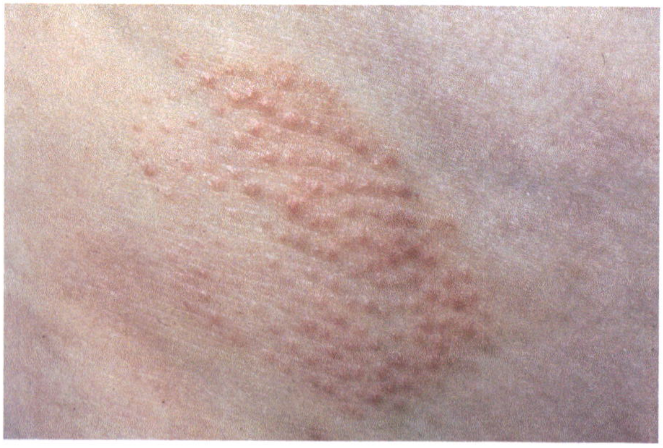

FIGURE 40.1 Keratosis spinulosa FST1. (Courtesy Dr. Richard Ashton, UK.)

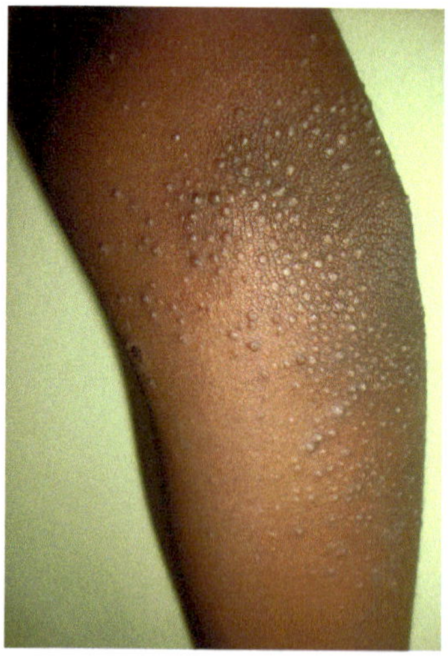

FIGURE 40.2 Keratosis spinulosa on the extensor surface of elbow in a 7-year-old boy FST5.

DOI: 10.1201/9781003479512-40

41
LICHEN NITIDUS

Introduction

Lichen nitidus is a variant of lichen planus and is characterized clinically by the presence of pinpoint to pinhead-sized papules. They are asymptomatic and skin-colored, with a flat, shiny surface. They remain discrete, although they are closely grouped. They appear on any part of the body, but the sites of predilection are the forearms, penis, abdomen, chest, and buttocks. On the palms or soles, lichen nitidus appears as confluent hyperkeratosis resembling chronic fissured eczema, or there may be multiple, distinctive, minute papules. Koebner phenomenon, lesions along scratch marks, is common. Nail pitting and rough nails may coexist with lichen nitidus. An actinic lichen nitidus has been documented in which lesions appear on sun-exposed areas.

Epidemiology

Observed in children of both sexes.

Associated diseases

Lichen nitidus has been described in association with Crohn's disease, trisomy 21, congenital megacolon, and Niemann–Pick disease type B.

Clinical characteristics in light skin (Fitzpatrick skin types I–III)

Lichen nitidus is a rare disease of middle-aged persons (Figures 41.1 to 41.3). There is no gender predilection; however, generalized forms apparently occur more frequently in women. Its etiology is unknown.

Lichen nitidus is characterized by small, flat-topped, slightly elevated, polygonal papules with a mother-of-pearl-like shine on their surface. On more pigmented skin, such as the penis shaft, they appear lighter. Itch is not characteristic. There may be an isomorphic effect to scratch (Koebner phenomenon). Nail changes are rare and seen as onychorrhexis or thickening.

Histopathology is very characteristic: A circumscribed granuloma with some giant cells is located in the papillary dermis, thinning the overlying epidermis, which may show vacuolar basal cell degeneration. The marginal epidermis is acanthotic and collarette-like.

Treatment is difficult and often in vain. Spontaneous resolution may occur after years.

Clinical characteristics in dark skin (Fitzpatrick skin types IV–V)

Lichen nitidus is common in our setting, frequently identified in children 2–10 years of age, with equal incidence in both girls and boys (Figures 41.4 to 41.6). Skin-colored, flat-topped, shiny-surfaced asymptomatic tiny papules may appear on any area of the body.

Investigations

This is diagnosed clinically.

Treatments

None, reassurance only. They disappear spontaneously over time.

Further reading

Kanai C, Terao M, Tanemura A, et al. (2013). Generalized Lichen Nitidus in Russell-Silver Syndrome. *Pediatr Dermatol*;30(1):150–151.

Lauffer F, Eyerich K (2024). Lichen Planus and Lichenoid Disorders. In: Griffiths C, et al. (eds). *Rook's Textbook of Dermatology*, 10th ed. John Wiley & Sons Ltd., UK; 37.17.

Tilly JJ, Drolet BA, Esterly NB (2004). Lichenoid Eruptions in Children. *J Am Acad Dermatol*;51(4):606–624.

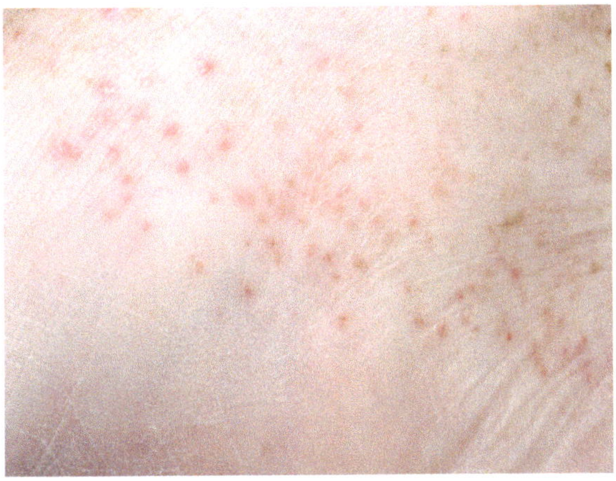

FIGURE 41.1 Lichen nitidus FST1. (Courtesy Prof. Ian Coulson, UK.)

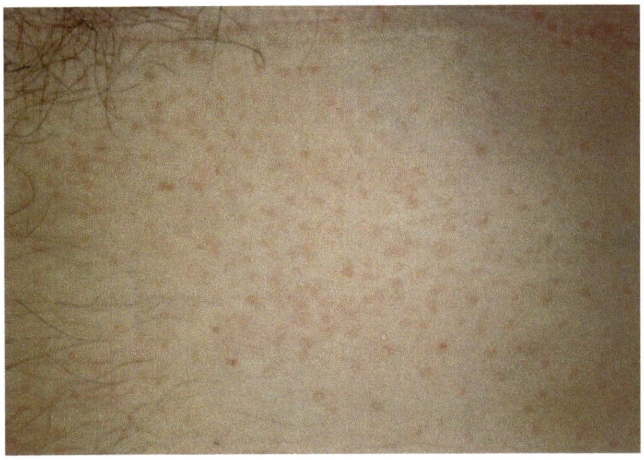

FIGURE 41.2 Lichen nitidus on lower abdomen FST1. (Courtesy Prof. Osvaldo Correia, Portugal.)

DOI: 10.1201/9781003479512-41

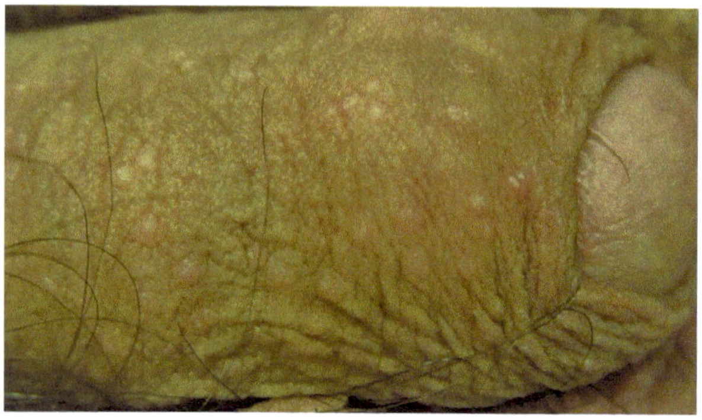

FIGURE 41.3 Lichen nitidus in a 48-year-old man's penile shaft FST2. (Courtesy Prof. Osvaldo Correia, Portugal.)

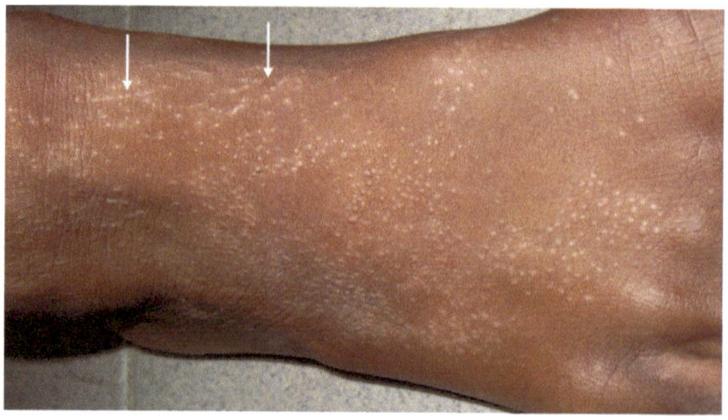

FIGURE 41.4 Lichen nitidus on the dorsum of the foot FST5. Note Koebner phenomena.

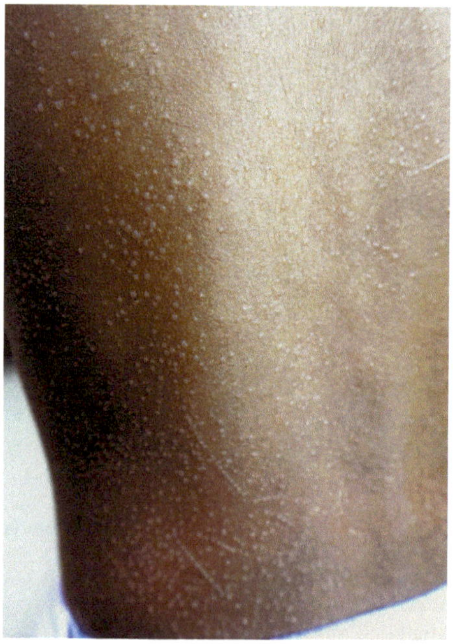

FIGURE 41.5 Lichen nitidus on the trunk in a 5-year-old boy FST5. Note Koebner phenomena.

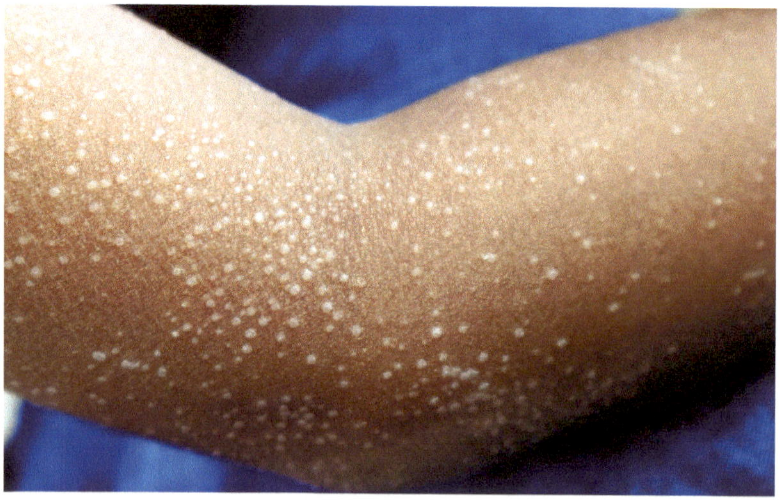

FIGURE 41.6 Lichen nitidus on the upper limb in a 5-year-old boy FST5.

42
LICHEN PLANOPILARIS OR FOLLICULAR LICHEN PLANUS

Introduction

Predominantly follicular lesions present in a patient with or without typical lichen planus (LP). Lichen planopilaris causes scarring alopecia on the affected sites, such as the scalp or trunk. A skin biopsy from these lesions shows the typical histopathology of LP. Graham Little–Piccardi–Lassueur syndrome comprises the triad of multifocal scalp cicatricial alopecia, non-scarring alopecia of the axillae and/or groin, and keratotic lichenoid follicular papules.

Frontal fibrosing alopecia is a scalp condition that affects elderly women in particular and frequently involves the eyebrows. It has been regarded by some authors as a clinically distinct variant of lichen planopilaris.

Associated diseases

Graham Little–Piccardi–Lassueur syndrome and frontal fibrosing alopecia

Clinical characteristics in light skin (Fitzpatrick skin types I–III)

Lichen planofollicularis is a variant of lichen planus with a predominantly folliculotropic lymphocytic infiltrate. It occurs mainly on the scalp and leads to irreversible scarring alopecia (Figures 42.1 and 42.2). Itching is not very marked. On the scalp, smooth, slightly depressed, whitish hairless areas develop that exhibit marginal follicular-bound papules with small, firm hyperkeratosis on top through which the hair shafts pierce. Once the hair follicle is destroyed, the inflammation stops. The bald spots may show erythema at their margin as a sign of activity. Pigmentation is not an obvious feature.

The small hairless spots of pseudopelade Brocq are probably small lesions of lichen planofollicularis of the scalp.

Lichen planofollicularis on the trunk and extremities in combination with scalp involvement and nail dystrophy is called Graham Little-Piccardi-Lassueur syndrome.

Frontal fibrosing alopecia is an enigmatic cicatricial disease leading to almost complete hair loss in front of the frontal hairline and rarely other areas, including the eyebrows. Despite its histological proximity to lichen plano-follicularis, its treatment is that of androgenetic alopecia.

Clinical characteristics in dark skin (Fitzpatrick skin types IV–V)

Dark gray to blackish papules of 1–2 mm diameter appear on the affected areas (Figures 42.3 to 42.5). These papules surround hair follicles at these sites. On the scalp, scarring alopecia is evident upon presentation.

Investigations

This is diagnosed clinically.

Histopathology is similar to typical LP with a perivascular and perifollicular lymphocytic infiltrate in the reticular dermis and mucinous perifollicular fibroplasia within the upper dermis, with an absence of interfollicular mucin and superficial perifollicular wedge-shaped scarring.

Treatments

- The first-line treatment is potent topical corticosteroids (e.g., 0.05% clobetasol propionate ointment twice daily) or intralesional steroids that can provide symptomatic relief.
- Systemic treatment is usually required in all but the mildest of cases. Hydroxychloroquine is the most frequently prescribed first option. Methotrexate, mycophenolate mofetil, and ciclosporin are considered second-line options.
- Systemic steroids are rarely used in the long term, but short courses can be of value in rapidly progressive disease.
- Platelet-rich plasma (PRP), Janus kinase (JAK) inhibitors, and pioglitazone (a PPAR-γ agonist) have been tried with variable success.
- JAK inhibitors, such as tofacitinib, phosphodiesterase-4 inhibitors, such as apremilast, and biologics targeting the interleukin-23/interleukin-17 pathway are novel therapeutic options, resulting in a dramatic change in the treatment landscape of LP (Tekin et al. 2024).

Further reading

Kannangara AP (2021). Lichen Planus and Lichenoid Disorders. In: Ranawaka RR, et al. (eds). *Atlas of Dermatoses in Pigmented Skin*. Springer, Singapore; 497–501.

Pedrosa AF, Duarte AF, Ventura F, et al. (2017). Frontal Fibrosing Alopecia: A Cross-Sectional Study of 108 Patients Followed at a Single Center. *J Dermatol Case Rep*;11(3):35–42.

Tekin B, Xie F, Lehman JS (2024). Lichen Planus: What Is New in Diagnosis and Treatment? *Am J Clin Dermatol*;97(2):208–29.

DOI: 10.1201/9781003479512-42

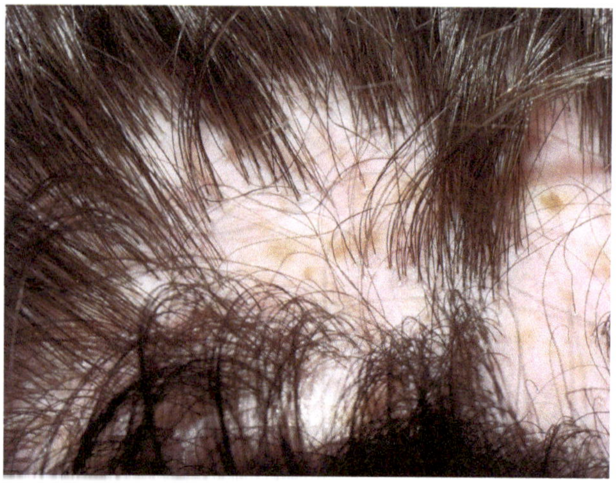

FIGURE 42.1 Lichen planopilaris on the scalp FST1. (Courtesy Prof. Ian Coulson, UK.)

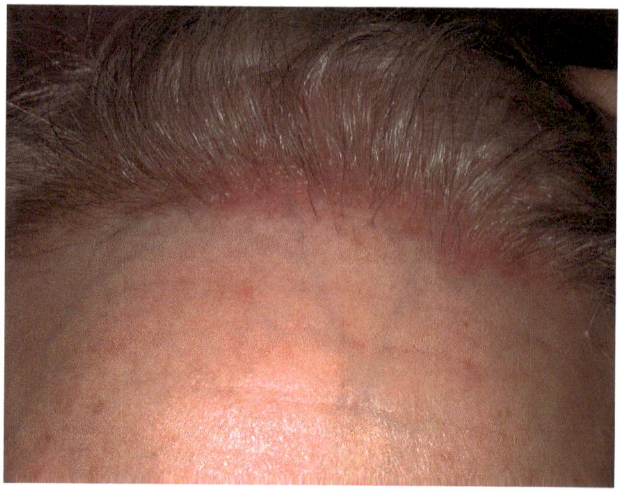

FIGURE 42.2 Frontal fibrosing alopecia, in an adult woman FST1. (Courtesy Prof. Ian Coulson, UK.)

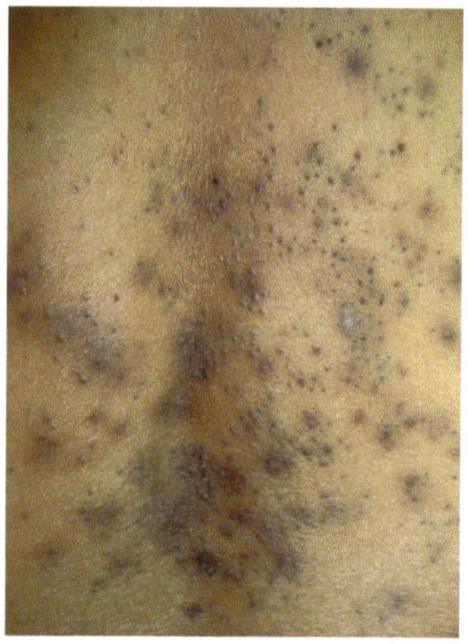

FIGURE 42.3 Lichen planopilaris on the back of the trunk in an adult man who had generalized LP (FST5).

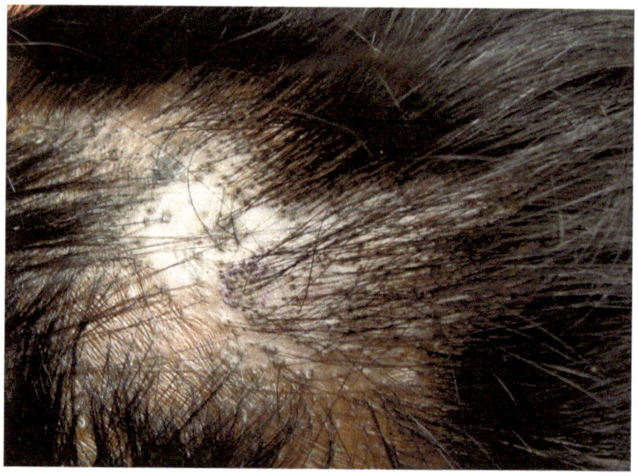

FIGURE 42.4 Lichen planopilaris on the scalp in an adult woman FST5.

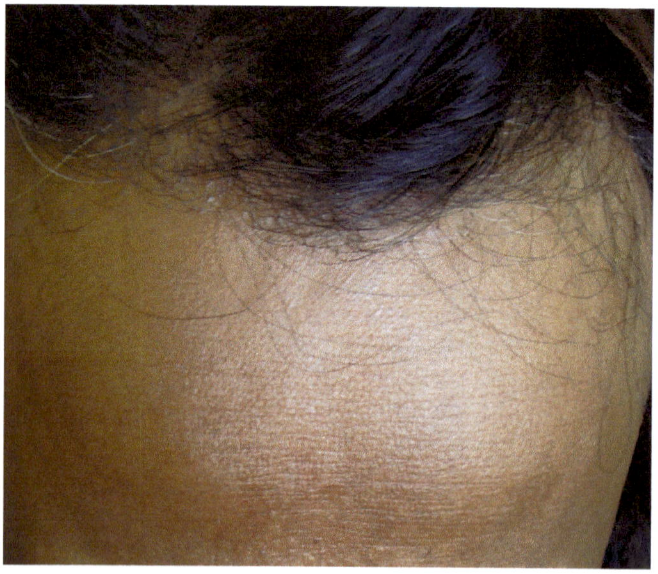

FIGURE 42.5 Frontal fibrosing alopecia, in an adult woman FST5. Note erythematous inflammation is not apparent in dark skin.

43
LICHEN PLANUS

Introduction

Lichen planus (LP) is thought to be a T-cell-mediated autoimmune disease, possibly targeting the basal keratinocytes. In most patients, cutaneous LP resolves spontaneously within 1–2 years without sequela. Pruritus is a fairly consistent feature in LP and ranges from occasional mild irritation to more or less continuous severe itching, which interferes with sleep and makes life almost intolerable; occasionally, pruritus is completely absent. Drugs such as antimicrobials, antihypertensives, antimalarials, antidepressants, anticonvulsants, diuretics, metals, non-steroidal anti-inflammatory drugs (NSAIDs), angiotensin converting enzyme (ACE) inhibitors, and beta-blockers may precipitate an LP-like eruption or lichenoid eruption. Dental amalgam and betel nut (in India and Southeast Asia) may induce oral LP.

Epidemiology

Prevalence is around 0.5–1% of the adult population and both men and women are equally affected. LP is not common in children.

Associated diseases

Squamous cell carcinoma may rarely arise on long-lasting cutaneous and anogenital LP lesions.

Patients with LP are five times as likely to test positive for Hepatitis C virus (HCV) as the general population, and those with HCV seropositivity are 2.5 to 4.5 times as likely to develop LP.

Clinical characteristics in light skin (Fitzpatrick skin types I–III)

LP in light skin is characterized by small polygonal, flat, violaceous papules that may be confluent and form larger plaques (Figures 43.1 to 43.5). Typically, the disease starts at the volar aspect of the wrist and then slowly extends to other cutaneous areas such as the lower back and ankle. Depending on the region involved, the clinical aspect may change. On the lower leg, LP may turn verrucous and itch severely. A bullous variant is rare. Ulcerative lesions may be excessively painful when localized on the soles of the feet. After applying a little oil on the surface of the LP plaques, dermatoscopy reveals a net of fine white lines, the Wickham striae.

LP of the scalp leads to scarring alopecia and is called LP follicularis or Graham Little–Lassueur syndrome. This may rarely affect other body sites as well.

Nail involvement is frequent, with about 10–15% of the LP individuals affected. The nails develop longitudinal ridging, surface defects, fissures, and finally pterygium until complete nail disappearance. Pigmentation in skin types I–III is rare, as is LP pigmentosus.

LP on the penis, particularly the glans, is often annular with a slightly atrophic center.

LP of the vulva is frequently erosive and may cause severe dyspareunia. It is often associated with oral lesions as vulvo-vaginal-gingival syndrome.

The oral mucosa is frequently involved; some claim oral LP is more frequent than cutaneous LP. The most characteristic mucosal form is a white net on the lining mucosa of the cheek, soft palate, and lips that usually remains asymptomatic and is often a chance observation. However, it may slowly develop into atrophic LP with dark red mucosa that tends to become erosive and ulcerated. The dorsum of the tongue may develop round white plaques that may become erosive after years. On the side of the tongue, the lesions may be erosive from the beginning. Atrophic, erosive, and ulcerated lesions may represent a precancerous condition.

Clinical characteristics in dark skin (Fitzpatrick skin types IV–V)

Common presentation is the firm, shiny, polygonal, 1–3 mm diameter papules and plaques with a violet to dark gray color (Figures 43.6 to 43.11). Fairer-skinned individuals may show redness in early lesions, but that is not a common feature in dark skin. Wickham striae (a tracery of thin white lines seen on the surface of the lesions) are barely visible in skin lesions, but more obvious in buccal mucosal lesions. LP resolves with post-inflammatory hyperpigmentation that may last months to years. Clinical variants such as annular lesions, lichen planopilaris, hypertrophic LP, linear lesions, bullous LP, ulcerative LP, and mucous membrane lesions have also been seen in dark-skinned individuals.

Investigations

This is diagnosed clinically.

Skin biopsy for histopathology if doubtful. The characteristic histological changes are best seen in biopsies of fully developed LP papules: Hyperorthokeratosis; focal thickening of the stratum granulosum; vacuolar degeneration of the stratum basale; colloid bodies, alteration to loss of rete ridges resulting in a sawtooth appearance; and a dense epidermotropic band of lymphocytes infiltrating the dermis along the dermo-epidermal

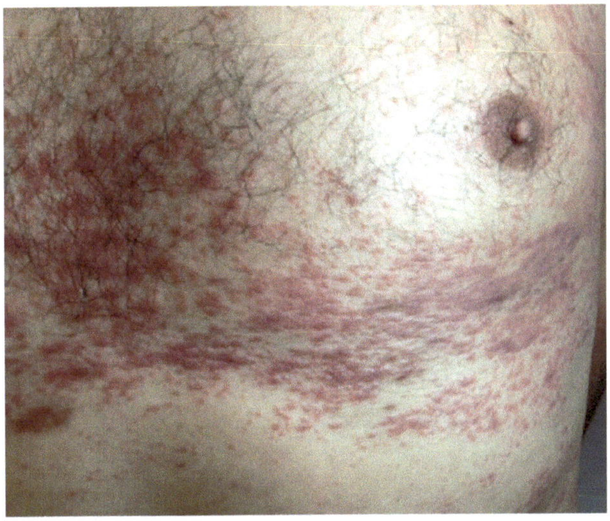

FIGURE 43.1 Lichen planus FST1. (Courtesy Dr. Carlo Enrico Urbani, Italy.)

DOI: 10.1201/9781003479512-43

junction (interface dermatitis). The hydropic basal layer degeneration may be so pronounced that a vesicular aspect develops. The hyperkeratosis can take on a verrucous aspect. Idiopathic LP (almost) never has eosinophils, whereas drug-induced LP may have eosinophils. Pigmentary incontinence with dermal melanophages is characteristic, particularly in skin of color.

Treatments

Treatment of LP depends on the localization, clinical form, and severity. For cutaneous LP, which can clear spontaneously within 1–2 years, the aim of treatment is to reduce pruritus and time to resolution. Topical or systemic corticosteroids are recommended as first-line treatment.

- Limited cutaneous LP:
  - Very potent (clobetasol propionate ointment 0.05%) or potent topical corticosteroids in less severe forms and during maintenance therapy.
- Topical tacrolimus 0.1% was found to be equally effective, with fewer side effects especially on the face, neck, genitals, and flexures, but it is more expensive.
- Widespread cutaneous LP:
  - Prednisolone 0.5–1 mg/kg per day until improvement.
  - Acitretin 30 mg per day for 8 weeks.
- PUVA or UVB: Two to three times a week, alone or with systemic retinoids (Re-PUVA).
- Tofacitinib has been shown to be very effective, as well as other Janus kinase inhibitors.
- Nail lichen planus is an emergency as scarring sequelae are permanent. Perilesional injections of triamcinolone 10 mg/mL are recommended for a few digits, intramuscular injections are recommended if many digits are involved.
- Scarring alopecia may also be treated with injections.

Further reading

Alaizari NA, Al-Maweri SA, Al-Shamiri HM, et al. (2016). Hepatitis C Virus Infections in Oral Lichen Planus: A Systematic Review and Meta-Analysis. *Aust Dent J*;61(3):282–287.

Huang MY, Armstrong AW (2023). Janus-Kinase Inhibitors in Dermatology: A Review of Their Use in Psoriasis, Vitiligo, Systemic Lupus Erythematosus, Hidradenitis Suppurativa, Dermatomyositis, Lichen Planus, Lichen Planopilaris, Sarcoidosis and Graft-versus-Host Disease. *Indian J Dermatol Venereol Leprol*;90(1):30–40.

Lauffer F, Eyerich K (2024). Lichen Planus and Lichenoid Disorders. In: Griffiths C, et al. (eds). *Rook's Textbook of Dermatology*, 10th ed. John Wiley & Sons Ltd., UK; 37.1.

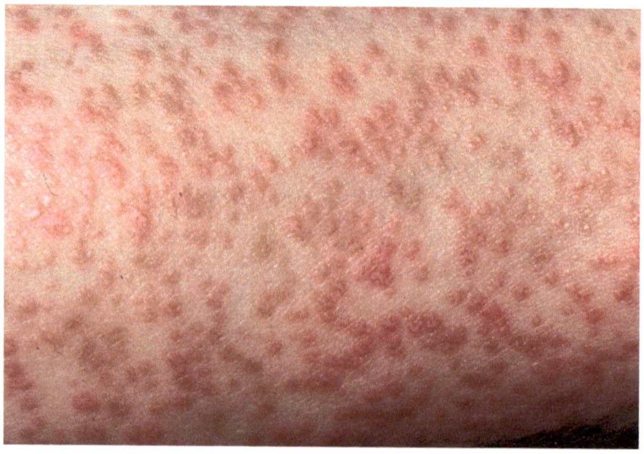

FIGURE 43.2 Lichen planus FST1. (Courtesy Dr. Richard Ashton, UK.)

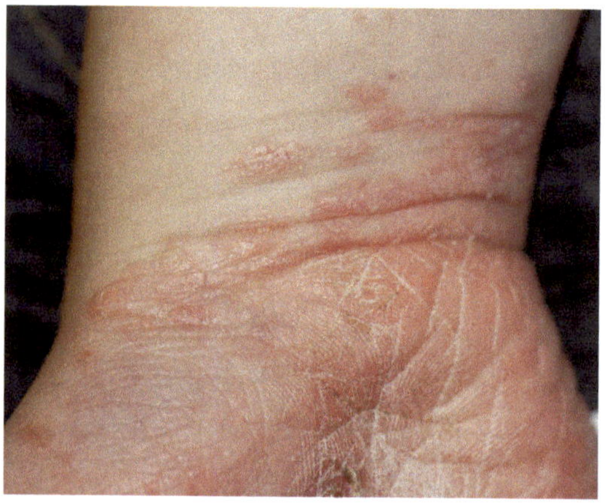

FIGURE 43.3 Lichen planus on the wrist FST1. (Courtesy Prof. Ian Coulson, UK.)

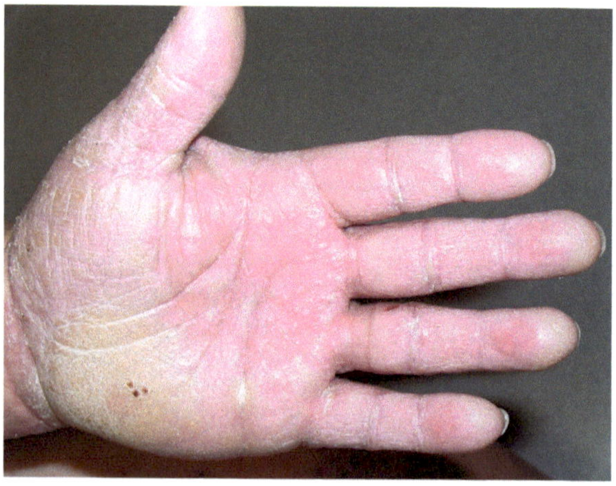

FIGURE 43.4 Lichen planus on palm FST1. (Courtesy Prof. Ian Coulson, UK.)

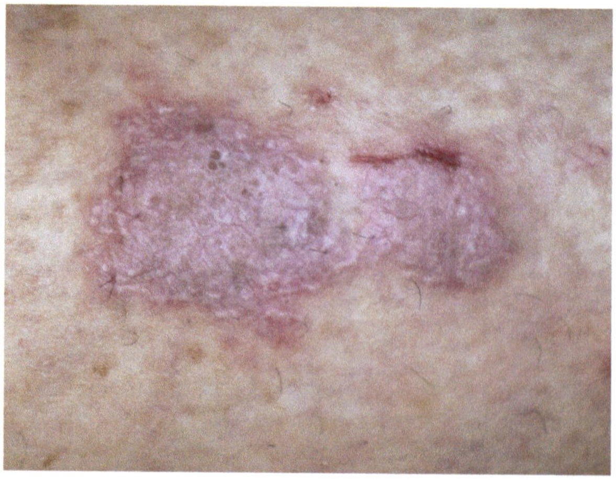

FIGURE 43.5 Wickham striae in lichen planus FST1. (Courtesy Prof. Ian Coulson, UK.)

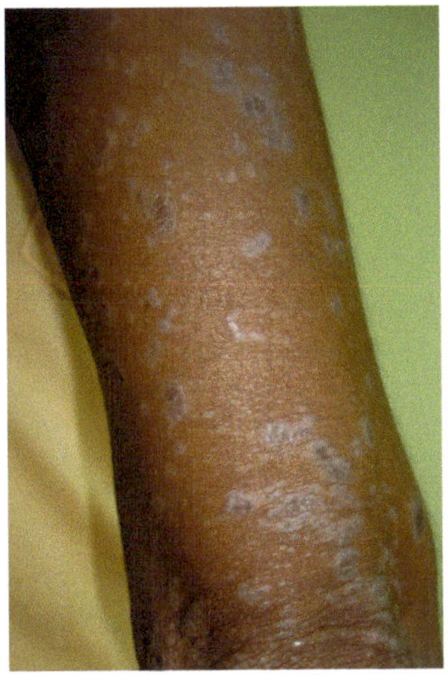

FIGURE 43.6 Classic clinical presentation of lichen planus is the firm, shiny, polygonal, 1–3 mm diameter papules and plaques with a violet to dark gray color FST5.

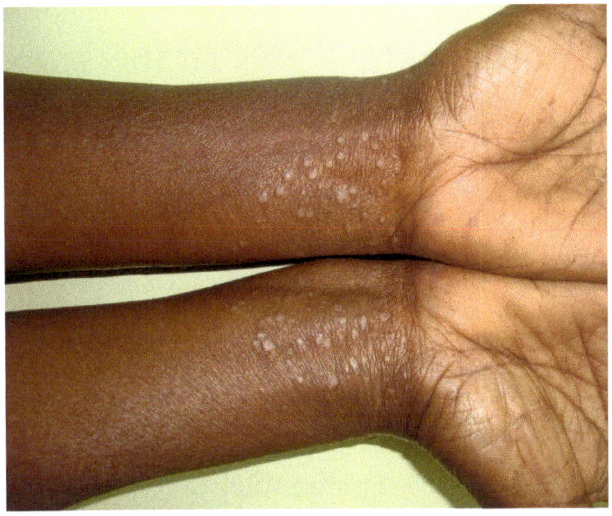

FIGURE 43.7 Lichen planus can affect any part of the body surface, but is most often seen on the volar aspect of the wrists, the lumbar region and around the ankles FST5.

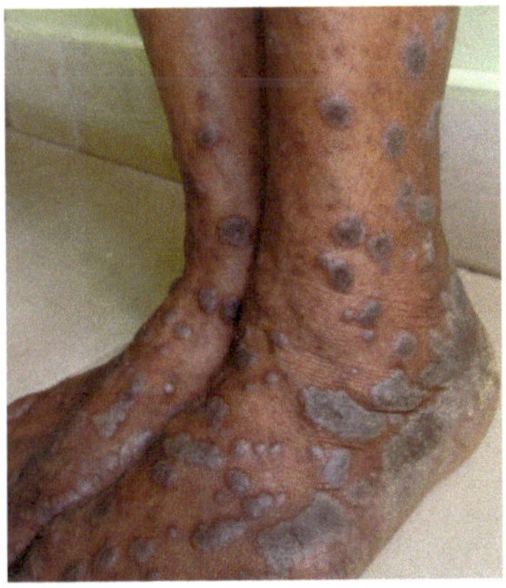

FIGURE 43.8 Hypertrophic lichen planus FST5. The ankles and shins are the commonest sites for hypertrophic lesions.

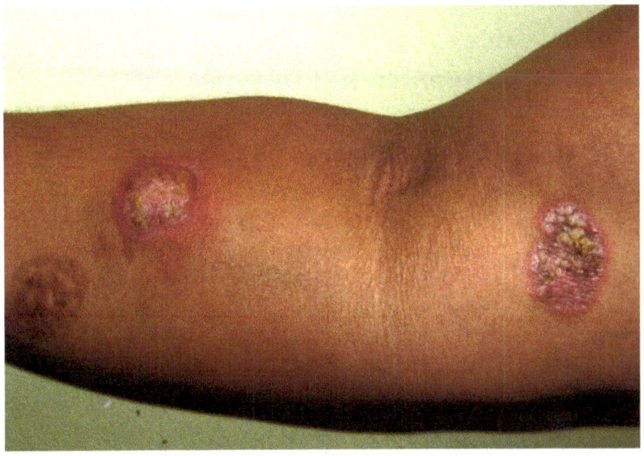

FIGURE 43.9 Ulcerative lichen planus in a 39-year-old woman FST5. Histopathology done twice for confirmation as this was not clinically suggestive of LP. This heal leaving post-inflammatory hyperpigmentation.

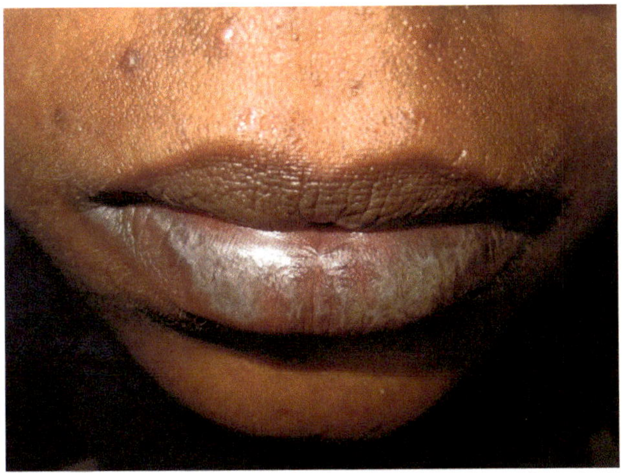

FIGURE 43.10 Lichen planus on the lips FST5.

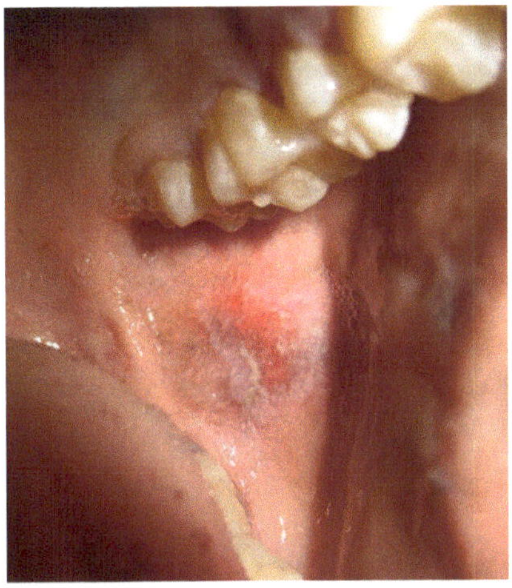

FIGURE 43.11 Lichen planus on buccal mucosa showing Wickham's striae FST5.

44
LICHEN PLANUS PIGMENTOSUS

Introduction

Lichen planus pigmentosus (LPP) is a clinical variant of lichen planus. This pigmentary disorder is seen in South Asia or the Middle East and may or may not be associated with typical lichen planus (LP) papules. The slate gray to brownish-black macular hyperpigmentation involves chiefly the face, neck, and upper limbs, although it can be more widespread. It is mostly diffuse, but reticular, blotchy, and perifollicular forms are seen. LPP alone is asymptomatic, but if it is associated with LP, itchiness may be a feature.

Epidemiology

Seen in South Asia and the Middle East.

Associated diseases

LPP may be associated with typical lLP.

Clinical characteristics in light skin (Fitzpatrick skin types I–III)

LPP is virtually not observed in light-skinned individuals. It is a variant of LP whose particular feature of pigmentation is closely linked to the degree of skin pigmentation (Figure 44.1). LP exhibits vacuolar degeneration of the epidermal basal layer where the bulk of the melanocytes are located. When the basal cells degenerate, melanocytes may drop down into the dermis or get destroyed, leading to marked pigmentary incontinence clinically seen as slate gray to brown pigmentation.

Clinical characteristics in dark skin (Fitzpatrick skin types IV–V)

Slate gray to brownish-black macular hyperpigmentation is not uncommon in our setting and may or may not be associated with typical LP. This is clinically distinguishable from ashy dermatoses (Figures 44.2 and 44.3).

Investigations

This is diagnosed clinically.

Treatments

- Diluted topical steroids give good results in relieving hyperpigmentation and mild pruritus.
- Generalized LPP significantly improved with the daily administration of Tofacitinib (Janus kinase inhibitor) at a dosage of 15 mg (Araghi et al. 2024).
- Q-switched Nd-YAG laser gives complete to near-complete resolution of pigment without many complications (Shah et al. 2019).

Further reading

Araghi F, Beyki F, Rakhshan A, et al. (2024). Generalized Lichen Planus Pigmentosus and a New Management Approach. *Clin Case Rep*;12(6):e8829.

Bhat RM, Mathanda TR, Jayaprakash CS, et al. (2017). Clinical, Histopathological Characteristics and Immunohistochemical Findings in Lichen Planus Pigmentosus. *Indian J Dermatol*;62(6):612–617.

Kannangara AP (2021). Lichen Planus and Lichenoid Dermatoses. In: Ranawaka RR, et al. (eds). *Atlas of Dermatoses in Pigmented Skin*. Springer, Singapore; 497–501.

Piguet V, Breathnach SM, Cleach LL (2016). Lichen Planus and Lichenoid Disorders. In: Griffiths C, et al. (eds). *Rook's Textbook of Dermatology*, 9th ed. Wiley-Blackwell Science, Oxford, UK; 37.8.

Shah DSD, Aurangabadkar DS, Nikam DB (2019). An Open-Label Non-Randomized Prospective Pilot Study of the Efficacy of Q-Switched Nd-YAG Laser in Management of Facial Lichen Planus Pigmentosus. *J Cosmet Laser Ther*;21(2):108–115.

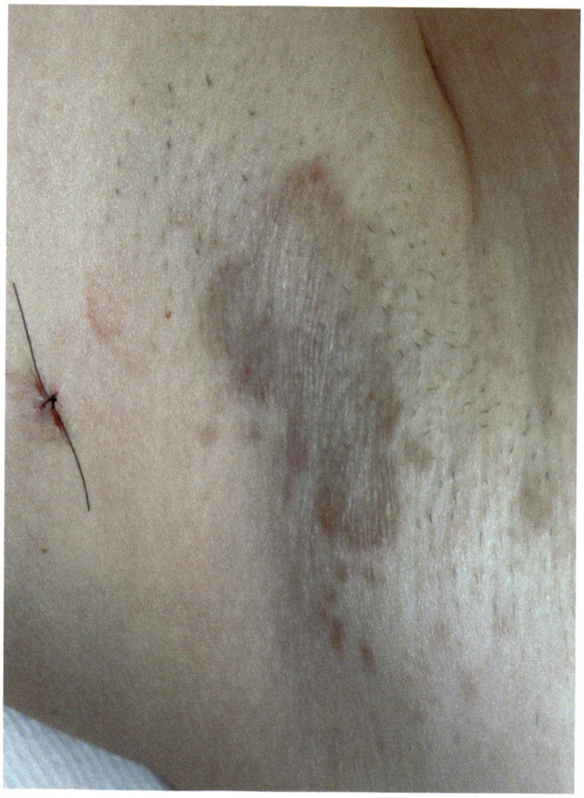

FIGURE 44.1 Lichen planus pigmentosus in the axilla FST1. (Courtesy Prof. Ian Coulson, UK.)

DOI: 10.1201/9781003479512-44

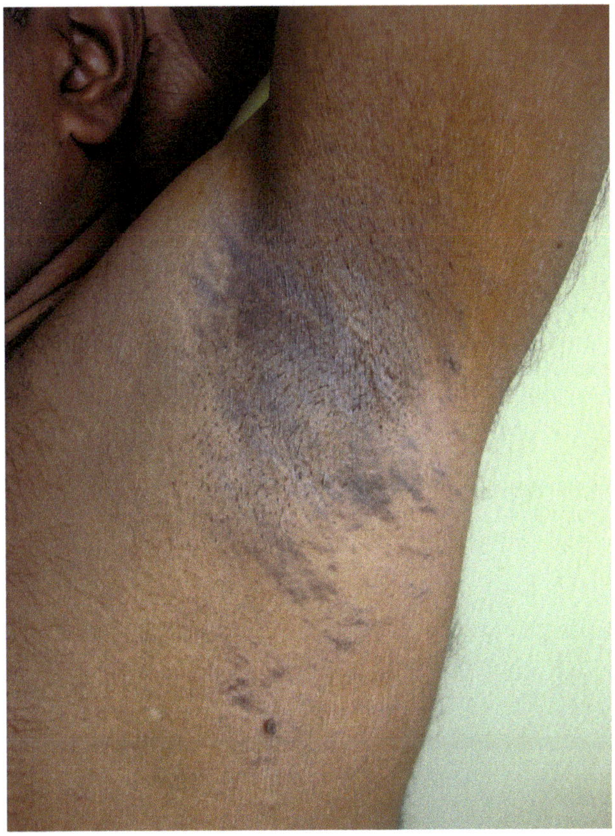

FIGURE 44.2 Lichen planus pigmentosus shows striking predominance of lesions at intertriginous sites, especially the axillae. This man had typical lichen planus on limbs FST5.

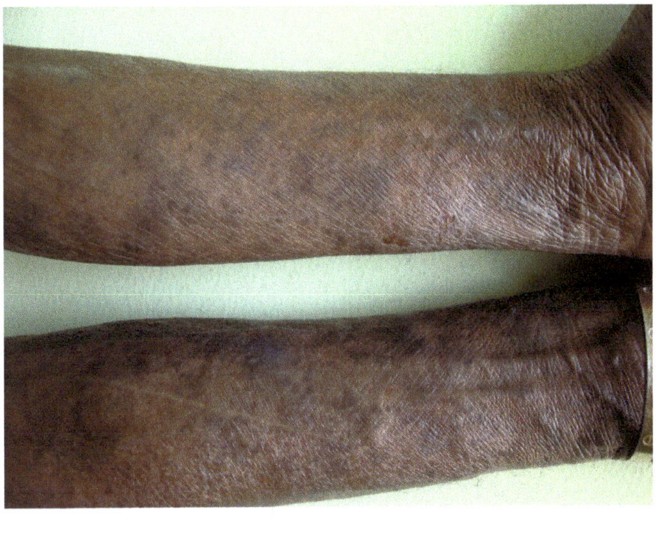

FIGURE 44.3 Lichen planus pigmentosus on forearms in a man who had typical lichen planus on other sites FST5.

45
LICHEN SCLEROSUS

Introduction

Lichen sclerosus (LS) is a common inflammatory dermatosis of the anogenital skin: Penis, vagina, and perianal skin. However, extragenital disease is also not uncommon. Rarely, oral lesions may appear. LS may present as secondary phimosis (non-retractile foreskin), paraphimosis (foreskin fixed in retraction), meatal 'pin hole' narrowing, and urinary retention in men. Itching, discomfort, dyspareunia, and constipation are the presenting symptoms in women. Perianal lesions are common in women and may not develop in men. Both men and women may describe itching, burning, bleeding, tearing, splitting, rash, hemorrhagic blisters, and dyspareunia. Itching is the earliest manifestation in female genital LS; 15–20% of cases are extra-genital LS, and they manifest as atrophic leukodermic patches or plaques.

Epidemiology

LS may occur at any age but is more common in prepubertal girls and post-menopausal women, and is 6–10 times more common in females.

Associated diseases

Dysplasia, carcinoma *in situ*, or of a frank squamous cell carcinoma are well-recognized complications.

Associated with other autoimmune disorders, commonly thyroid disease.

Clinical characteristics in light skin (Fitzpatrick skin types I–III)

Lichen sclerosus et atrophicans (LSA) is a fairly common, chronic, often progressive disease characterized by the development of atrophic white spots predominantly in the anogenital area, and rarely on other regions of the body (Figures 45.1 to 45.4). There are two age groups: Disease onset between 5 and 10 years of age and in the fifth and sixth decades.

Genital lesions are seen in both genders and lead to different signs and symptoms: In boys and men, mainly the prepuce is involved and may shrink to cause phimosis or paraphimosis, or when the tip of the glans is affected (balanitis xerotica obliterans) the urethral meatus becomes stenotic, leading to micturition difficulties. In girls and women, the labia minora become atrophic, turn white, and may finally disappear. Particularly in young girls, there may be bleeding into the lesional skin, raising concern of child abuse.

Extragenital lesions often start with small white spots that may coalesce (historical term: White spot disease).

All lesions develop a more or less pronounced atrophy with fine wrinkling of the skin when it is raised between the fingers. Spotty hyperkeratosis may develop and should be biopsied.

Occasionally, LSA coincides with morphea.

Balanitis keratotica et micacea praeblastomatosa is mainly observed in elderly men after long-term LSA. In women, LSA of the vulva is apparently associated with a higher risk of vulva carcinoma.

Clinical characteristics in dark skin (Fitzpatrick skin types IV–V)

Vitiligoid LS is a very common presentation of LS in dark skin (Figures 45.5 to 45.8). It appears in both adults and children, and in both sexes. They present with a clinical appearance of leukoderma on genital areas; itching is a frequent complaint; no other areas of vitiligo. Since itching is not a feature of autoimmune vitiligo, that directs us to perform a skin biopsy which shows histological features of LS. In fear of vitiligo, these patients present early for treatment. Vitiligoid LS has a very good prognosis with complete clearance without sequelae if they present early for treatment.

Investigations

Exclusive oral or genital depigmentation is a common problem, and histological evaluation is essential to differentiate vitiligoid LS from true vitiligo.

Treatments

- Soap substitute and a barrier preparation to avoid contact with soap, urine, and pubic hair.
- An ultrapotent topical corticosteroid, clobetasol propionate 0.05%, is the first-line treatment and should be used under supervision. The risk of herpes simplex and wart reactivation should be kept in mind.
- Secondary candida and bacterial infections should be treated.
- Topical calcineurin inhibitors (tacrolimus or pimecrolimus as steroid-sparing alternatives) are as effective as topical steroids and have fewer side effects. However, the treatment should be a short course due to the risk of neoplastic change.
- Surgery: Appropriate surgery to relieve symptoms is usually circumcision in men. In women, surgery is only indicated for the management of functional problems caused by post-inflammatory scarring, premalignant lesions, and malignancy.

Further reading

Arif T, Fatima R, Sami M (2022). Extragenital Lichen Sclerosus: A Comprehensive Review. *Australas J Dermatol*;63(4):452–462.

Attili VR, Attili SK (2008). Vitiligoid Lichen Sclerosus: A Reappraisal. *Indian J Dermatol Venereol Leprol*;74(2):118–21.

Bunker CB, Watchorn RE (2024). Dermatoses of the Male Genitalia. In: Griffiths C, et al. (eds). *Rook's Textbook of Dermatology*, 10th ed. John Wiley & Sons Ltd, UK; 109.15.

Dennin MH, Stein SL, Rosenblatt AE (2018). Vitiligoid Variant of Lichen Sclerosus in Young Girls with Darker Skin Types. *Pediatr Dermato*; 35(2):198–201.

Karawita A, Ranawaka RR (2021). Genital Dermatoses. In: Ranawaka RR, et al. (eds). *Atlas of Dermatoses in Pigmented Skin*. Springer, Singapore; 777.

DOI: 10.1201/9781003479512-45

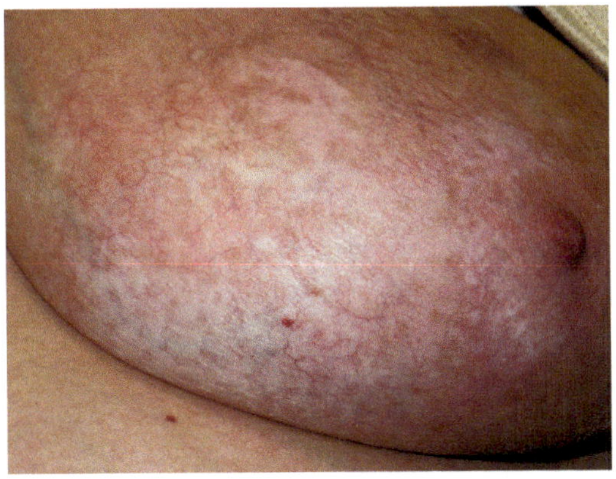

FIGURE 45.1 Lichen sclerosis on the breast FST1. (Courtesy Prof. Ian Coulson, UK.)

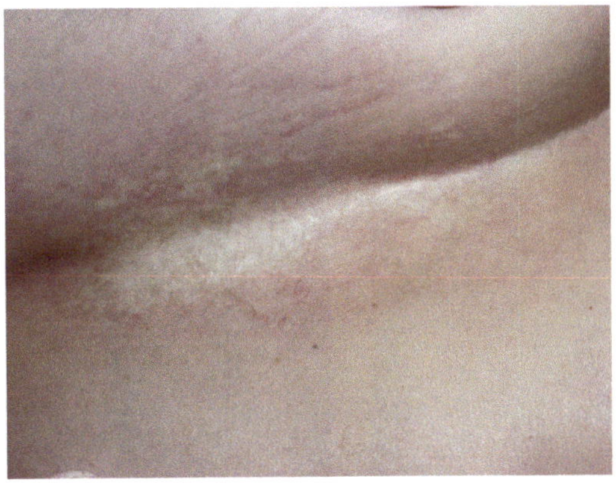

FIGURE 45.2 Localized lichen sclerosis on the submammary area after radiotherapy FST1. (Courtesy Prof. Ian Coulson, UK.)

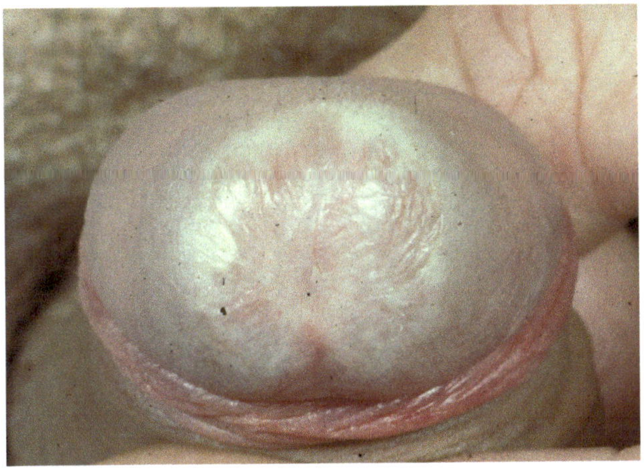

FIGURE 45.3 Meatal lichen sclerosis FST1. (Courtesy Prof. Ian Coulson, UK.)

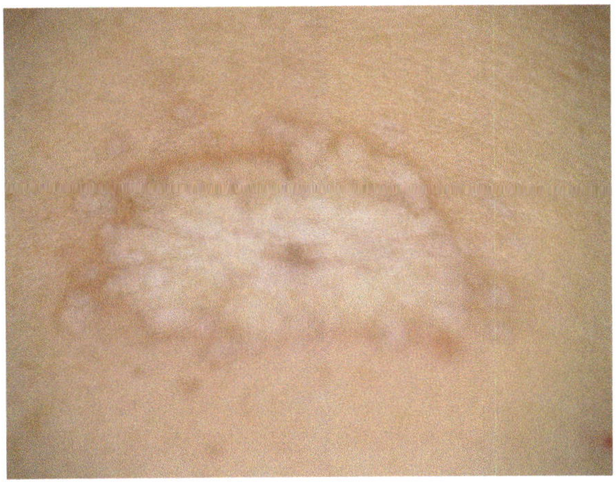

FIGURE 45.4 Extra-genital lichen sclerosus FST2. (Courtesy Prof. Ian Coulson, UK.)

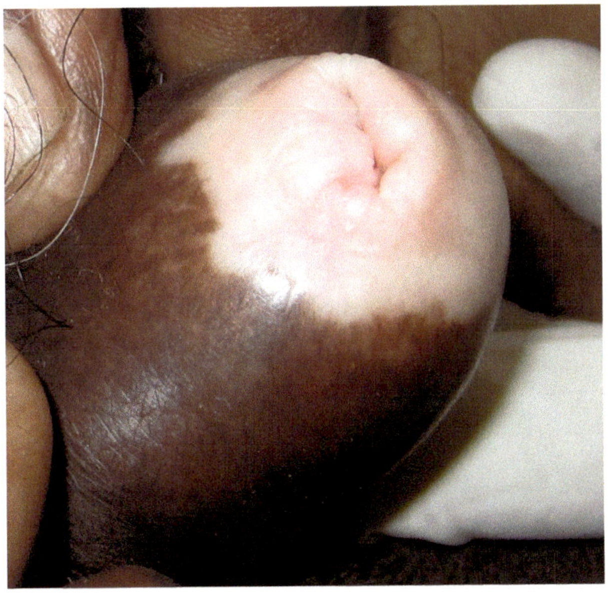

FIGURE 45.5 Meatal lichen sclerosis FST5; a 48-year-old man with vitiligoid lichen sclerosus. He has ignored this as a single patch of vitiligo in a hidden area; presented with phimosis.

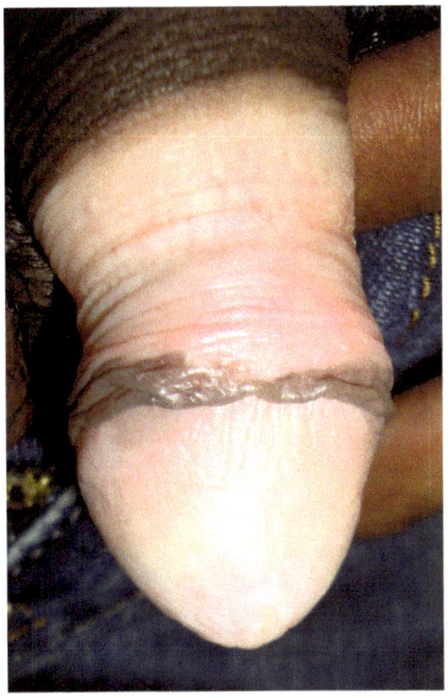

FIGURE 45.6 Lichen sclerosus in glans penis in a 34-year-old man. His vtiliginous lesion on glans penis has been ignored for years thinking that it is vitiligo on a covered area. He presented with paraphimosis.

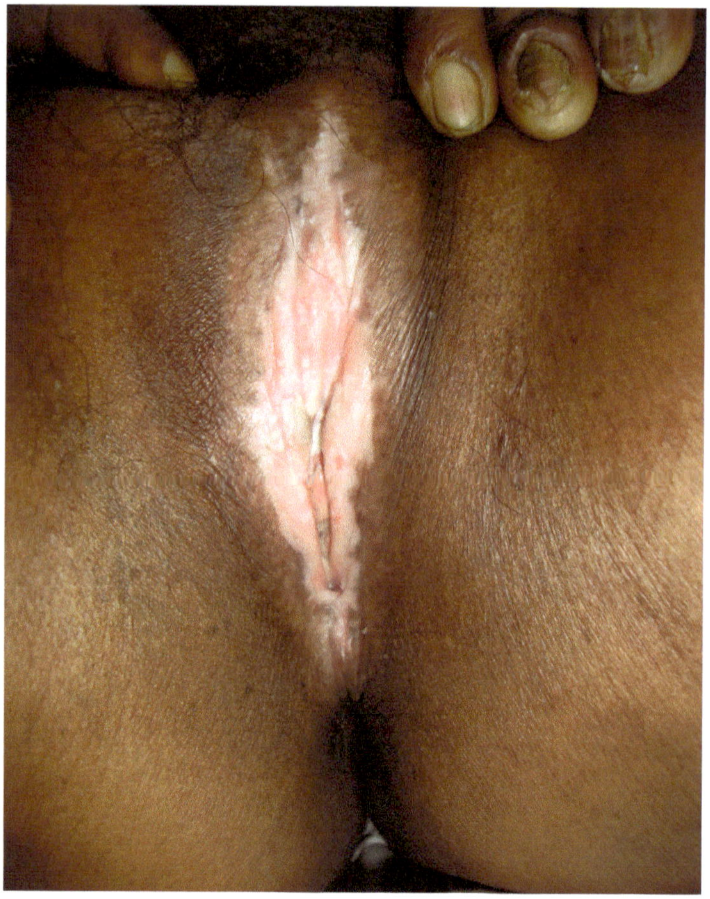

FIGURE 45.7 A 57-year-old woman with vitiligoid lichen sclerosus FST5. She presented to us with intractable itching, irritation, burning sensation, and dyspareunia.

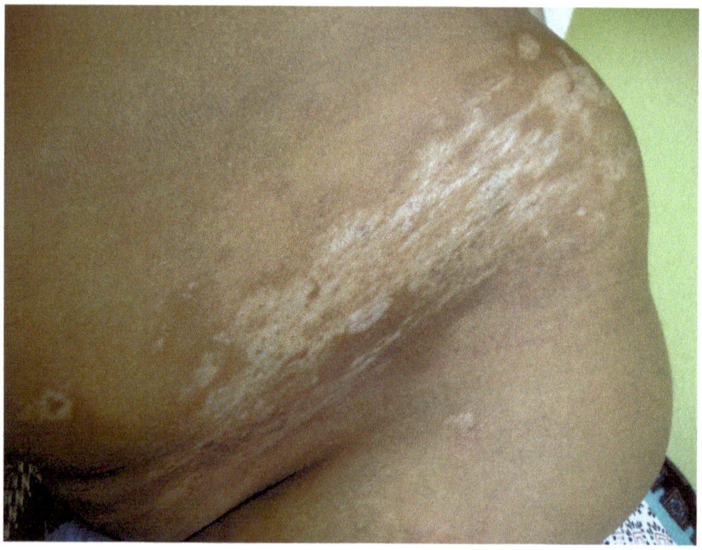

FIGURE 45.8 Extra-genital lichen sclerosus in a 35-year-old woman FST5. Skin biopsy was performed for confirmation and to exclude morphea and vitiligo.

46
LICHEN SIMPLEX CHRONICUS

Introduction

Lichen simplex chronicus (LSC) or neurodermatitis circumscripta is a highly pruritic, circumscribed plaque that is due to incessant scratching and rubbing. The affected skin becomes pigmented, thickened, and slightly scaly. The commonest sites are those that are conveniently reached: The nape of the neck, the sides of the neck, the lower legs and ankles, the scalp, the upper thighs, the vulva, pubis or scrotum, and the extensor forearms.

Epidemiology

LSC is seen at any age, but is more prevalent between 30 and 50 years of age, and is more common in women.

Associated diseases

LSC patients often have an atopic background. In fact, many consider it to be a localized form of atopic dermatitis.

Clinical characteristics in light skin (Fitzpatrick skin types I–III)

The lesional skin is thickened, lichenified, usually darker pigmented, and often shows areas of skin with scratch defects (Figure 46.1). Particularly on the lower legs, the lesions may take on a verrucous aspect. Secondary infection due to scratching is common.

Clinical characteristics in dark skin (Fitzpatrick skin types IV–V)

The lesion mimics lichenified eczema that is confined to one plaque on an accessible site. It is dark gray or blackish in color (Figures 46.2 and 46.3).

Investigations

This is a clinical diagnosis. However, lichen planus, lichen amyloidosus, and psoriasis need to be excluded clinically.

Histopathology reveals an acanthotic, hyperkeratotic epidermis with foci of parakeratosis, irregular hypergranulosis, mild spongiosis, broad elongated epidermal rete ridges, and pseudoepitheliomatous hyperplasia, giving it a psoriasiform aspect. Papillary fibrosis, as well as interstitial inflammatory infiltrates with histiocytes, lymphocytes, and some eosinophils, are seen in the superficial dermis.

Treatments

- The patient is educated on the nature of lichen simplex and the need to break the scratching habit.
- Treatment is aimed at breaking the itch–scratch cycle and suppression of pruritus, usually by topical or intralesional corticosteroids. The application of an occlusive dressing or an occlusive bandage will intensify the effect of topical steroids.
- Self-adhesive steroid-impregnated tape and some thin modern adhesive dressings are often helpful.
- Tacrolimus and pimecrolimus may be used as steroid-sparing topicals with H1 antihistamines.
- Topical capsaicin, intralesional corticosteroids, or UV phototherapy are second-line therapies.
- Gabapentin, pregabalin, and antidepressants systemically.

Further reading

Aschoff R, Wozel G (2007). Topical Tacrolimus for the Treatment of Lichen Simplex Chronicus. *J Dermatolog Treat*;18(2):115–157.

Boyd K, Shea SM, Patterson JW (2014). The Role of Capsaicin in Dermatology. *Prog Drug Res*;68:293–306.

Liao YH, Lin CC, Tsai PP, et al. (2014). Increased Risk of Lichen Simplex Chronicus in People with Anxiety Disorder: A Nationwide Population-Based Retrospective Cohort Study. *Br J Dermatol*;170(4):890–894.

Ranawaka RR (2021). Psychocutaneous Disorders. In: Ranawaka RR, et al. (eds). *Atlas of Dermatoses in Pigmented Skin*. Springer, Singapore; 629.

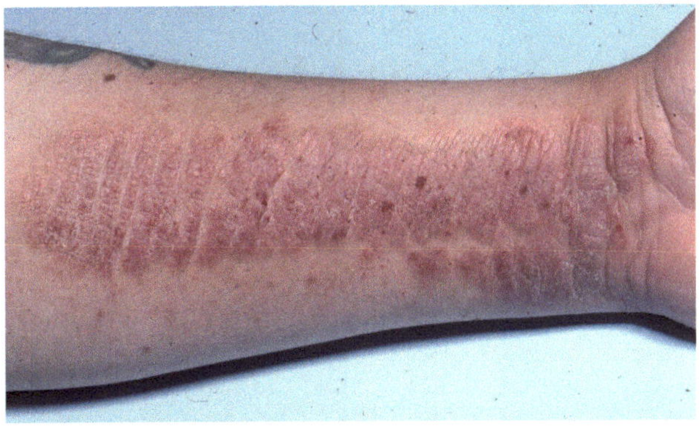

FIGURE 46.1 Lichen simplex chronicus FST1. (Courtesy Dr. Richard Ashton, UK.)

DOI: 10.1201/9781003479512-46

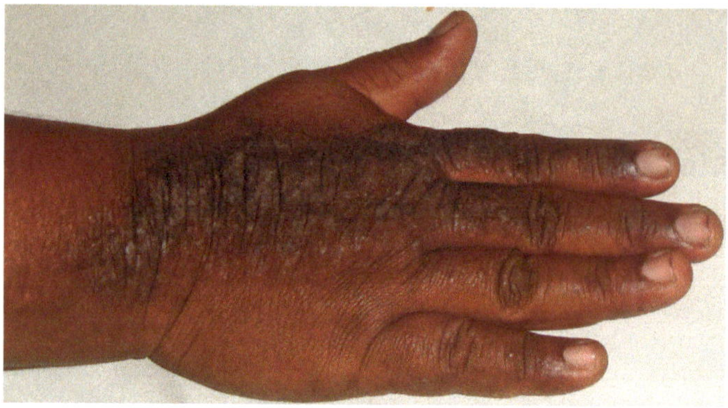

FIGURE 46.2 Lichen simplex chronicus in a 32-year-old woman. In darker skin, LSC appears as a blackish rash on an easily accessible site.

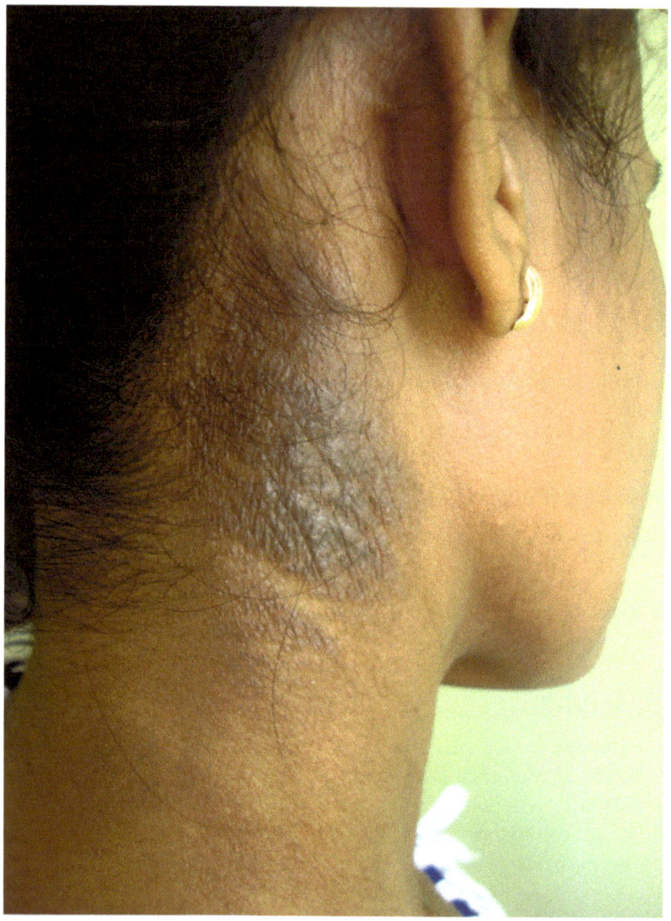

FIGURE 46.3 Lichen simplex chronicus in a 14-year-old girl. In darker skin LSC appears dark gray or blackish rash on accessible site.

47
LICHEN STRIATUS

Introduction

Lichen striatus is a self-limiting, asymptomatic inflammatory dermatosis in a linear distribution that develops along the lines of Blaschko. It has a sudden onset, usually unilateral, and is mostly asymptomatic but mild pruritus may be a feature. Within 2–3 weeks, it typically reaches its maximum extent and then it persists for years. It may extend the entire length of a limb or 'S' shape on the trunk in a Blaschko-linear distribution. Involvement of the nails may result in longitudinal ridging, splitting, onycholysis, or nail loss. Clinical variants have been reported as parallel linear bands, zosteriform patterns, or bilateral involvement. Usually, lichen striatus resolves spontaneously over 6–12 months, sometimes leaving hypo- or hyperpigmentary changes that can last for years. The etiology is not identified.

Epidemiology

Occurs as isolated lesions on the limbs in children aged 5–15 years. More common in females.

Associated diseases

Atopy was reported in approximately 43% of cases.

Clinical characteristics in light skin (Fitzpatrick skin types I–III)

Lichen striatus is an uncommon inflammatory disease characterized by its distribution along the lines of Blaschko. Crops of small lichenoid papules develop mostly on the extremities, rarely on the trunk (Figure 47.1). They eventually extend all along the entire extremity and often involve the nail, usually only one lateral third of it.

As the disease often remains asymptomatic, no treatment is necessary; if requested, topical steroids are the first choice.

The differential diagnosis comprises a number of other dermatoses that can occasionally be linear, such as linear lichen planus, linear psoriasis, linear eczema, etc.

Clinical characteristics in dark skin (Fitzpatrick skin types IV–V)

Sudden onset of skin-colored small, discrete papules in a typical linear distribution (Figure 47.2). Rapid extension over days or weeks and rapid coalescence to form a dull-brown, slightly scaly, irregular linear band, usually 2 mm to 2 cm in width. Erythema is not a feature in dark skin.

Investigations

This is diagnosed clinically.

Histopathology is variable and depends on the stage of the disease. Early lesions may show histopathology of chronic eczema – intercellular edema, spongiosis, acanthosis in variable degrees. Usually, lesions show a band-like infiltrate composed of lymphocytes and histiocytes with associated overlying epidermal changes, including parakeratosis and hyperkeratosis, resembling lichen planus.

Treatments

- No treatments are necessary in children with asymptomatic lesions.
- If troublesome itching occurs (usually adults), topical corticosteroids are the first line of management. Additionally, calcineurin inhibitors (1% tacrolimus or pimecrolimus ointment) are used.
- Nail involvement may respond to potent steroid cream under occlusion.

Further reading

Lauffer F, Eyerich K (2024). Lichen Planus and Lichenoid Disorders. In: Griffiths C, et al. (eds). *Rook's Textbook of Dermatology*, 10th ed. John Wiley & Sons Ltd., UK; 37.17.

Mu EW, Abuav R, Cohen BA (2013). Facial Lichen Striatus in Children: Retracing the Lines of Blaschko. *Pediatr Dermatol*;30(3):364–346.

Payette MJ, Weston G, Humphrey S, et al. (2015). Lichen Planus and Other Lichenoid Dermatoses: Kids Are Not Just Little People. *Clin Dermatol*;33(6):631–643.

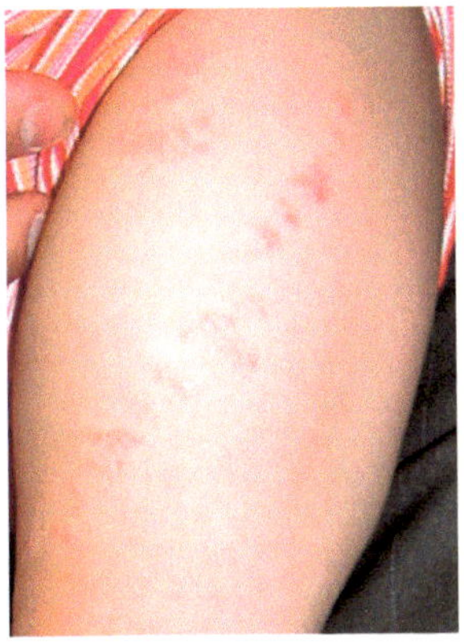

FIGURE 47.1 Lichen striatus along the leg FST1. (Courtesy Prof. Ian Coulson, UK.)

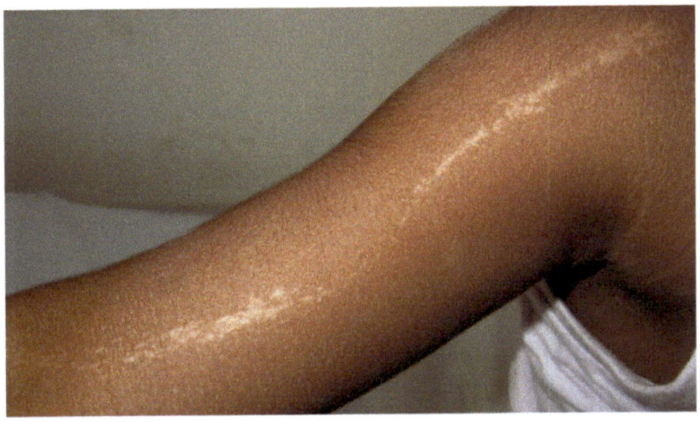

FIGURE 47.2 Lichen striatus along the upper limb in a 3-year-old girl FST5.

DOI: 10.1201/9781003479512-47

48
LICHENOID DRUG RASH

Introduction

Lichen planus (LP)-like drug eruptions are clinically indistinguishable from idiopathic LP although they are frequently more severe. Antimalarials, angiotensin-converting enzyme inhibitors, gold, beta-blockers, mercury, amalgam, lithium, non-steroidal anti-inflammatory drugs, methyldopa, penicillamine, quinidine, thiazide diuretics, and sulfonylureas are drugs implicated. Acute onset, severe, generalized eruption helps to advocate the drug-induced etiology. The onset of LP-like eruptions may appear months (even years) after the first exposure to the medication. Therefore, identifying the offending drug may be impossible in some patients.

Epidemiology

Drug-induced LP reactions represent approximately 10% of all LP cases.

Clinical characteristics in light skin (Fitzpatrick skin types I–III)

Lichenoid drug reactions are not uncommon (Figure 48.1). Clinically, they look like a disseminated LP and cannot be distinguished just by observation. However, a drug-induced lichenoid rash shows eosinophilia in biopsy specimens, which is not seen in classical LP. Furthermore, the trunk is more often involved, and the main localizations, such as the volar wrist, are not predominant. The development of the lesions is usually faster.

Clinical characteristics in dark skin (Fitzpatrick skin types IV–V)

The skin changes of LP-like drug eruptions may be non-specific or may resemble the classical small shiny papules and plaques with Wickham's striae, as in idiopathic LP (Figure 48.2). Rapid onset of severe generalized disease spreading to involve the whole body within days or weeks implies that the skin rash is triggered by drugs.

Investigations

Skin histology is essential for the investigation of lichenoid drug eruptions. Lichenoid drug eruptions show typical histological evidence of lichenoid change, including hyperkeratosis, hypergranulosis, 'sawtooth' acanthosis, and a band-like infiltrate in the superficial dermis. A higher frequency of necrotic keratinocytes and eosinophilia are the only distinguishing histological characteristics of drug-induced LP, as opposed to non-drug LP.

Treatments

- Withdrawal of the offending drug is essential if identified.
- Use of a potent or super-potent topical corticosteroid is usually effective in clearing the eruption.
- In severe cases, a short course of oral glucocorticoids helps to resolve the acute disease.

Further reading

Ardern-Jones MR (2024). Benign Cutaneous Adverse Reactions to Drugs. In: Griffiths C, et al. (eds). *Rook's Textbook of Dermatology*, 10th ed. John Wiley & Sons Ltd., UK; 117.7.

Bhanja DB, Sil A, Maiti A, et al. (2024). Clinical Profile of Patients with Lichenoid Drug Eruption: A Observational Study. *Indian J Dermatol*. 69(2):137–144.

Rijal H, Bouadi N, Molin S (2024). Onset of Pityriasis Lichenoides in Patients Treated with Biologic Therapy: A Systematic Review. *J Cutan Med Surg*;12034754241265714.

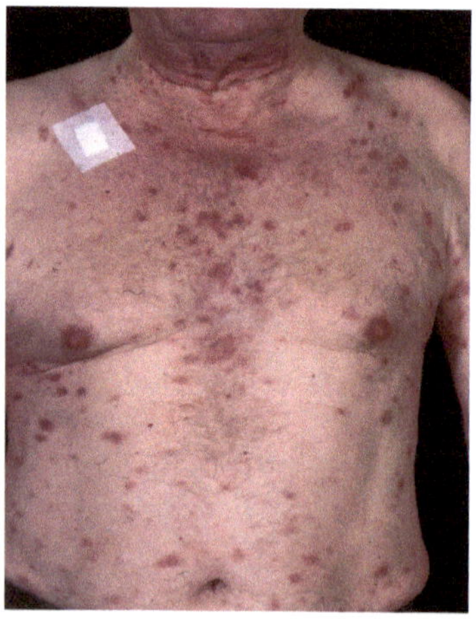

FIGURE 48.1 Lichenoid drug rash following ACE inhibitors FST1. (Courtesy Dr. Richard Ashton, UK.)

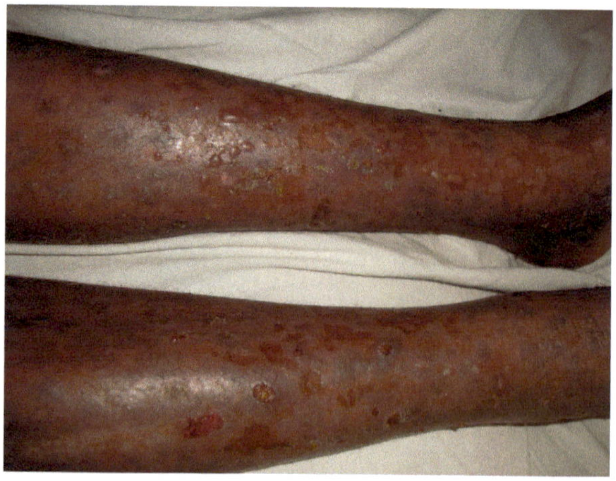

FIGURE 48.2 Severe generalized LP-like reaction in a 57-year-old woman FST5. This had appeared all over the body within a week. She had had antimalarials 3 months earlier and was the only possible causative drug identified.

DOI: 10.1201/9781003479512-48

49
LIVEDO RETICULARIS

Introduction

Livedo reticularis (LR) is a mottled, cyanotic discoloration of the skin, which has a characteristic network pattern and is accentuated by cold; it commonly occurs on the legs, but the arms and trunk may also be affected. Livedo reticularis may be physiological, idiopathic, or secondary to intravascular obstruction or vessel wall disease (then it is livedo racemosa).

Associated diseases

Physiological livedo reticularis (cutis marmorata) is a transient cyanotic mottling of the skin that occurs as a physiological response to cold exposure and disappears with warming. It is usually encountered in healthy infants and resolves during the first year of life.

Congenital livedo reticularis (cutis marmorata telangiectatica congenita) is a rare developmental defect, present at birth. The reticulated area is persistent and enhanced by cold, crying, and exercise. It may be accompanied by skin atrophy. Most improve during the first 2 years of life.

Idiopathic livedo reticularis occurs in young adults and middle-aged women in relation to winter or summer.

Secondary livedo racemosa occurs with vascular diseases, intravascular obstructions, infections, or drugs.

Differential diagnosis

This includes erythema ab igne, capillary nevi, and angioma serpiginosum.

Clinical characteristics in light skin (Fitzpatrick skin types I–III)

There is a transient or persistent pattern of reddish-blue to purple, net-like cyanosis of the skin, mainly on the lower leg, rarely on the thighs and trunk (Figures 49.1 and 49.2). It is far more common in young females, and there may also be Raynaud's disease concomitantly or later in the course of the condition. Typically, gently pressing on the cyanotic area causes blanching and a slow reappearance of the color from the periphery to the center, called the iris phenomenon. The hands and feet are often cold and sweaty, even in summer. This is thought to be the consequence of disruptions in the flow of blood through the skin occurring in various physiologic and pathologic states. It can manifest idiopathically (physiological LR) or from vascular disease (pathologic LR) and tenderness or pain are generally absent. Palpation of the skin does not reveal any resistance, in contrast to livedo racemosa (livedoid vasculopathy), which represents a vascular disease and is palpable.

In fair-skinned individuals, physiologic LR, also called cutis marmorata, typically manifests in response to colder temperatures. It is characteristically seen in preterm infants and neonates.

The skin lesions of primary LR do not correlate with environmental temperatures.

The differential diagnosis comprises secondary LR that may be associated with hematological and autoimmune disorders, infections, neurological conditions, and medications such as amantadine, gemcitabine, and minocycline.

Clinical characteristics in dark skin (Fitzpatrick skin types IV–V)

Bluish or purplish lace-like pattern on the surface of the skin. This is not easily visible in darker skin (Figure 49.3). Ulceration of the dark areas occurs rarely, but if present, suggests significant large-vessel vasculitis or intraluminal thrombosis of livedo racemosa.

Investigations

Laboratory investigations are done to assess underlying medical problems; thrombophilia screen, autoimmune screen, full blood count, metabolic panel, serum protein electrophoresis, ultrasound, and echocardiography may be required to look for sources of emboli.

Histopathology shows normal skin and cutaneous vessels in typical LR, whereas classical vascular changes with fibrin thrombi may be found in the depth of the skin in livedo racemosa, particularly in Sneddon syndrome. They are not always obvious, so serial sections and often several biopsies, both from the pale center as well as the cyanotic periphery, may be necessary to find them.

Treatments

- Treat the underlying condition.
- The appearance of LR is reversible if the underlying cause is treated.

Further reading

Algarin YA, Pariser R (2024). Painful, Tender, Localized, Idiopathic Livedo Reticularis. *Cureus*;16(1):e52311.

Bilgic A, Ozcobanoglu S, Bozca BC, et al. (2021). Livedoid Vasculopathy: A Multidisciplinary Clinical Approach to Diagnosis and Management. *Int J Womens Dermatol*;7:588–599.

DOI: 10.1201/9781003479512-49

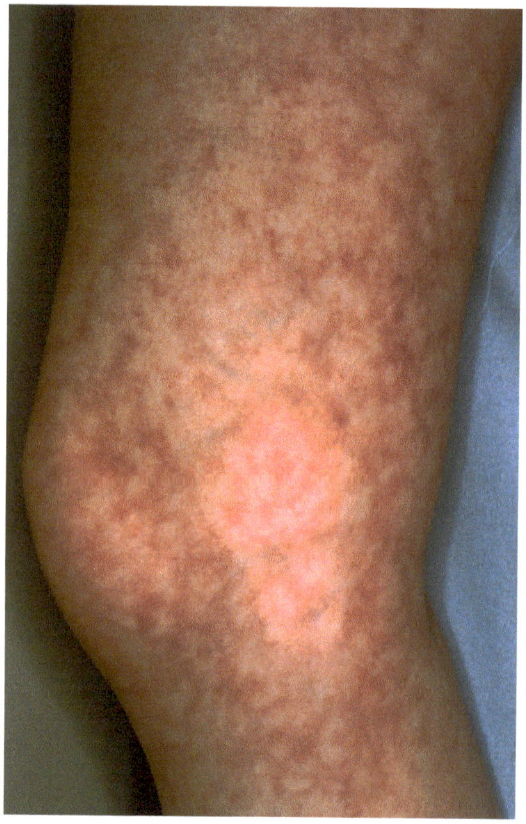

FIGURE 49.1 Livedo reticularis in a hepatitis C positive person FST1. (Courtesy Prof. Ian Coulson, UK.)

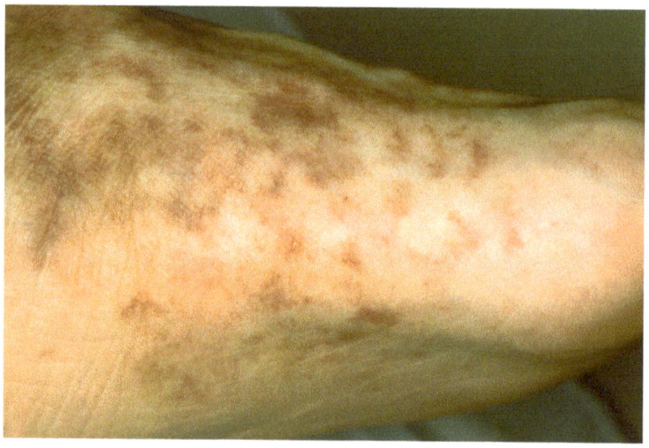

FIGURE 49.2 Livedo reticularis in lupus anticoagulant person FST1. (Courtesy Prof. Ian Coulson, UK.)

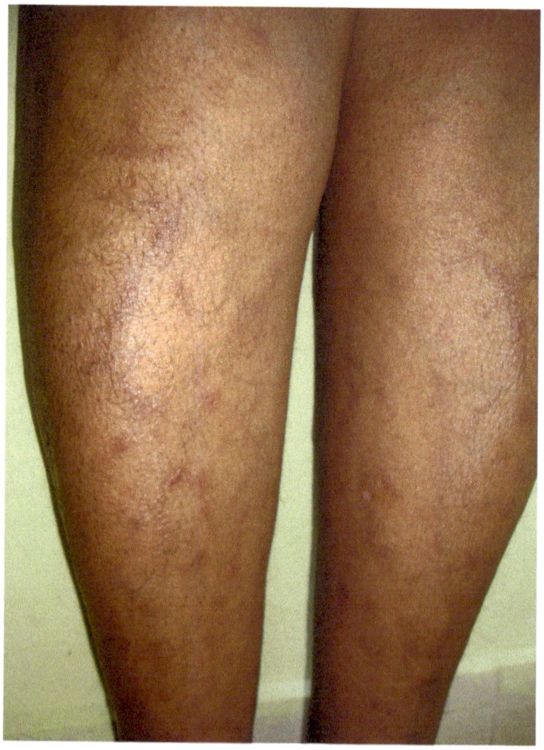

FIGURE 49.3 Livedo reticularis; erythematous, bluish or purplish lace-like pattern on the surface of the skin in a 37-year-old woman FST5.

50
DISCOID LUPUS ERYTHEMATOSUS

Introduction

Lupus erythematosus (LE) is an autoimmune inflammatory disease usually divided into two main types: Discoid LE (DLE) and systemic LE (SLE), with a third group, subacute cutaneous LE (SCLE). DLE most frequently involves the face and scalp, and is characterized by well-defined scaly patches of variable size, which heal with atrophy, scarring, and pigmentary changes. Most patients have localized DLE (disease limited to the head and neck), but a few have disseminated DLE (more extensive disease). DLE lesions heal with scarring.

Epidemiology

DLE can occur at any age, but peak is in the fourth decade in females and slightly later in males. It affects twice as many females as males.

Associated diseases

Porphyria, pemphigus, myasthenia gravis, and thymoma are associated with DLE.

Clinical characteristics in light skin (Fitzpatrick skin types I–III)

Chronic DLE is predominantly localized in the face and can cause severe mutilations if untreated (lupus [Latin] means wolf) (Figures 50.1 and 50.2). It is thought to be an autoimmune disease with a strong influence of sun exposure. Serological tests are negative. Most patients are young adults; however, as the disease persists, one may also see their patients over many years. Women are more often affected, at a ratio of 2–3:1. Delayed provocation by sun exposure is frequent. The most common localization is the face, with a butterfly-type rash on the cheeks, dorsum of the nose, forehead, and temples. The ears and scalp may be involved with marked atrophy and cicatricial alopecia. The upper chest may also show lesions. First, a red plaque develops that slowly extends centrifugally with central scarring and hyperkeratosis. They are firmly attached as they are anchored in the follicle openings. Stroking over a lesion with the free margin of the nail usually elicits pain. In the long run, the lesions become atrophic and scarred, often with irregular depigmentation.

Several variants are known: Disseminated superficial DLE develops many superficial plaques on the body, LE tumidus with a dense and deep inflammatory infiltrate, LE profundus with painful deep lesions reaching into the subcutaneous fat, LE hypertrophicus with almost verrucous hyperkeratosis. Chilblain lupus is a variant with frostbite-like lesions on acral skin, mainly the toes.

Histopathology is characteristic and pathognomonic.

Clinical characteristics in dark skin (Fitzpatrick skin types IV–V)

Well-defined erythematous and hypo- or hyperpigmented patches. It is well demarcated with a hyperpigmented border (Figures 50.3 and 50.4).

Investigations

This is diagnosed clinically.

Skin biopsy in doubtful cases is recommended; the histological hallmark of cutaneous lupus is interface dermatitis, with lymphocytic infiltration and a thickened basal membrane in PAS stain.

Treatments

- Early diagnosis and active treatment are important to avoid irreversible, long-term sequelae such as scarring.
- Topical steroids and long-term synthetic antimalarials are still the mainstay of therapy.
- Sun protection is essential.

Further reading

Dutz J, Khosravi-Hafshejani T (2024). Lupus Erythematosus. In: Griffiths C, et al. (eds). *Rook's Textbook of Dermatology*, 10th ed. John Wiley & Sons Ltd., UK; 51.12.

Liang KR, Lee C, Hilts A, et al. (2024). Resolution of Discoid Lupus Alopecia with Systemic Hydroxychloroquine and Topical Pimecrolimus Combination Therapy. *Cureus*;16(6):e63419.

Mallawaarachchi K (2021). Autoimmune Connective Tissue Disease. In: Ranawaka RR, et al. (eds). *Atlas of Dermatoses in Pigmented Skin*. Springer, Singapore; 563–586.

Ocon A, Avalos Sugastti E, et al. (2024). Impressive Resolution of Refractory Hypertrophic Discoid Lupus Erythematosus with Anifrolumab. *BMJ Case Rep*;17(6):e258487.

DOI: 10.1201/9781003479512-50

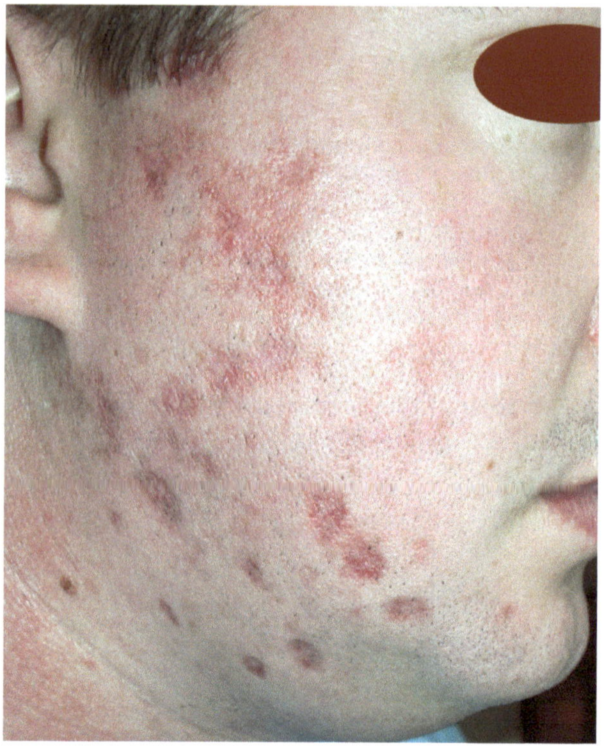

FIGURE 50.1 Discoid lupus erythematosus on the face FST1. (Courtesy Prof. Ian Coulson, UK.)

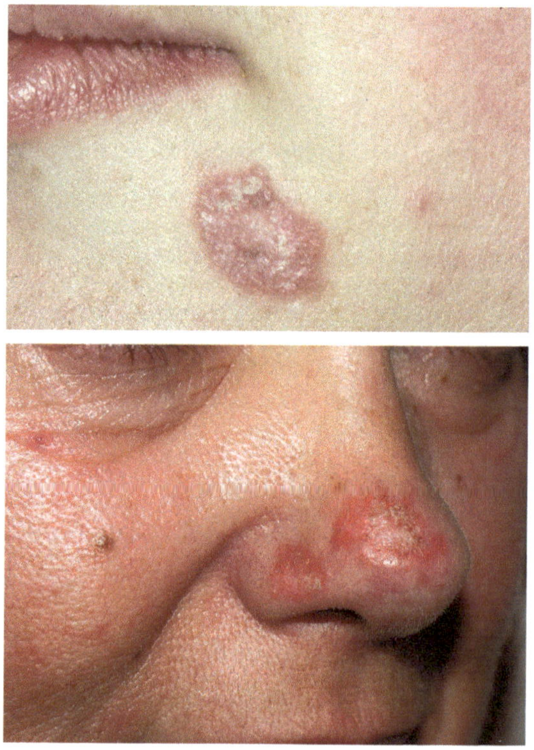

FIGURE 50.2AB Discoid lupus erythematosus on the cheek and on the nose FST1. Close-up view. (Courtesy Prof. Ian Coulson, UK.)

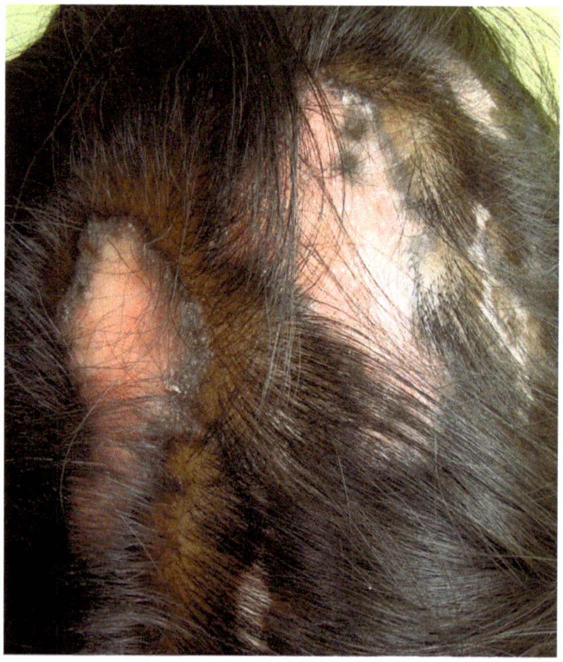

FIGURE 50.3 Discoid lupus erythematosus on the scalp in a 29-year-old woman FST5. Patchy scarring alopecia showing an erythematous plaque surrounded by well-demarcated hyperpigmented border.

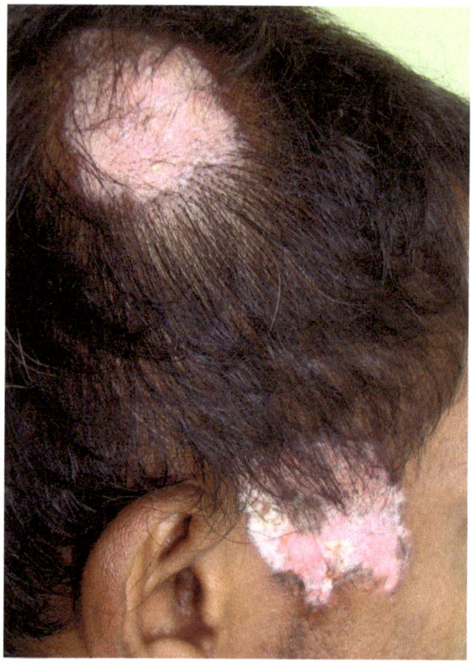

FIGURE 50.4 Discoid lupus erythematosus on the scalp and face in a 42-year-old man FST5. Patchy scarring alopecia showing an erythematous plaque surrounded by well-demarcated hyperpigmented border.

51
SYSTEMIC LUPUS ERYTHEMATOSUS

Introduction

Systemic lupus erythematosus (SLE) is a systemic disease characterized by multisystem organ inflammation, most commonly affecting the skin, joints, and vasculature, and associated with immunological abnormalities. The main clinical features include fever, rashes, and arthritis, but renal, pulmonary, cardiac, and neurological involvement may occur, with increased mortality. SLE most commonly presents with fever (90%), arthritis and arthralgia (90%), skin lesions (87%), renal involvement (67%), and lymphadenopathy (50%).

Epidemiology

Common in women in a 15:1 ratio or more, and onset is in early adult life, 18–35 years of age.

Associated diseases

Kindreds have an increased incidence of other autoimmune diseases, such as thyroid disease and rheumatoid arthritis.

Clinical characteristics in light skin (Fitzpatrick skin types I–III)

SLE is a severe autoimmune disease potentially affecting all organ systems. The skin lesions typically start with a butterfly rash, a symmetrical erythema of the cheeks connected with a reddening over the bridge of the nose but sparing the nasolabial folds (Figures 51.1 and 51.2). It may spread to larger areas of the face, upper trunk, and extremities. These skin lesions are characteristically photosensitive and may thus raise the challenge of distinguishing it from dermatomyositis. The oral mucosa may be erythematous, tends to become erosive, sometimes being similar to acute oral mucosal lichen planus. Diffuse alopecia is often an extreme burden for young women.

The differential diagnoses involve facial erysipelas (cellulitis), a streptococcal infection, rosacea that usually leaves the bridge of the nose uninvolved, pellagra which is characterized by the '4 Ds' dermatitis, diarrhea, dementia, and death, and dermatomyositis that starts with heliotropic edema around the eyes and muscular weakness.

Clinical characteristics in dark skin (Fitzpatrick skin types IV–V)

Erythematous rash on the malar area of the face (butterfly rash) is characteristic but can be very subtle in darker skin. Asymptomatic palatal ulcer is common in SLE and should be looked for (Figures 51.3 and 51.4).

Diffuse, non-scarring alopecia, known as telogen effluvium, in more than 60% of cases. The alopecia can be chronic and associated with disease activity, leading to coarse, dry, and fragile hair along the peripheral hairline during a systemic flare is so-called 'lupus hair.'

Investigations

- This is mainly diagnosed clinically.
- Immunoserology tests are the diagnostic mainstay.
- Skin biopsy is secondary.

Treatment

- Avoid sun exposure.
- Synthetic antimalarials in mild cases.
- Systemic steroids in moderate to severe cases.
- Full immunosuppression for all severe cases: Oral steroids, cytostatics, etc.
- Despite intensive therapy, some cases run a fatal course.

Further reading

Guffroy A, Jacquel L, Guffroy B, et al. (2024). CAR-T Cells for Treating Systemic Lupus Erythematosus: A Promising Emerging Therapy. *Joint Bone Spine*;91(5):105702.

Khorasanchi A, Korman AM, Manne A, et al. (2024). Immune Checkpoint Inhibitor-Induced Subacute Cutaneous Lupus Erythematosus: A Case Report and Review of the Literature. *Front Med*;11:1334718.

Lin L, Ren R, Xiong Q, et al. (2024). Remodeling of T-Cell Mitochondrial Metabolism to Treat Autoimmune Diseases. *Autoimmun Rev*;Jun;23(6):103583.

Pecher AC, Hensen L, Lengerke C, et al. (2024). The Future of CART Therapeutics to Treat Autoimmune Disorders. *Mol Diagn Ther*;Sep;28(5):593–600.

DOI: 10.1201/9781003479512-51

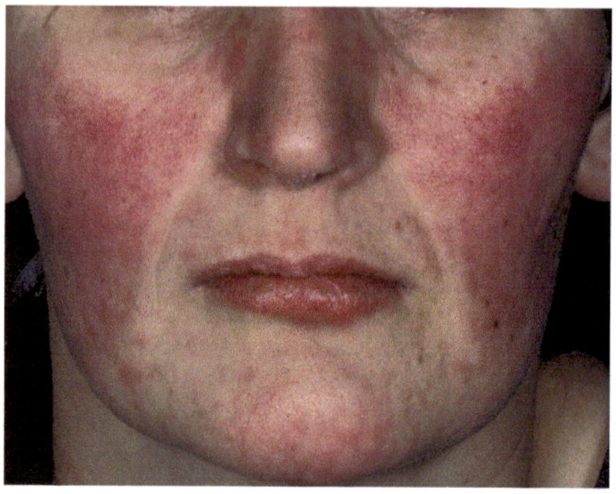

FIGURE 51.1 Malar rash in systemic lupus erythematosus FST1. (Courtesy Dr. Richard Ashton, UK.)

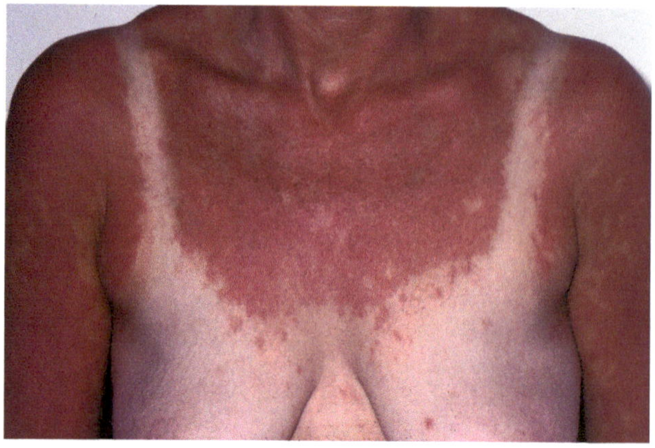

FIGURE 51.2 Photosensitive rash in systemic lupus erythematosus FST1. (Courtesy Dr. Richard Ashton, UK.)

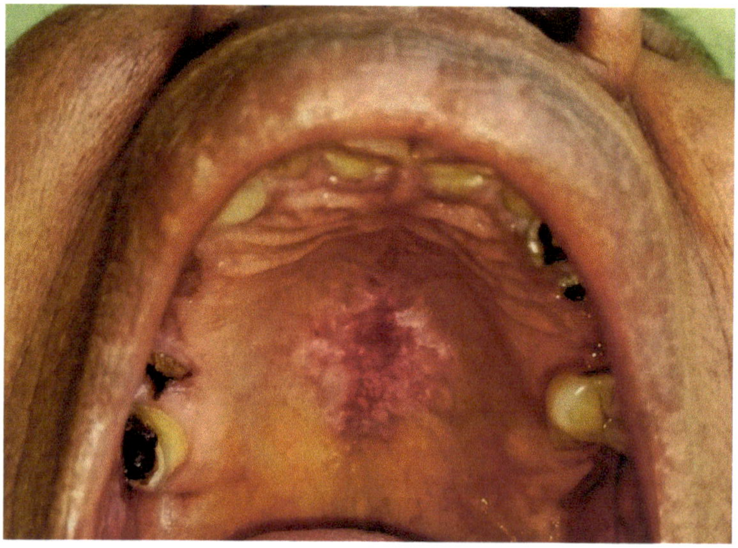

FIGURE 51.3 Asymptomatic palatal ulcer in SLE.

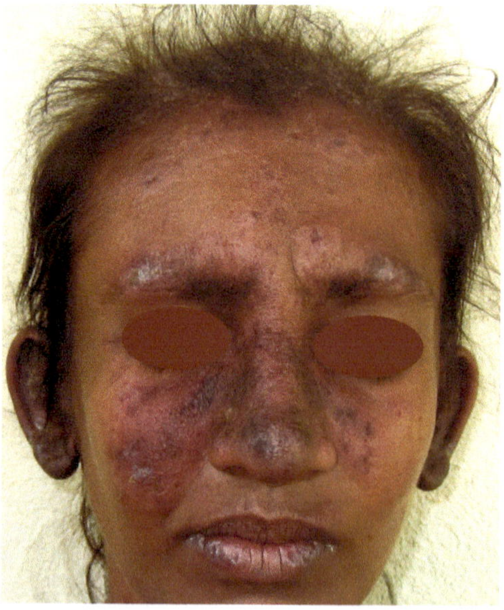

FIGURE 51.4 Butterfly rash (photosensitive rash on malar area of the face), diffuse non-scarring alopecia, and lupus hair (coarse dry and fragile hair) in a 37-year-old woman with SLE (FST5).

52
SUBACUTE CUTANEOUS LUPUS ERYTHEMATOSUS

Introduction

Subacute cutaneous lupus erythematosus (SCLE) is a specific 'subset' of lupus which comprises approximately 10% of patients with LE. Patients have mainly cutaneous disease and usually have a good prognosis with a limited degree of systemic involvement. Arthritis is the most frequent feature, while fever, malaise, and central nervous system involvement occur, but renal disease is mild and infrequent.

Drug-induced SCLE is common (about 65% of SCLE); antihypertensive agents, such as thiazides and calcium channel blockers, and terbinafine are the most common causes. Compared with idiopathic disease, it occurs in older patients (mean age 59 years) and is generally milder, but involves the face and shows bullous and erythema multiforme-like patterns.

Epidemiology

SCLE predominantly affects adults of all ages, but is reported in children too. Female predominance (85%).

Associated diseases

Associated with other autoimmune diseases: Sjögren syndrome, rheumatoid arthritis, Sweet syndrome, Crohn's disease, etc.

Clinical characteristics in light skin (Fitzpatrick skin types I–III)

SCLE is a rare form of lupus erythematosus (LE) that is somehow grouped in between chronic discoid LE and systemic LE. Serological immune phenomena are positive but not to the extent of systemic LE.

There is a butterfly rash on the face and often large circinate or gyrate lesions on the trunk (Figures 52.1 and 52.2). They do not usually heal with scarring, in contrast to discoid lupus erythematosus (DLE).

Clinical characteristics in dark skin (Fitzpatrick skin types IV–V)

Non-scarring papulosquamous eruption (two-thirds of patients) or annular polycyclic lesions (one-third of patients) (Figure 52.3). The lesions usually occur above the waist and particularly around the neck, on the trunk, and on the outer aspects of the arms. Patients may have a history of previous sun-induced skin problems, and often classical polymorphic light eruption.

Investigations

This is diagnosed clinically.

1. Antibodies to the Ro/SS-A antigen are an almost universal finding in this subset of lupus (in approximately 80%).
2. Homogeneous ANAs are found in approximately 60%.
3. Skin biopsy to differentiate from photosensitive rash or DLE.
4. Investigate fully to exclude evidence of internal organ disease in systemic lupus erythematosus (SLE).

Treatments

- Must avoid ultraviolet (UV) light exposure; use sunscreens.
- Topical or intralesional corticosteroids, or topical pimecrolimus and tacrolimus, are first line of therapy.
- Antimalarial drugs are often helpful; either hydroxychloroquine (HCQ) or chloroquine. HCQ is safer from an ophthalmological point of view and requires less monitoring. Mepacrine (quinacrine) does not have ocular side effects but does induce a yellow discoloration of the skin.
- Patients that don't respond to antimalarials may respond to oral corticosteroids or methylprednisolone, acitretin, isotretinoin, dapsone, methotrexate (oral, intravenous, and subcutaneous), thalidomide, mycophenolate mofetil, intravenous immunoglobulin, or etanercept.

Further reading

Dutz J, Khosravi-Hafshejani T (2024). Lupus Erythematosus. In: Griffiths C, et al. (eds). *Rook's Textbook of Dermatology*, 10th ed. John Wiley & Sons Ltd., UK; 51.12.

Fijałkowska A, Kądziela M, Żebrowska A (2024). The Spectrum of Cutaneous Manifestations in Lupus Erythematosus: A Comprehensive Review. *J Clin Med*;13(8):2419.

Kurz B, Ivanova I, Drexler K, et al. (2024). Rapid Clinical Improvement of Refractory Subacute Cutaneous Lupus Erythematosus with Oral Tyrosine Kinase 2 Inhibitor Deucravacitinib: A Case Report. *J Eur Acad Dermatol Venereol*;38(5):e434–e436.

Mallawaarachchi K (2021). Autoimmune Connective Tissue Diseases. In: Ranawaka RR, et al. (eds). *Atlas of Dermatoses in Pigmented Skin*. Springer, Singapore; 563–586.

DOI: 10.1201/9781003479512-52

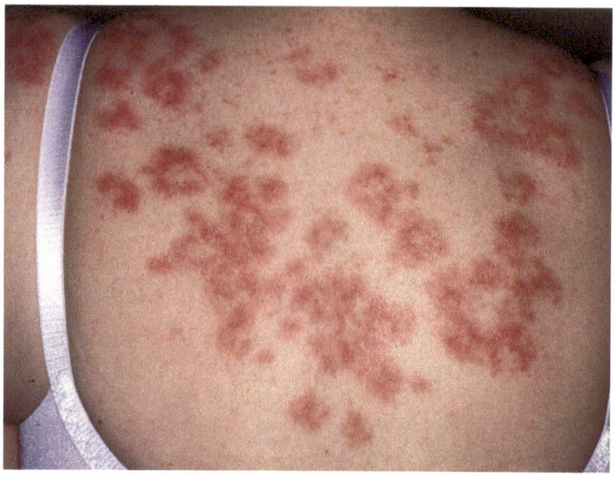

FIGURE 52.1 Subacute cutaneous lupus erythematosus in FST1. (Courtesy Prof. Ian Coulson, UK.)

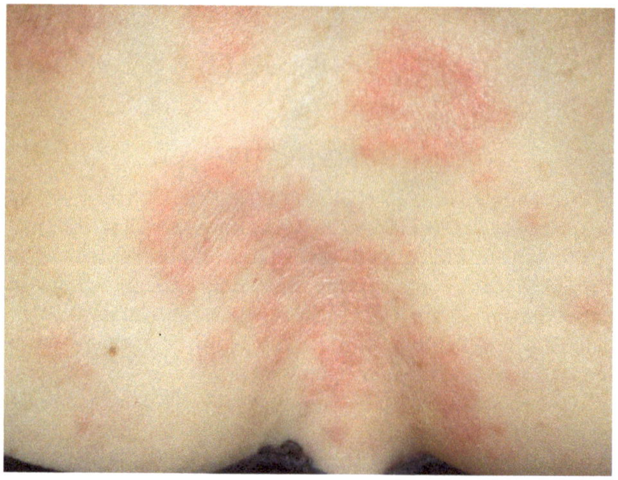

FIGURE 52.2 Subacute cutaneous lupus erythematosus in FST1 closer view. (Courtesy Prof. Eckart Haneke, Germany.)

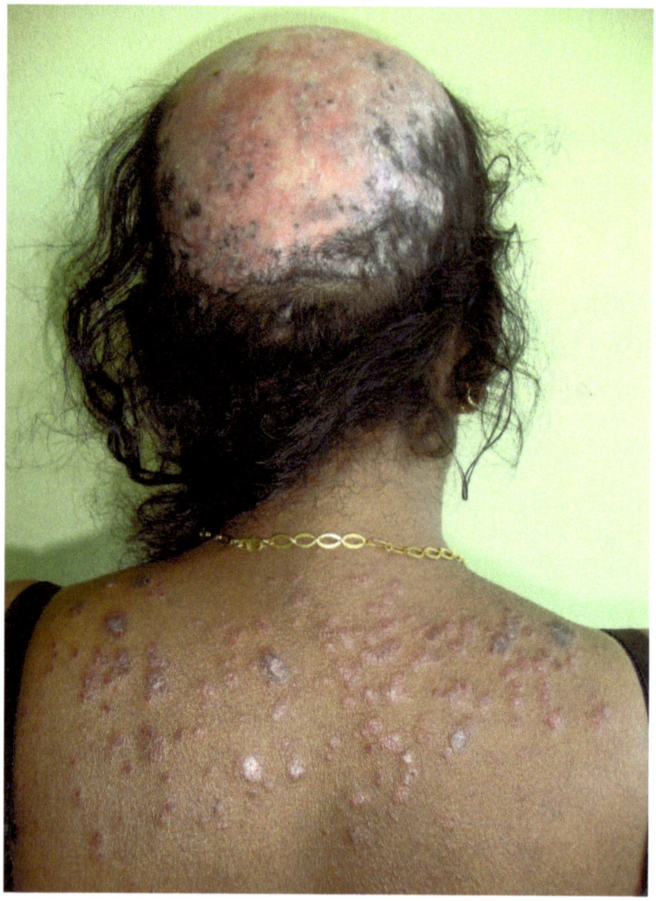

FIGURE 52.3 DLE on the scalp and subacute cutaneous lupus erythematosus on the trunk in a 47-year-old woman FST5.

53
MELANOMA

Introduction

Melanoma is a malignant tumor arising from melanocytes. About 75–80% of cutaneous melanomas originate from normal skin. Only 20–25% of melanomas are thought to develop in association with a cutaneous melanocytic nevus. Melanoma represents 4% of skin cancers but accounts for 80% of skin cancer deaths. White, fair-skinned (Fitzpatrick I–III) populations are mainly affected, whereas incidence rates are low in dark-skinned populations.

Epidemiology

The highest incidence rates are recorded in Australia and New Zealand, whereas the lowest rates are found in Asia and Africa. Diagnosis is done at any age except very early in life (0.6% of melanoma is diagnosed under the age of 20) with a median age at diagnosis of around 60.

Associated diseases

For large congenital melanocytic nevi (largest diameter >20 cm), the lifetime risk of melanoma transformation has been estimated to be between 5 and 15%.

Clinical characteristics in light skin (Fitzpatrick skin types I–III)

Four different types of melanoma are distinguished (Figures 53.1 to 53.4): *Superficial spreading melanoma* (SSM) usually but not exclusively occurring in skin that is occasionally sun-exposed and prone to sunburns, *lentigo maligna melanoma* (LMM) occurring in chronically sun-exposed skin of the head and neck and rarely other body regions, *nodular melanoma* (NM) developing in all body regions, and *acral lentiginous melanoma* (ALM) involving the palms, soles, and nails; however, the latter is now recognized to be two different types based on epidemiological, prognostic, and genetic features.

SSM develops from a tiny brown spot or papule to a plaque-like lesion often characterized by a multicolored aspect of a light brown, brown, black, bluish, purple plaque sometimes with obvious areas of spontaneous involution that may appear white, gray, or bluish. After months to years of this horizontal growth, a nodule may arise that soon tends to become eroded and ulcerated, indicating the vertical growth phase. The SSM is often found on the nape of the neck, back, upper extremities, and thighs.

Lentigo maligna is the forerunner of LMM. It is a brown spot with an irregular outline in skin that is chronically exposed to sunlight. With time, often years or decades, a slightly infiltrated nodular or plaque-like area develops that still may take years to enter a vertical growth phase and start troubling the patient. This melanoma type may involve large areas of the face, dorsa of the hands, forearms, and neck.

NM is the form with the worst prognosis. It is often located on the face but may occur anywhere. At diagnosis, it usually already shows a high Breslow index, indicating a poor prognosis. It may present as a bleeding nodule with a black or brown color, but may also be completely amelanotic. Often, patients present with existing metastatic disease.

ALM is a rare form of melanoma in light-skinned individuals, accounting for approximately 7–8% of all cutaneous melanomas. It usually starts as a grayish-brownish spot on the palm or sole that is overlooked for years. When noticed by the patient it is not taken seriously, either by the patient or the consulted physician. Melanomas of decade-long growth may cover almost an entire sole of the foot. Finally, a shallow ulceration develops, indicating vertical growth.

Melanoma of the nail unit makes up almost 2% of cutaneous melanomas in fair-skinned people; however, they are as frequent in absolute numbers in light and dark skin. Roughly three-quarters of nail melanomas start with a brown streak in the nail extending from the cuticle into the free margin of the nail plate. Periungual pigmentation in association with a melanonychia is called Hutchinson's sign. As with common ALM, the diagnosis is often made very late and therefore the prognosis is generally worse than in all other melanoma types.

There are more rare types of skin melanoma: Animal-type melanoma (pigmented epithelioid melanocytoma) with deep pigmentation often seen on the scalp and trunk, melanoma developing in a congenital nevus, mucosal melanoma, etc.

Clinical characteristics in dark skin (Fitzpatrick skin types IV–V)

All types of melanomas are rare in dark skin (Figures 53.5 to 53.7). Out of the varied types, acral lentiginous melanoma and subungual melanomas are the common presentations in dark skin.

An acral lentiginous melanoma (a pigmented stain on the soles and palms) is the most common presentation in dark skin. Its initial presentation is a discrete dark brown or black macule, often described as a 'dirty-like stain,' with indistinct borders on the soles of patients usually aged over 60 years. This type represents 2–10% of melanomas in white populations and 60–72% in black populations. Because of the discrete localization and as a benign pigmentation on the soles is frequent, the diagnosis is often delayed by years. At later stages, a nodule or ulceration can develop and would be confused with warts or trophic ulceration.

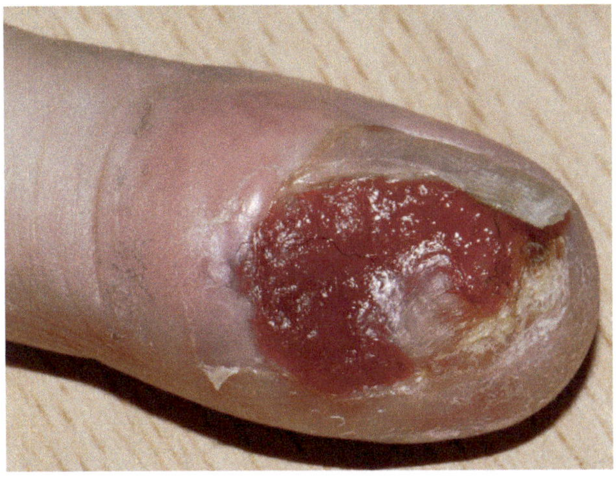

FIGURE 53.1 Malignant melanoma in nail fold FST1. (Courtesy Prof. Ian Coulson, UK.)

DOI: 10.1201/9781003479512-53

Subungual melanomas (melanoma in the nail area) represent approximately 2–3% of the melanomas in white-skinned but a higher proportion in dark-skinned populations. The first sign is a brown to black linear discoloration in the nail, hard to differentiate from benign melanonychia, which is quite common in dark skin. Later, Hutchinson's sign (pigmentation in the adjacent skin) and inflammatory or pigmented paronychia appear; however, it can be difficult to distinguish from onychomycosis, paronychia, nevus, and pyogenic granuloma.

Mucosal, ocular, and amelanotic melanoma have also have been reported in darker-skinned individuals, but are rare.

Investigations

Analytical examination and algorithms: This is the most commonly described diagnostic clue, known as the ABCDEF algorithm, which assumes that if a 'nevus' is *A*symmetrical, with irregular *B*orders, and inhomogeneous *C*olor, with a *D*iameter over 6 mm; recent *E*volution, and a positive melanoma *F*amily history, it may be considered as a potential melanoma.

Dermatological periodic monitoring of high-risk population: This can be performed either by full body clinical examination, by comparison with reference total body photographs or by computerized dermoscopy which permits an individual nevus follow-up. Such monitoring is highly efficacious, but quite time-consuming.

Education on self-detection and skin self-examination.

Histopathological diagnosis is still the gold standard for melanoma diagnosis.

Treatments

- Wide local excision.
- Sentinel lymph node biopsy in patients with Breslow index over 0.75 (1) mm.
- Therapeutic total lymph node dissection (TLND) of metastases to regional lymph nodes.
- Adjuvant systemic therapy – immunotherapy, targeted therapy, neo-adjuvant therapy, and chemotherapy.

Further reading

Duarte AF, Sousa-Pinto B, Azevedo LF, et al. (2021). Clinical ABCDE Rule for Early Melanoma Detection. *Eur J Dermatol*;31(6):771–778.

Duarte AF, Sousa-Pinto B, Barros A, et al. (2018). Lentigo Maligna – Not Always a Face and Neck Disease of the Elderly. *Dermatology*;234(1–2):37–42.

Ferrara G, Gianotti R, Cavicchini S, et al. (2013). Spitz Nevus, Spitz Tumor, and Spitzoid Melanoma: A Comprehensive Clinicopathologic Overview. *Dermatol Clin*;31(4):589–98, viii.

Sondak VK, Messina JL (2024). Melanoma in Pediatric and Young Adult Patients. *Curr Oncol Rep*;26(7):818–825.

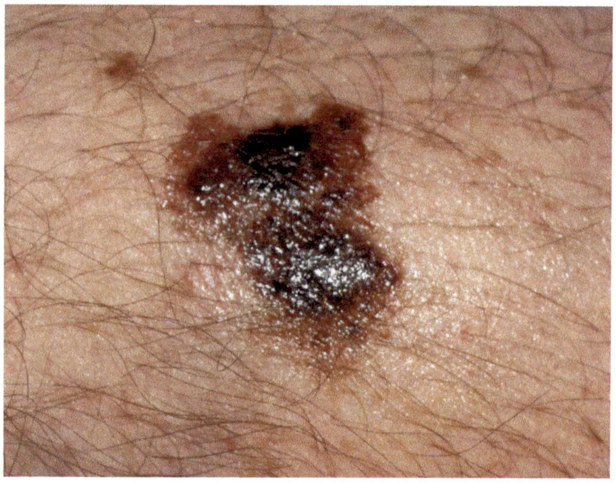

FIGURE 53.2 Superficial spreading malignant melanoma FST1. (Courtesy Prof. Ian Coulson, UK.)

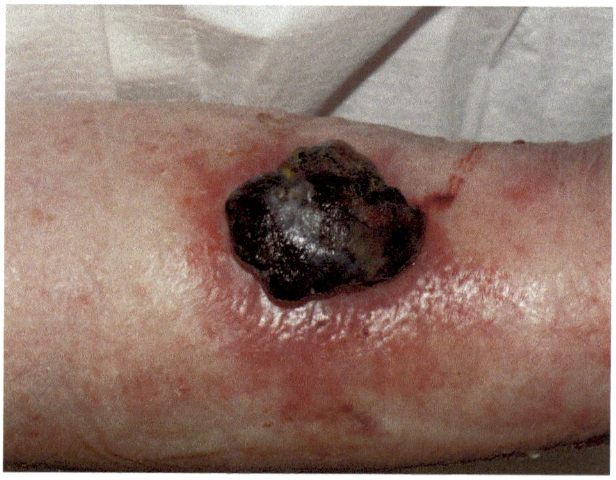

FIGURE 53.3 Nodular melanoma FST1. (Courtesy Prof. Ian Coulson, UK.)

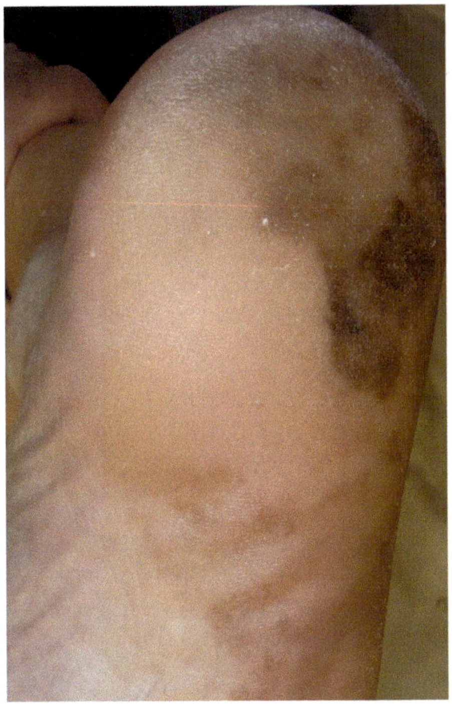

FIGURE 53.4 Acrolentiginosis melanoma in FST1. (Courtesy Prof. Eckart Haneke, Germany.)

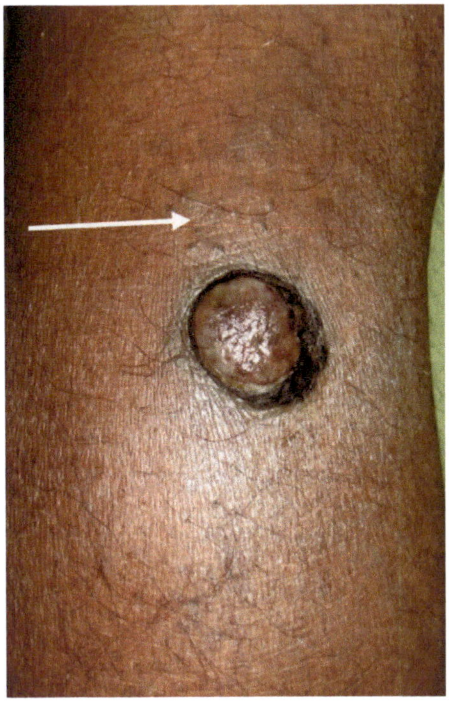

FIGURE 53.5 A 65-year-old man presented with this nodule at the left popliteal fossa. Note the satellite lesions, which we did not notice at the time of excision of the lump. This was melanoma spread to a distant site.

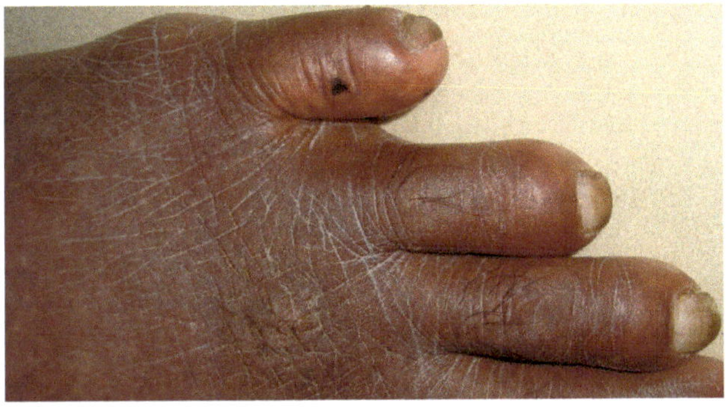

FIGURE 53.6 After extensive search, the primary site of the melanoma was found at the fifth toe.

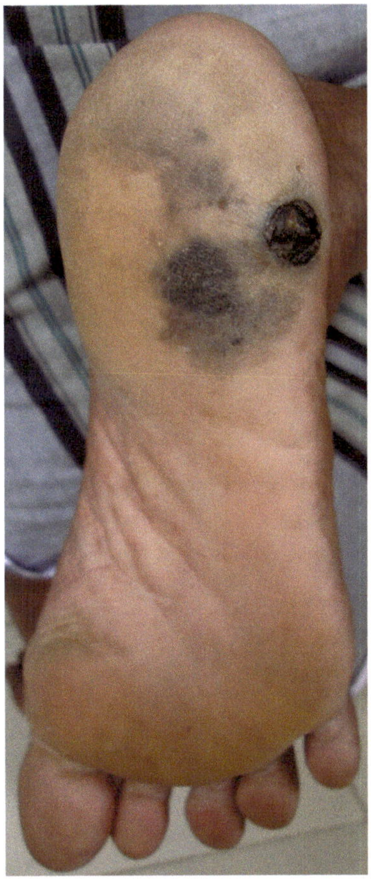

FIGURE 53.7 An acral lentiginous melanoma (a pigmented stain on the soles) is the commonest presentation in dark skin FST5.

54
MELANONYCHIA

Introduction

Melanonychia is a brown to black discoloration of the nail plate and is a common cause of nail plate pigmentation. Melanonychia refers to the Greek word *melas*, meaning black (or brown) color, and *onyx* meaning nail. The pigment referred to is conventionally melanin. It may involve single or multiple nails, both in finger and toenails. Drug exposure, skin diseases, onychomycosis, and racial pigmentation typically involve multiple nails, while lentigines, nail matrix nevus, and melanoma involve single nails.

In three-quarters of the cases, melanoma of the nail apparatus starts in the matrix and presents as longitudinal melanonychia. Hutchinson's sign describes the presence of pigment on the proximal, lateral, or distal nail fold. It represents the radial in-situ growth of melanoma. Although this sign is highly suggestive of melanoma, it is not pathognomonic. Melanoma of the nail apparatus is rare but associated with a poor prognosis.

Longitudinal melanonychia is a rare presentation in onychopapilloma, onychomatricoma, squamous cell carcinoma, basal cell carcinoma, and lichen planus (transient or permanent longitudinal melanonychia). In AIDS, longitudinal melanonychia may be seen in untreated cases as well as in those receiving zidovudine.

Epidemiology

Melanonychia is a common cause of nail discoloration, accounting for nearly half of the cases of chromonychia. Longitudinal melanonychia is the most common morphological pattern. Only one-third of patients with longitudinal melanonychia seek medical advice.

Associated diseases

Melanoma of the nail apparatus may present as longitudinal melanonychia. Approximately half of patients with Laugier–Hunziker–Baran syndrome also develop multiple longitudinal melanonychia.

Chemotherapy-induced melanonychia is very common.

Clinical characteristics in light skin (Fitzpatrick skin types I–III)

In light-skinned Caucasians, melanonychia is much less frequent than in people of color. It may be present at birth, develop during childhood, adolescence, or in adult life. Whereas melanonychia in children remains benign despite an often worrisome clinical appearance, a recently acquired longitudinal brown band in the nail of a person over 25–30 years is suspicious and requires an accurate diagnostic procedure. The thumb, big toe, index, and middle fingernails are particularly at risk, although melanomas may occur on any digit. The intensity of the color is not a marker of malignancy. A suspicious streak is usually asymmetrical with various color shades and irregular lines that make up the band. Race is **not** a risk factor. Any streak wider than one-third of the nail is highly suspicious. A triangular melanonychia with a proximal base being wider than the distal end is a sign of horizontal growth of the melanocytic focus in the matrix. The nature of the pigment is easy to determine: A nail clipping can be sent for histopathology, and a Fontana stain shows intracellular granular pigment if it is melanin. The Hutchinson sign, periungual pigmentation, is easier to see in light-skinned people. Even the slightest nail dystrophy in association with melanonychia is an indicator of malignancy.

Dermatoscopy is not necessary to make the diagnosis of longitudinal melanonychia but can help to identify micro-Hutchinson and pseudo-Hutchinson signs.

Clinical characteristics in dark skin (Fitzpatrick skin types IV–V)

Racial pigmentation is very common in our settings where multiple nails are involved. Chemotherapy-induced melanonychia is common with cyclophosphamide, hydroxyurea, docetaxel, and doxorubicin (Ranawaka 2009). Furthermore, longitudinal melanonychia in children and young adults is also not uncommon and is frequently due to a nail matrix nevus. In the middle-aged and elderly this should arouse the suspicion of acral lentiginous melanoma, which is the most common melanoma in dark skin (the author has not come across this in over 18 years of experience).

Investigations

Nail matrix biopsy in suspected malignancy. Nail matrix biopsies are most useful for longitudinal melanonychia as it originates in the distal matrix. Since examination of the entire pigmented lesion is required, only excisional biopsies should be performed.

The dermoscopic pattern of melanoma in the nail apparatus is well established; a brown background with brown to black lines that are unevenly pigmented, irregularly spaced, of variable thickness, and with or without interruption of parallelism.

Intraoperative dermoscopy and reflectance confocal microscopy (RCM) have recently been advocated for better

DOI: 10.1201/9781003479512-54

visualization of nail matrix pigmentation during exploratory nail surgery for melanonychia.

Treatments

Management decides on the eitiology of melanonychia.

Further reading

Ani O, Xu W, Chang B, et al. (2024). Clinical and Histopathological Investigation of Pediatric Melanonychia: A Single-Center Retrospective Case Series. *Ann Plast Surg*;92(4S Suppl 2):S87–S90.

Gradinaru TC, Mihai M, Beiu C, et al. (2020). Melanonychia – Clues for a Correct Diagnosis. *Cureus*;12(1):e6621.

Haneke E (2021). Eleven Myths on Nail Melanoma. *EMJ Dermatology*;9(1):83–86.

Haneke E, Ranawaka RR (2021). Disorders of Nails. In: Ranawaka RR, et al. (eds). *Atlas of Dermatoses in Pigmented Skin.* Springer, Singapore; 723–764.

Ranawaka RR (2009). Patterns of Chromonychia During Chemotherapy in Patients with Skin Type V and Outcome after 1 Year of Follow-up. *Clin Exp Dermatol*;34(8):e920–e926.

Singal A, Bisherwal K (2020). Melanonychia: Etiology, Diagnosis, and Treatment. *Indian Dermatol Online J*;11(1):1–11.

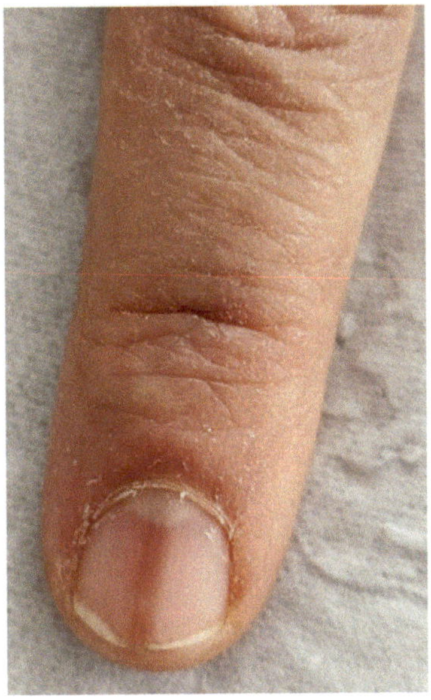

FIGURE 54.1 Melanonychia FST1. (Courtesy Prof. Nooshin Bagherani, Iran.)

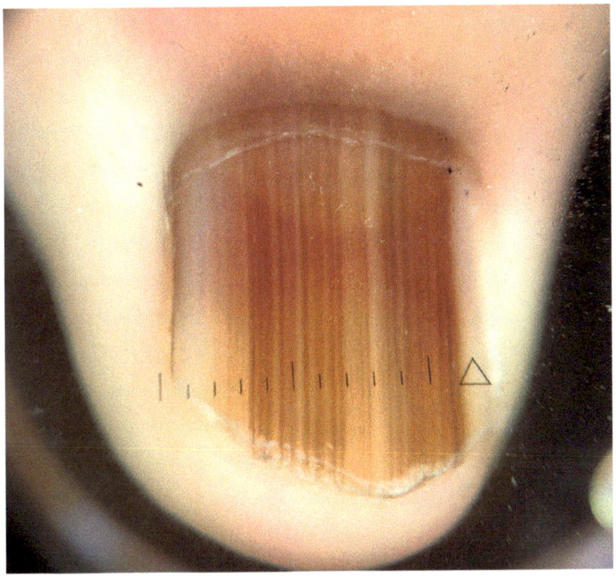

FIGURE 54.2 Melanonychia FST1 dermoscopy showing regular longitunal streaks. (Courtesy Prof. Ian Coulson, UK.)

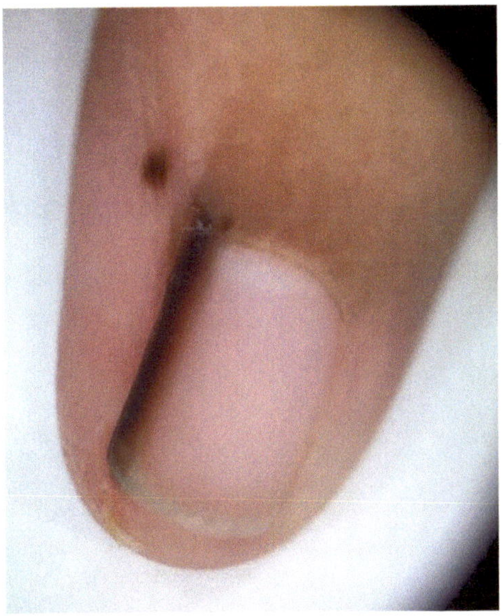

FIGURE 54.3 Recurrent longitudinal melanonychia due to a melanocytic nevus of the matrix FST2. (Courtesy Prof. Eckart Haneke, Germany.)

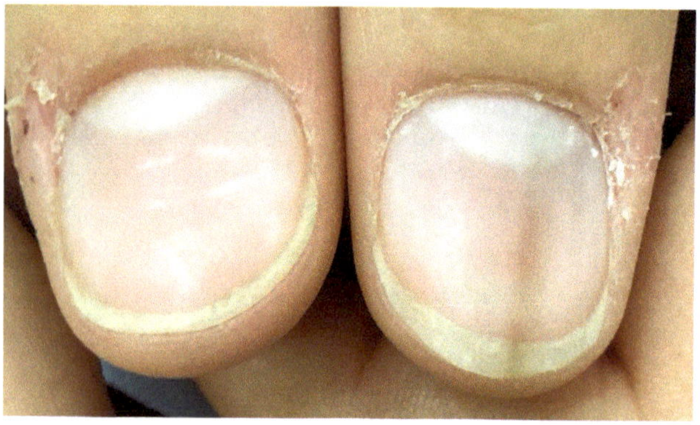

FIGURE 54.4 Thumb nail of a 15-year-old girl with a functional melanonychia due to picking of the nail region (perionychotillomania). (Courtesy Prof. Eckart Haneke, Germany.)

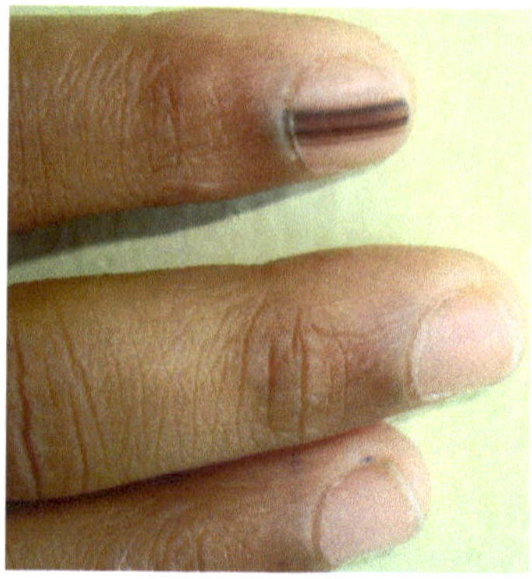

FIGURE 54.5 Longitudinal melanonychia in a 17-year-old girl due to a nail matrix nevus FST5.

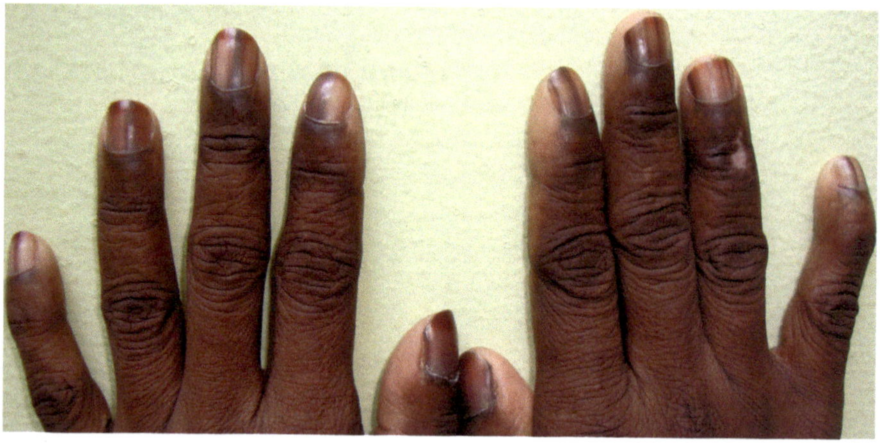

FIGURE 54.6 Racial pigmentation typically involves multiple nails, and is common in dark skin FST5.

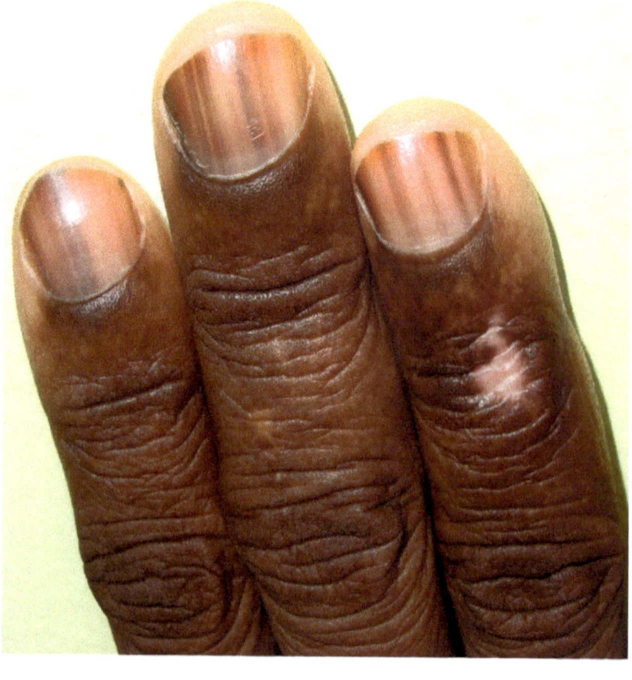

FIGURE 54.7 Racial pigmentation closer view FST5.

55
FRICTIONAL MELANOSIS

Introduction

Friction melanosis (FM) is an acquired pigmentary disorder reported in adults, clinically characterized by diffuse hyperpigmentation on bony prominences. Venkataram et al. in 2018 in India showed that the arm was the most common site of involvement, followed by the forearm, upper back, legs, chest, neck, and shoulder. Al-Aboosi et al. in 2004 reported a similar problem in Jordanian young adults, primarily affecting the skin regions over the osseous prominences, especially the clavicular zone and upper back. All the participants in his study had a history of rubbing their skin repeatedly with scrub pads (loofah) or bathroom towels. Even though the role of friction has been proposed to be the causative factor in the etiology, friction is not noted in all cases.

Epidemiology

Both adult men and women are equally affected. It is uncommon in children.

Associated diseases

Common in overweight or obese middle-aged adults. Observed in both men and women.

Clinical characteristics in light skin (Fitzpatrick skin types I–III)

Friction melanosis is rare but does exist in light-skinned persons. It is not only classical friction through rubbing but may also be chronic or chronic-repeated pressure. In obese women, the bra may cause brown stripes over the shoulders. Devout Muslims may show a pigmented spot on their mid-forehead, often with skin induration.

Rubbing from shoes may cause frictional melanonychia of the big toe and particularly the little toe.

Reassurance is usually sufficient.

Clinical characteristics in dark skin (Fitzpatrick skin types IV–V)

This is a very common asymptomatic cosmetic issue in our settings (Figure 55.1). Even though adult women seek treatments, this is equally prevalent in adult men. It is mostly noted in overweight or obese individuals. Well-demarcated darkly pigmented diffuse macular areas are observed over bony prominences, most commonly over the ulnar bone on the forearms. Other bony prominences, such as elbows, knees, lateral malleolus, and lateral border of the foot, are frequently involved. It is mostly bilateral but may not be symmetrical.

Investigations

This is diagnosed clinically.

Histopathology shows basal layer pigmentation, acanthotic epidermis, condensation of collagen, and pigmentary incontinence in the dermis. Absence of amyloid is important to exclude macular amyloidosis.

Treatments

Depigmenting agents, with or without keratolytics such as diluted topical steroids, 1% topical tacrolimus ointment, or topical steroids with 3–4% salicylic acid, and glycolic acid preparations, give good results after 2–3 months of application.

Further reading

Al-Aboosi M, Abalkhail A, Kasim O, et al (2004). Friction Melanosis: A Clinical, Histologic, and Ultrastructural Study in Jordanian Patients. *Int J Dermatol*;43(4):261–264.

Venkataram M, Shashikant M, B A. (2018). Frictional Melanosis and Its Clinical and Histopathological Features. *Iranian J Dermatol*;21(4):124–127.

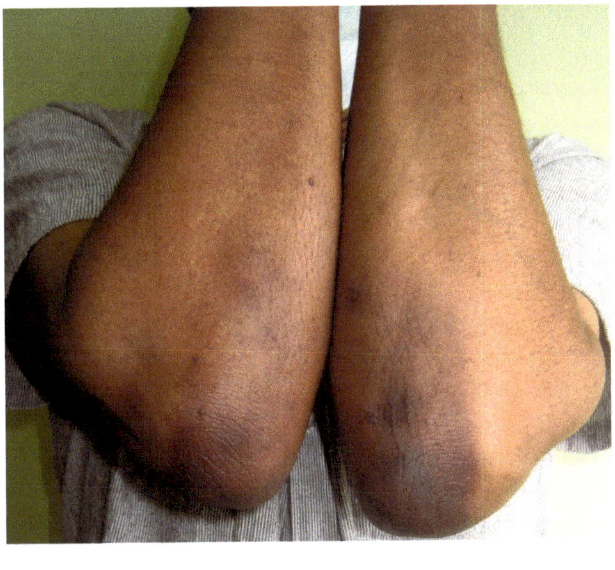

FIGURE 55.1 Frictional melanosis in a 45-year-old man FST5. Hyperpigmentation is bilateral but not symmetrical, appears on elbows and border along the ulnar bone.

DOI: 10.1201/9781003479512-55

56
HAIR DYE MELANOSIS

Introduction

Hair dye-induced hyperpigmentation is common in Sri Lanka. Dark-skinned individuals use either black or dark brown color to conceal their gray hair. Prolonged use of these causes gray-black pigmentation on the anterior margin of the scalp, forehead, helix of the ear, and zygomatic area. This hyperpigmentation is uniformly spread over the affected area.

Epidemiology

Only seen among middle-aged men and women of 55–65 years of age. In their mid-70s, people accept gray hair and usually give up hair coloring, therefore this condition is not seen among the elderly.

Associated diseases

Contact dermatitis to hair dye should be considered to exclude post-inflammatory hyperpigmentation.

Clinical characteristics in light skin (Fitzpatrick skin types I–III)

The author has not seen this in over 50 years of practice in light-skinned persons.

Clinical characteristics in dark skin (Fitzpatrick skin types IV–V)

Gray-black pigmentation on the anterior scalp, forehead, helix of the ear, and zygomatic area (Figure 56.1). This is asymptomatic. Hyperpigmentation is uniformly spread over the affected area and blends with the adjacent normal skin.

Investigations

This is diagnosed clinically.

Treatments

- Topical retinoic acids or triple therapy (a combination of three medicines: hydroquinone, mometasone, and tretinoin, which treats melasma).
- Laser therapy.

Further reading

Meghana V, Gopinath H, Karthikeyan K, et al. (2020). Face and Neck Pigmentary Alterations in Hair Dye Users: A Cross-Sectional Study from South India. *Indian Dermatol Online J*;11(5):760–765.

Woo YR, Kim JS, Lim JH, et al. (2018). Acquired Diffuse Slate-Grey Facial Dyspigmentation Due to Henna: An Unrecognized Cause of Pigment Contact Dermatitis in Korean Patients. *Eur J Dermatol*;28(5):644–648.

Palaniappan V, Karthikeyan K, Anusuya S (2023). Dermatological Adverse Effects of Hair Dye Use: A Narrative Review. *Indian J Dermatol Venereol Leprol*;Jul 27:1–17.

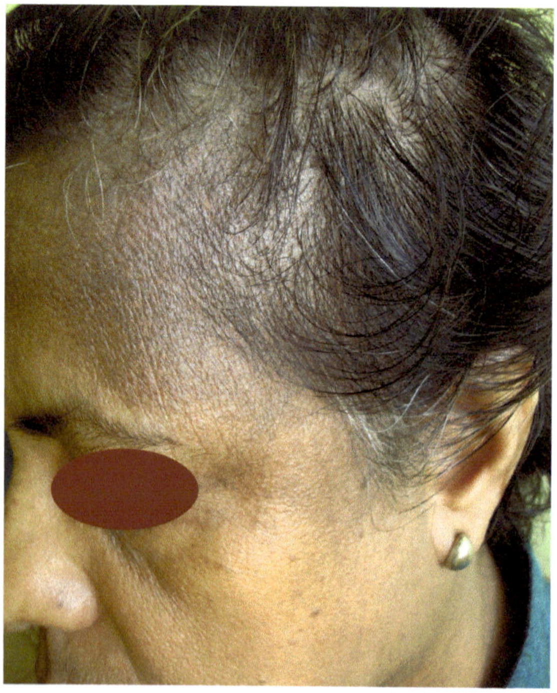

FIGURE 56.1 Hair dye melanosis in a 62-year-old woman FST5.

DOI: 10.1201/9781003479512-56

57
MATURATIONAL MELANOSIS

Introduction

Maturational melanosis is a very common finding in middle-aged men and women in Sri Lanka and in South India. Most of them are obese and 40–60 years of age. Most have one or more obesity-related medical problems such as diabetes, hypertension, cardiac diseases, fatty liver, or abnormal lipids. The case reports from India show a direct relationship with maturational melanosis and metabolic syndrome (Sonthalia 2020, Sidharth 2018).

Absence of acanthosis nigricans (AN) on other areas of the body, absence of dermoscopy features of AN, and differing histopathology help to differentiate from facial AN (Panda 2017).

Epidemiology

Seen in middle age, 45–60 years, obese men and women, and more common in men. It is a common cosmetic problem in South India and Sri Lanka.

Associated diseases

Associated with central obesity and metabolic syndrome.

Clinical characteristics in light skin (Fitzpatrick skin types I–III)

This is a condition described in the Indian dermatological literature in middle-aged persons with metabolic syndrome. The author has not seen it in fair-skinned individuals of normal weight or those suffering from obesity.

Clinical characteristics in dark skin (Fitzpatrick skin types IV–V)

Patients present with asymptomatic, granular-surfaced, dark brown to blackish pigmentation on the zygomatic areas of the face (Figures 57.1 and 57.2). Mostly, the involvement is bilateral and usually not symmetrical. The lesion has ill-defined borders, merging with the surrounding normal skin, and a rough surface with a finely granulated pattern in the center.

Investigations

This is diagnosed clinically.

Histopathology is used to exclude other clinical mimics such as macular amyloidosis, facial acanthosis nigricans, or friction melanosis. Histopathology shows increased basal layer melanocytes, mild epidermal hyperplasia, and papillomatosis, but no dermal inflammation or amyloid deposits (Sidharth S 2018).

Investigate for metabolic syndrome: HbA1C, liver transaminases, lipid profile, check blood pressure, and cardiac status.

Treatments

Topical lightening agents (e.g., kojic acid, azelaic acid, arbutin, retinoic acid) have been tried with favorable clinical responses.

Further reading

Panda S, Das A, Lahiri K, et al. (2017). Facial Acanthosis Nigricans: A Morphological Marker of Metabolic Syndrome. *Indian J Dermatol*;62(6):591–597.

Ranawaka RR (2021). Facial Melanosis. In: Ranawaka RR, et al. (eds). *Atlas of Dermatoses in Pigmented Skin*. Springer, Singapore; 803–822.

Sidharth S, Rashmi S, Shekhar N (2018). Maturational Hyperpigmentation: Clinico-Dermoscopic and Histopathological Profile of a New Cutaneous Marker of Metabolic Syndrome. *Pigment International*;5(1):54–56.

Sonthalia S, Agrawal M, Sharma P, et al. (2020). Maturational Hyperpigmentation: Cutaneous Marker of Metabolic Syndrome. *Dermatol Pract Concept*;10(2):e2020046.

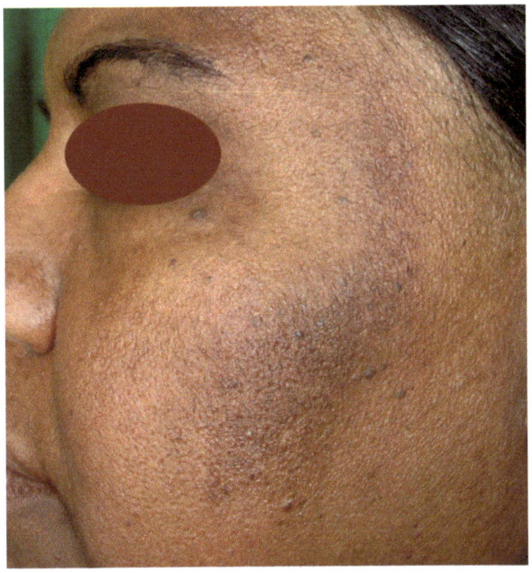

FIGURE 57.1 Maturational melanosis in a 52-year-old obese (BMI 32.5) woman FST5.

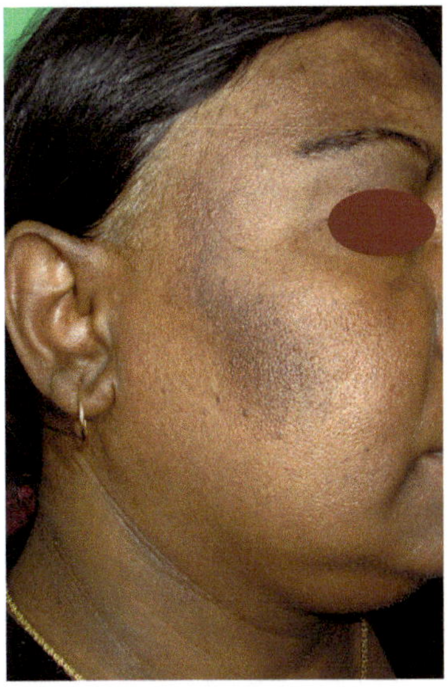

FIGURE 57.2 Same woman's right side of the face FST5. This is bilateral in most and may not be symmetrical. Note, even though she is obese her acanthosis nigricans is not significant.

DOI: 10.1201/9781003479512-57

58
SEBORRHEIC MELANOSIS

Introduction

Sebomelanosis is a very common skin problem and a major cosmetic concern in young adults with dark skin (Fitzpatrick skin type IV–V) who have seborrhea (oily skin) on the face. The localized darkening occurs on seborrheic areas of the face, namely, the alar grooves, angles of the mouth, and labio-mental crease. This is a distressing cosmetic problem in young adults.

Epidemiology

It presents in African, Asian, and Hispanic skin, in young adults aged 20–40, with both sexes equally affected.

Associated diseases

Most patients have mild to moderate dandruff and marked seborrhea on the face and scalp, but no associated seborrheic dermatitis or acne.

Clinical characteristics in light skin (Fitzpatrick skin types I–III)

This condition depends on the individual's ability to produce pigment and is uncommon in persons with fair skin.

Clinical characteristics in dark skin (Fitzpatrick skin types IV–V)

Mostly asymptomatic, but some complain of mild itching and a burning sensation. Brownish-to-grayish hyperpigmented thin plaques over the centrofacial areas (alar creases, sides of the nose, labio-mental crease, angles of the mouth, and to a lesser extent, the transverse nasal line). The lesions appear greasy and velvety with faint perilesional erythema (Figures 58.1 to 58.4).

There is no involvement of the forehead, beard, retroauricular area, or trunk (vs seborrheic dermatitis). And there is no associated acne or seborrheic dermatitis in these patients.

Investigations

This is diagnosed clinically.

Treatments

Topical anti-inflammatory/fungistatic agents effective in seborrheic dermatitis should be considered first, to allow any inflammatory component to subside; e.g., topical calcineurin inhibitors – 0.1% tacrolimus ointment, 1% pimecrolimus cream; mild topical steroids and 2% ketoconazole cream combinations.

- Topical lightening agents (e.g., kojic acid, azelaic acid, arbutin, retinoic acid) may be added at a later stage.
- The patient must be counseled regarding the slow treatment response, chronicity, and innocuous nature of the condition.

Further reading

Ranawaka RR (2021). Facial Melanosis. In: Ranawaka RR, et al. (eds). *Atlas of Dermatoses in Pigmented Skin*. Springer, Singapore; 803–822.

Vashisht KR, Garg S (2022). Seborrheic Melanosis: A Unique Under-Recognized Entity in Ethnic Skin. *J Clin Aesthet Dermatol*;15(1):15–16.

Verma SB, Vasani RJ, Chandrashekar L, et al. (2017). Seborrheic Melanosis: An Entity Worthy of Mention in Dermatological Literature. *Indian J Dermatol Venereol Leprol*;83(3):285–289.

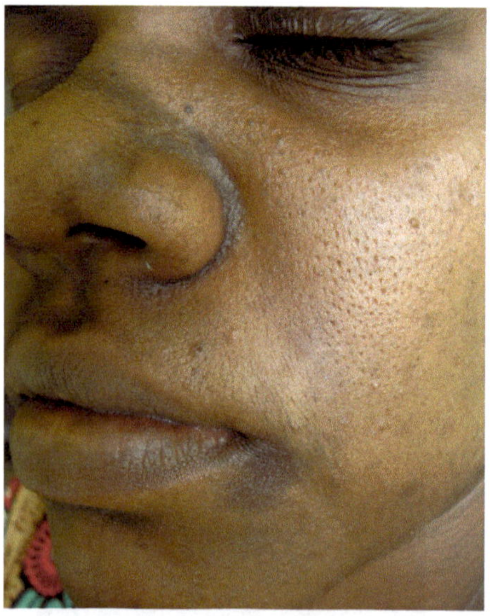

FIGURE 58.1 A 24-year-old woman with sebomelanosis FST5. Note oily skin and absence of acne. Hyperpigmented thin plaques over the alar creases, sides of nose, labio-mental crease, angles of mouth (and also transverse nasal band).

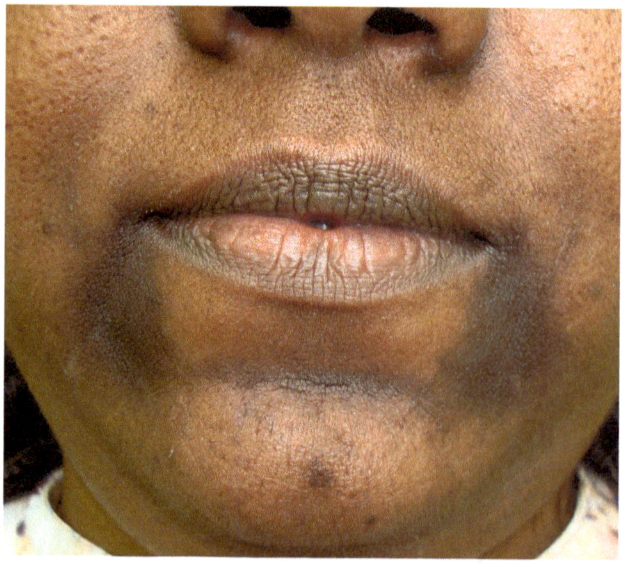

FIGURE 58.2 A 29-year-old woman with sebomelanosis FST5. Note oily skin and absence of acne. Hyperpigmented thick plaques over the alar creases, sides of nose, labio-mental crease, and angles of mouth.

DOI: 10.1201/9781003479512-58

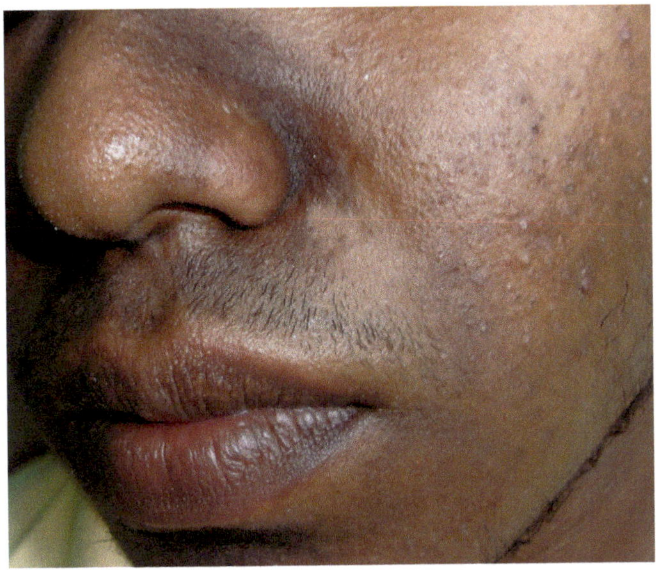

FIGURE 58.3 A 29-year-old man with sebomelanosis FST5. Note oily skin and absence or very mild acne. Hyperpigmented thick plaques over the alar creases, sides of nose, labio-mental crease.

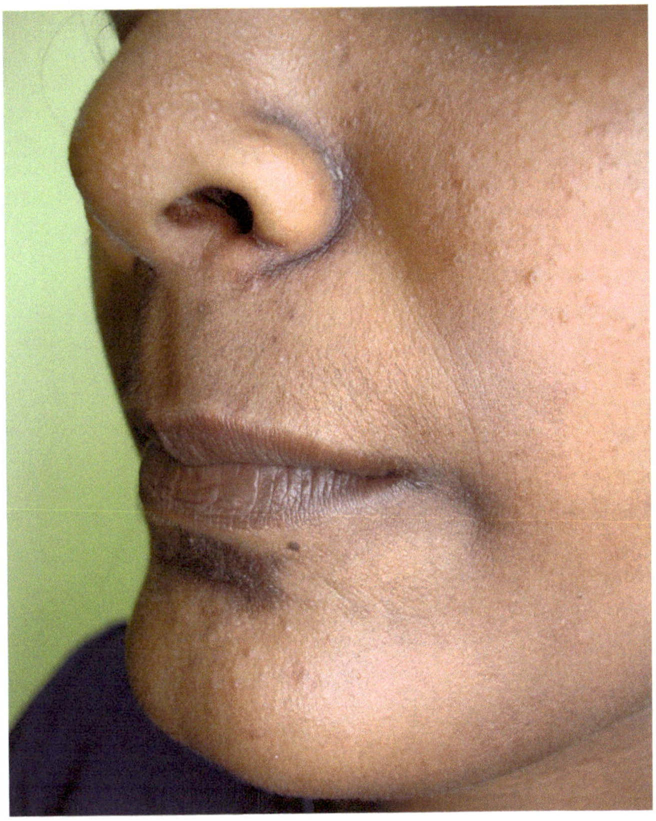

FIGURE 58.4 A 32-year-old woman with sebomelanosis FST5. Note oily skin and absence acne. Hyperpigmented thick plaques over the alar creases, sides of nose, labio-mental crease, and sides of the mouth.

59
MELASMA

Introduction

Melasma, or chloasma, is the most common cause of facial melanosis and is manifested by hyperpigmented macules on the face, which become more pronounced after sun exposure.

Epidemiology

Mostly starts between the ages of 20 and 40 years and 90% occur in women. More common in light brown skin types: Latin Americans, and those from the Middle East or Asia.

Associated diseases

Common in pregnancy and associated with oral contraceptive pills.

Clinical characteristics in light skin (Fitzpatrick skin types I–III)

Melasma is an unwanted spotted to patchy pigmentation, mainly of the face, with a serious negative impact on the affected individual, mainly women (Figure 59.1 and 59.2). When it begins in pregnancy, it is often called chloasma. Melasma is strongly dependent on sun exposure and hormonal factors, with genetic factors and skin irritation most probably adding to its development. Most pigmented patches occur in the centrofacial, malar, and mandibular areas. There are no other symptoms than cosmetic embarrassment.

Clinical characteristics in dark skin (Fitzpatrick skin types IV–V)

Dark brown pigmentation affects mainly the malar regions, forehead, nasal brim, and upper lip (Figures 59.3 and 59.4). The pigmentary changes are usually bilateral and are frequently symmetrical.

Investigations

This is a clinical diagnosis.

A Wood's lamp examination can be helpful in identifying the depth of melanin pigmentation and determining the type of melasma (epidermal, dermal, or mixed). Epidermal melasma shows enhanced color contrast with a Wood's lamp examination. Dermal melasma often shows less color contrast with a Wood's lamp. Dermal melasma is generally less responsive to therapy, especially to topical modalities.

Treatments

Although there are many different treatment options, all therapies are somehow delicate. Women often try to force the therapeutic effect, achieving the opposite. Any harsh treatment may result in a severe relapse after a short improvement; this is particularly true for many lasers. Vitamin D may be an option to the common depigmenting agents.

Treatment of melasma can be difficult due to the refractory and recurrent nature of the condition.

- Hydroquinone is the most extensively studied depigmenting agent for the treatment of melasma. It inhibits tyrosinase, an enzyme critical to the pigment-producing pathway in melanocytes.
- Topical retinoid therapy has also been used as monotherapy for melasma but with only moderate efficacy.
- Triple combination therapy, comprised of hydroquinone, a retinoid, and a corticosteroid, is a highly effective and safe treatment for melasma.
- Dual therapy (e.g., hydroquinone 2% plus glycolic acid 10%) may be used but can cause severe irritation.
- Pregnancy-related melasma tends to improve spontaneously postpartum, and treatment may not be necessary.
- Sun protection using broad-spectrum sunscreen (SPF > 50) is advised in all patients before and after any mode of therapy.
- Chemical peels, alone or in combination with topical treatments.
- Laser therapy, intense pulsed light therapy, adjuvant to topical treatment: Be extremely cautious!
- Dermabrasion.

Further reading

Bolanca I, Bolanca Z, Kuna K, et al. (2008). Chloasma: The Mask of Pregnancy. *Coll Antropol*;32(Suppl 2):139–141.

Chen Q, Liu L, Zhang Y (2024). Vitamin D and Wound Healing: Assessing Skin Barrier Function and Implications for Chloasma Treatment. *Int Wound J*;21(1):e14541.

DOI: 10.1201/9781003479512-59

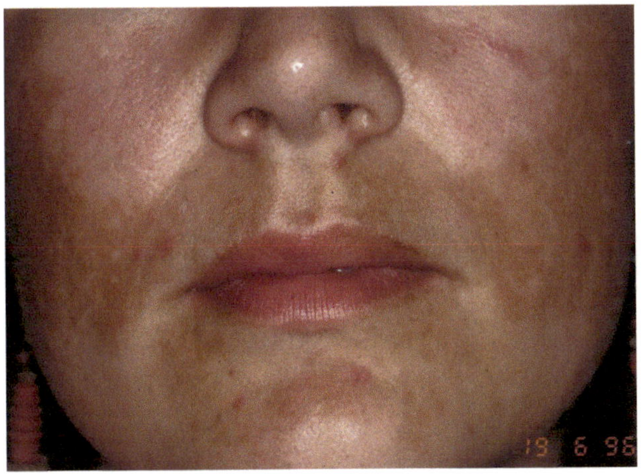

FIGURE 59.1 Melasma FST1. (Courtesy Dr. Richard Ashton, UK.)

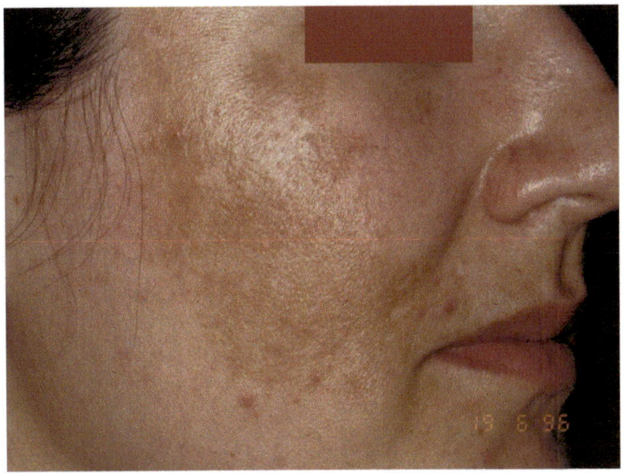

FIGURE 59.2 Melasma FST2. (Courtesy Dr. Richard Ashton, UK.)

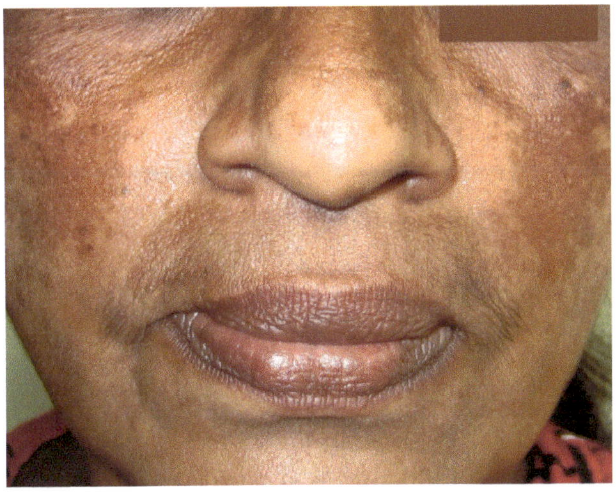

FIGURE 59.3 Melasma FST5.

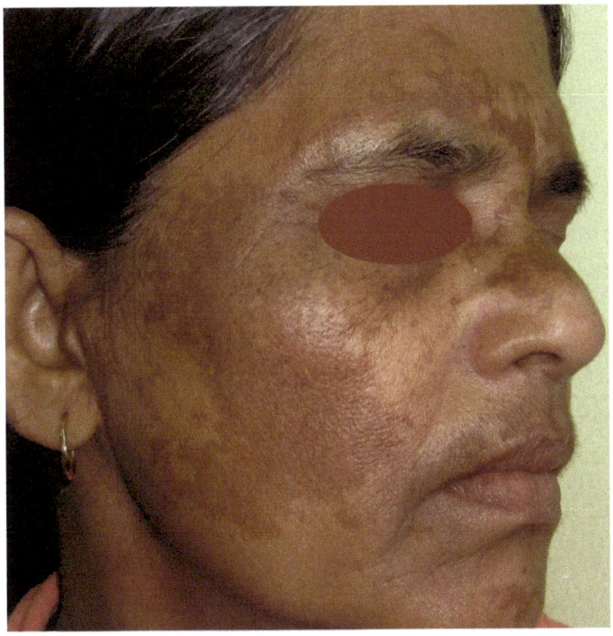

FIGURE 59.4 Melasma in a 51-year-old woman FST5.

60
MILIA OR KERATIN CYSTS

Introduction

Milia are small subepidermal keratin cysts. These commonly appear *de novo*, but secondary milia due to second-degree burns, epidermolysis bullosa, porphyria cutanea tarda, bullous lichen planus, following dermabrasion, chemical peels, in areas of chronic topical corticosteroid-induced atrophy, and radiotherapy are not uncommon.

Epidemiology

Milia are quite common at all ages.

Associated diseases

Rombo syndrome: A rare familial disorder with vermiculate atrophoderma, milia, hypotrichosis, trichoepitheliomas, basal cell carcinomas, and peripheral vasodilation with cyanosis.

Clinical characteristics in light skin (Fitzpatrick skin types I–III)

Milia are very common asymptomatic tiny keratin cysts mostly occurring on the face, particularly on the zygoma and around the eyes (Figure 60.1). In skin types I–III, they are usually ivory-colored and firm. Gently lifting the surface with an injection needle allows the contents to be taken out; it looks like a tiny whitish lesion the size of a grain of sand.

Clinical characteristics in dark skin (Fitzpatrick skin types IV–V)

Very common in all ages, and mostly women seek treatment. Elderly women present with numerous milia due to a delay in pursuing treatments (Figures 60.2 and 60.3). These are asymptomatic and are only of cosmetic concern. Small subepidermal papules of 1–2 mm in diameter, yellowish brown and sometimes translucent. They are usually noticed only on the face. They feel soft and release their keratinous contents when punctured.

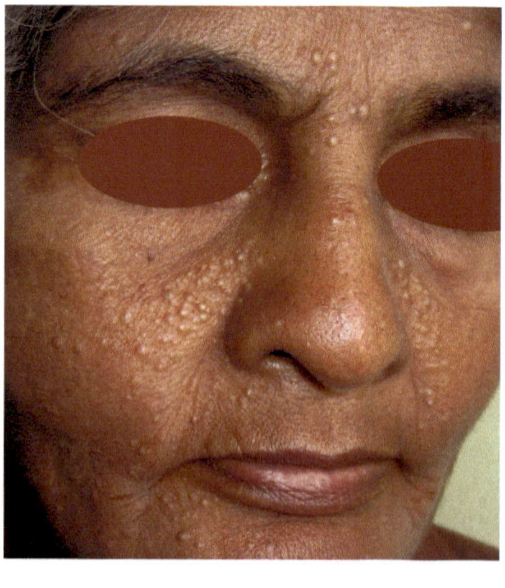

FIGURE 60.2 Multiple asymptomatic milia or keratin cysts in a 62-year-old woman FST5.

Investigations

This is a clinical diagnosis.

Treatments

- Incision of the overlying epidermis and expression of the contents are curative. Recurrence is uncommon.
- Spontaneous disappearance occurs in many milia in infants.
- Laser ablation, puncturing the milia, electrodesiccation, and topical tretinoin may be effective.

Further reading

Madan V, Seaton E (2024). Cutaneous Cysts. In: Griffiths C, et al. (eds). *Rook's Textbook of Dermatology*, 10th ed. John Wiley & Sons Ltd., UK; 133.4.

Rodrigues FT, Cabral GCCC, Alvim PFMF, et al. (2024). Milia en plaque on the Shoulder as an Early Manifestation of Mycosis Fungoides. *Dermatol Online J*;Mar 15;30(1).

Snyder KAM, Voelckers AD (2024). Newborn Skin: Part I. Common Rashes and Skin Changes. *Am Fam Physician*;109(3):212–216.

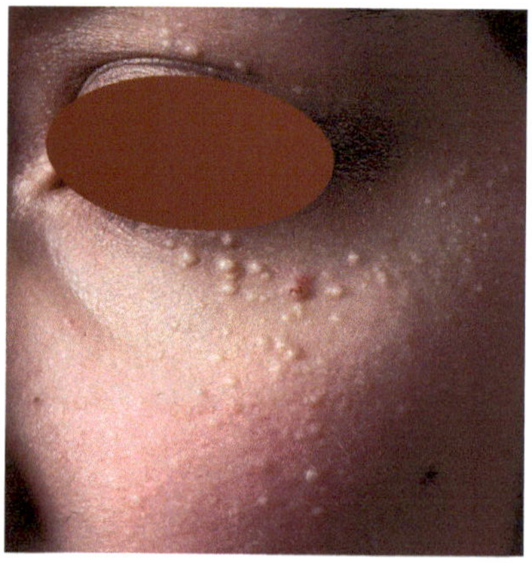

FIGURE 60.1 Milia FST1. (Courtesy Dr. Richard Ashton, UK.)

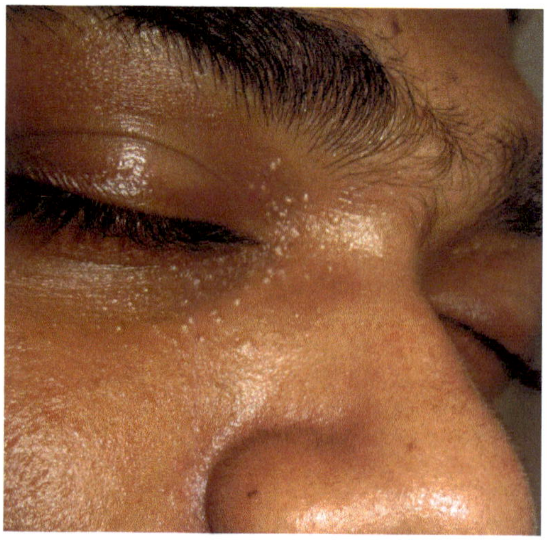

FIGURE 60.3 Milia around the eye in a 29-year-old man FST5.

DOI: 10.1201/9781003479512-60

61
MILIARIA OR SWEAT RASH

Introduction

Miliaria is a common skin condition that arises due to the occlusion or disruption of eccrine sweat ducts in hot, humid conditions, resulting in a leakage of sweat into the epidermis or dermis. It is classified into four subtypes: *miliaria crystallina*, *miliaria rubra*, *miliaria profunda*, and *miliaria pustulosa*.

Epidemiology

Miliaria crystallina occurs commonly in infants due to a delay in patency developing in the sweat ducts. Miliaria rubra, or sweat rash, is very common in tropical hot humid climates.

Clinical characteristics in light skin (Fitzpatrick skin types I–III)

Miliaria, in the types mentioned above, is rarely seen by dermatologists in cold and temperate climates (Figure 61.1). Miliaria crystallina is a benign, self-resolving skin condition that results from the superficial obstruction of sweat ducts in the stratum corneum. It is most commonly seen in neonates but is also observed in adults exposed to high heat and humidity, such as in febrile illnesses or tropical environments. It usually appears suddenly as a water-drop rash.

Miliaria rubra results from sweat duct obstruction in the spinous layer of the epidermis. It may be pruritic.

Miliaria profunda is rare and mainly seen in persons who tend to recurrently develop miliaria rubra or have recently relocated to a warm, hot climate. As the terms imply, miliaria crystallina looks like clear water droplets, whereas miliaria rubra resembles tiny red papules. In miliaria pustulosa, there is pustular progression of vesicles.

These so-called eccrine miliaria should not be confused with miliaria apocrina, the hallmark of Fox–Fordyce disease, which is mainly localized in apocrine gland-bearing skin like axillae, perimamillary, and genito-anal areas.

Clinical characteristics in dark skin (Fitzpatrick skin types IV–V)

Miliaria rubra is the most common form in hot humid climates, in which typical lesions develop on the body, especially in areas of friction with clothing and in flexures. The lesions are uniformly minute erythematous papules in very large numbers. Erythema may be obscured in darker skin (Figures 61.2 and 61.3). These produce intense discomfort in the form of an unbearable pricking sensation. In infants, lesions commonly appear on the occluded skin of the neck, groin, and axillae.

Miliaria crystallina presents as clear, thin-walled vesicles, 1–2 mm in diameter without an inflammatory areola, are usually symptomless and develop in crops, mainly on the trunk. The vesicles soon rupture and are followed by superficial, branny desquamation.

Investigations

This is a clinical diagnosis.

Treatments

- Control the local environment (remove excess bedding, fans, air conditioning).
- Cool the skin (with damp compresses, cool showers) will resolve this early.
- Avoid tight or excessive clothing.
- Menthol (e.g., 0.5% menthol in aqueous cream) and calamine lotion will help with skin cooling.
- Topical antibiotics if there is a secondary infection.
- Mild topical steroids for erythema and itching in miliaria rubra.
- Removal to a cooler climate and prophylactic oral vitamin C if this is recurrent in infancy.

Further reading

Coulson IH, Wilson NJE (2024). Disorders of the Sweat Glands. In: Griffiths C, et al. (eds). *Rook's Textbook of Dermatology*, 10th ed. John Wiley & Sons Ltd., UK; 92.12.

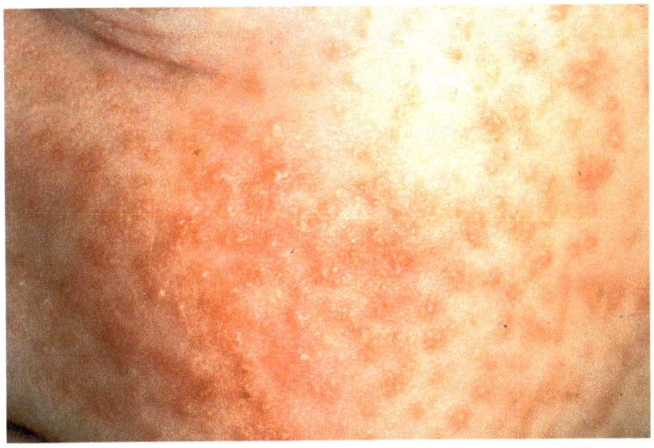

FIGURE 61.1 Miliaria. (Courtesy Dr. Richard Ashton, UK.)

DOI: 10.1201/9781003479512-61

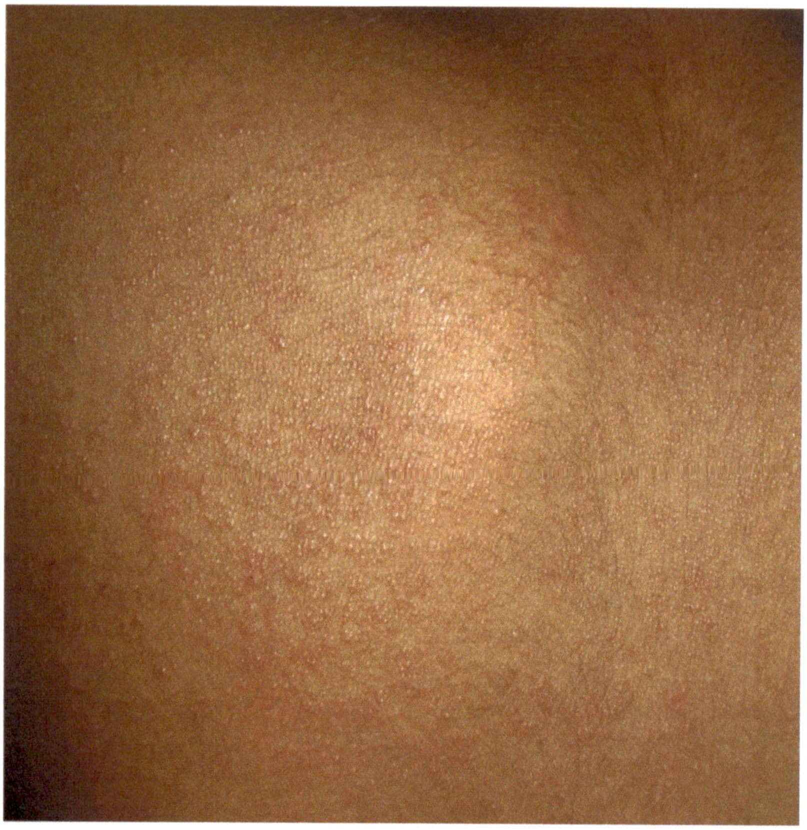

FIGURE 61.2 Miliaria rubra in a 7-year-old child FST5. Note the minute uniform erythematous papules in very large numbers where the patient complains of a pricking sensation.

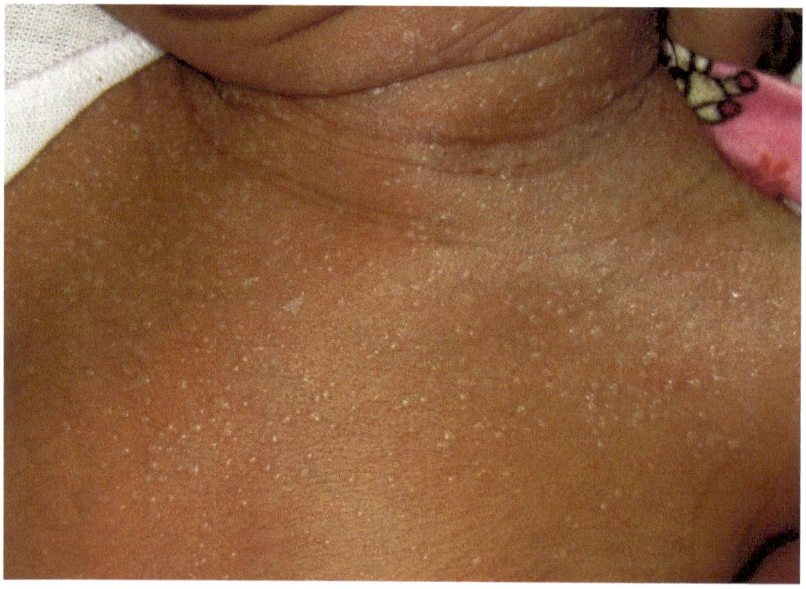

FIGURE 61.3 Miliaria crystallina in a newborn (2-day-old) infant FST5.

62
ADULT COLLOID MILIUM

Introduction

Colloid milium and colloid degeneration of the skin present as yellowish, translucent papules, nodules, or plaques on light-exposed skin. These dermal papules are 1–5 mm in diameter, yellowish-brown, and sometimes translucent. They develop slowly in irregular groups in areas exposed to sunlight. They feel soft and may release their gelatinous contents when punctured. There are several clinical variants, of which the most common is adult colloid milium, which manifests as multiple milia-like papules on light-exposed skin. The most frequently involved sites are the face, especially around the orbits, the dorsa of the hands, the back and sides of the neck, and the ears.

Epidemiology

Reported from fair-skinned, outdoor workers living in sunny climates, a rare juvenile form manifests before puberty and is often familial. The nodular form is even rarer.

Associated diseases

Associated with sun-damaged skin and actinic elastosis, the nodular variant may be associated with melanoma.

Clinical characteristics in light skin (Fitzpatrick skin types I–III)

Ivory to yellowish-colored dome-shaped nodules are seen in sun-exposed areas (Figure 62.1). They may coalesce to form ill-defined plaques. The main differential diagnoses are nodular amyloidosis and Favre–Racouchot disease, also called actinic acne with cysts and comedones, which shows multiple solitary open black comedones located bilaterally on the zygoma region of the cheeks and temples. In addition, yellowish, smooth-surfaced papulonodular lesions are present in close association with the comedones. These lesions are clustered on both sides of the malar and periorbital areas, giving a cobblestone appearance due to severe actinic elastosis.

Histopathology of colloid milium shows large, pale-stained, PAS-positive, Congo red-negative globules of amorphous material in the papillary dermis.

Clinical characteristics in dark skin (Fitzpatrick skin types IV–V)

We encounter colloid milium mostly in elderly women (possibly more women who seek treatments), and this is not rare in our settings in the elderly (Figures 62.2 and 62.3). The most frequently involved site is the face and periorbital area. In dark skin, these lesions present with larger plaque-like lesions that are hyperpigmented and blackish.

Investigations

Histopathology is the appearance of colloid globules at the tips of the dermal papillae. There is characteristically a subepidermal uninvolved Grenz zone. The colloid is usually eosinophilic but may be basophilic. In the larger, plaque-like lesions, the colloid change occurs diffusely throughout the dermis.

Treatments

Dermabrasion and long-pulsed Er:YAG laser have claimed good results, but no completely satisfactory intervention has been found.

Further reading

Azimi SZ, Zargari O, Rudolph RI (2017). Nodular Colloid Milium Mimicking Keloid. *J Cosmet Dermatol*;16(4):e45–e47.

Fahy CMR, Lovell CR (2024). Acquired Disorders of Dermal Connective Tissue. In: Griffiths C, et al. (eds). *Rook's Textbook of Dermatology*, 10th ed. John Wiley & Sons Ltd., UK; 94.5.

Siadat AH, Mokhtari F (2013). Colloid Milium. *Adv Biomed Res*;2:28.

Zeng YP, Nguyen GH, Fang K, et al. (2016). A Split-Face Treatment of Adult Colloid Milium Using a Non-Ablative, 1550-nm, Erbium-Glass Fractional Laser. *J Eur Acad Dermatol Venereol*;30(3):490–491.

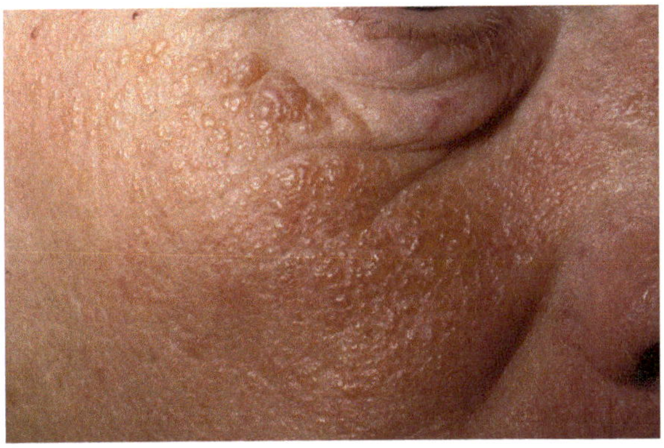

FIGURE 62.1 Adult colloid milium FST2. (Courtesy Dr. Richard Ashton, UK.)

DOI: 10.1201/9781003479512-62

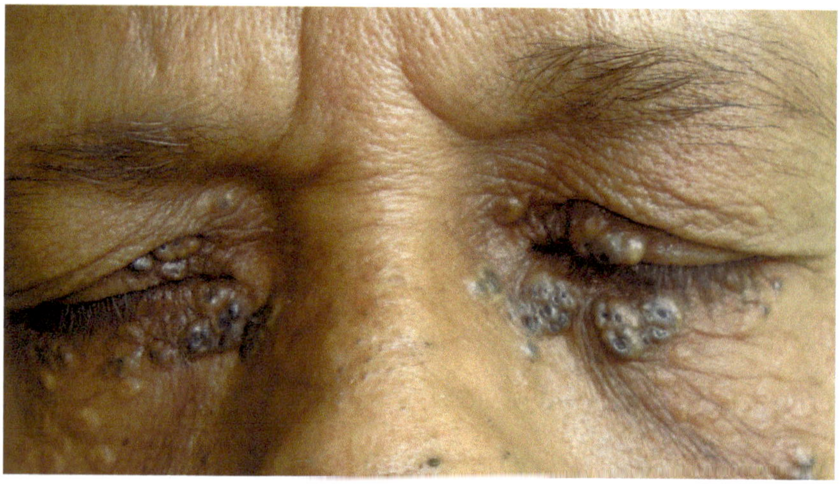

FIGURE 62.2 Adult colloid milium in a 65-year-old woman FST5.

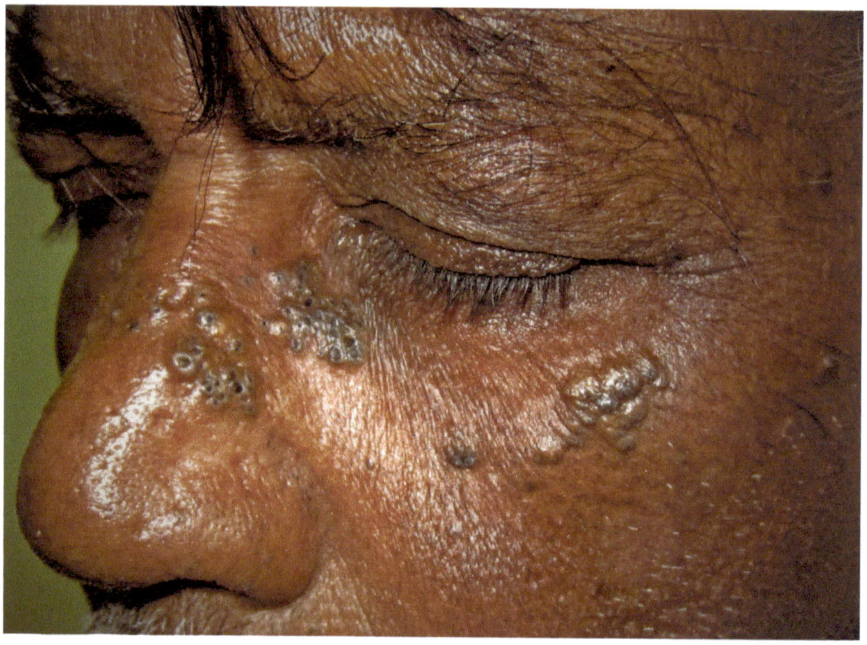

FIGURE 62.3 Adult colloid milium in a 62-year-old man FST5.

63
MOLES OR ACQUIRED MELANOCYTIC NEVI

Introduction

Acquired melanocytic nevi are benign neoplasms of melanocytic nevus cells that begin to proliferate at the dermal–epidermal junction (junctional nevus), and over time tend to migrate into the dermis while a component remains in contact with the basal layer (compound nevus). At the end stage of this process, all the nevus cells are completely detached from the overlying epidermis (intradermal nevus). A junctional nevus is a uniformly pigmented brown macule, with a diameter of 2–10 mm. A compound nevus is a slightly raised, oval or round papule with a symmetrical shape. This nevus is also pigmented with shades of brown. Intradermal (or dermal) nevi are skin-colored to brown, dome-shaped nodules that can be larger than junctional nevi. Their surface is usually smooth but can also appear papillomatous. Larger nevi often contain hair.

Pre-existing nevi may darken in pregnancy due to increased circulating levels of melanocyte-stimulating hormones and high circulating levels of sex hormones. This can lead to anxiety and concern about possible malignant melanoma. These changes may reverse following delivery. However, true malignant transformation of nevi is a very rare event.

Epidemiology

Acquired melanocytic nevi are the most common neoplasms among white people and are usually multiple. The number of acquired melanocytic nevi increases from childhood to midlife and decreases progressively thereafter. There is no sex predilection.

Associated diseases

The presence of multiple acquired melanocytic nevi indicates a risk for melanoma in white skin. White patients with more than 100 nevi have a sevenfold increased melanoma risk.

Clinical characteristics in light skin (Fitzpatrick skin types I–III)

Acquired melanocytic nevi may display a huge array of different clinical features. Most are light to dark brown, round or oval; some are dome-shaped, some are papillomatous and soft, while others firm and hairy (Figures 63.1 to 63.3). The majority of these nevi are found on the upper half of the body. Some individuals have hundreds of melanocytic nevi of various sizes, shapes, and colors. As they are at an increased risk for melanoma development, regular nevus controls and counts are recommended; they should be photographically documented and stored so that they can be compared at regular time intervals. Some software performs an automatic comparison of these nevi and alerts the clinician in case of any suspicious change.

The attempt to remove all nevi has not been successful and probably does not decrease the melanoma risk, as it is not the preexistent nevus that undergoes malignant degeneration.

Some nevi in particular localizations such as palms, soles, genitals, knees, and hairy scalp may display worrisome histopathological features, and a clinico-pathological correlation is therefore warranted.

Clinical characteristics in dark skin (Fitzpatrick skin types IV –V)

Moles are very common benign lesions on dark-skinned individuals (Figures 63.4 to 63.6). Both junctional nevi and compound nevi appear black in color, while intradermal nevi are dark brown to black-colored, dome-shaped nodules. Their surface is usually smooth but can also appear papillomatous. One or a few hair shafts may project from the nevus surface. Melanoma is never reported within moles in darker-skinned individuals. However, acral lentiginous melanoma can be frequently mistaken for a pigmented nevus and may lead to a delayed diagnosis.

Investigations

This is a clinical diagnosis.

Early excisional biopsy is recommended for anyone presenting with a suspicious pigmented lesion.

Treatments

No treatment is required. Surgical removal is performed only for aesthetic purposes.

Further reading

Shah SA, Jahnke MN (2024). Nevi: When to Refer. *Curr Opin Pediatr*;36(4):411–417.

Snyder KAM, Voelckers AD (2024). Newborn Skin: Part II. Birthmarks. *Am Fam Physician*;109(3):217–221.

Stefanaki I, Sgouros D, Stratigos A (2024). Benign Melanocytic Proliferations and Melanocytic Naevi. In: Griffiths C, et al. (eds). *Rook's Textbook of Dermatology*, 10th ed. John Wiley & Sons Ltd., UK; 131.22.

Wong CSM, Chan MWM, Shek SYN, et al. (2024). Evaluation of a Novel Dermal Cooling System for the Treatment of Benign Pigmented Lesions in Asians. *Lasers Surg Med*;56(6):541–550.

DOI: 10.1201/9781003479512-63

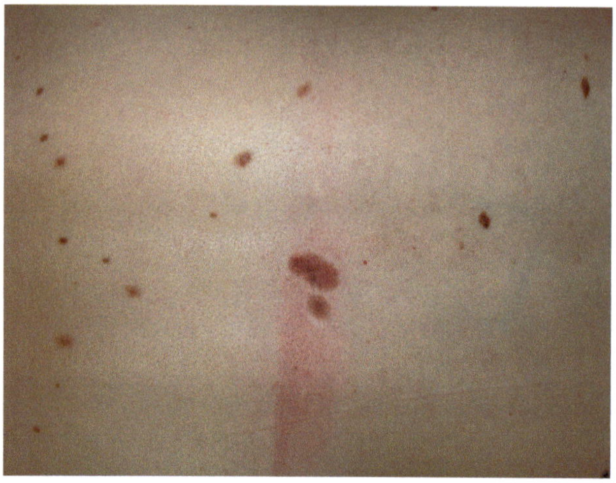

FIGURE 63.1 Atypical nevus FST1. (Courtesy Prof. Ian Coulson, UK.)

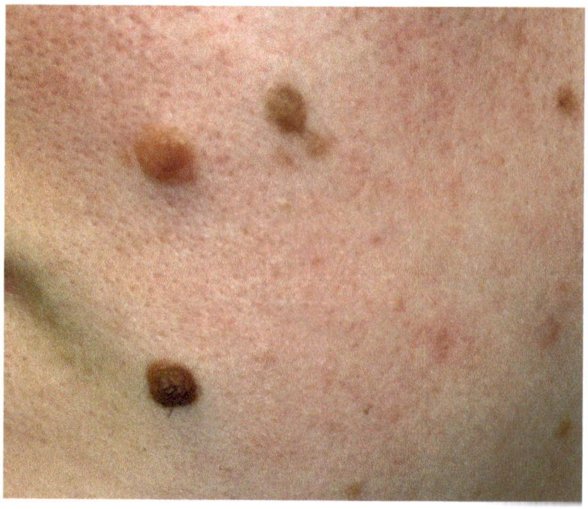

FIGURE 63.2 Compound nevus and junctional nevus FST1. (Courtesy Dr. Richard Ashton, UK.)

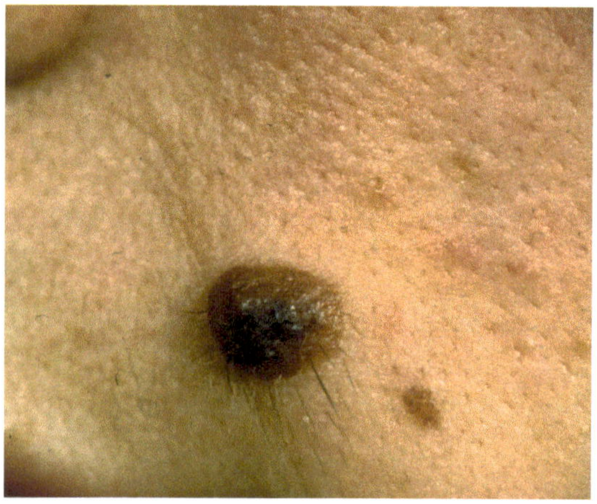

FIGURE 63.3 Compound nevus FST1. (Courtesy Dr. Richard Ashton, UK.)

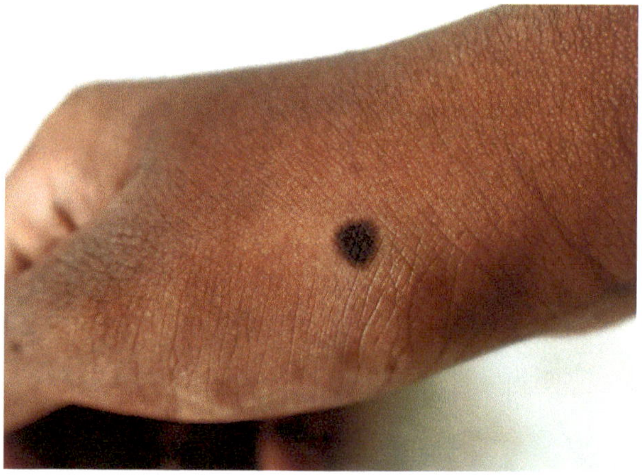

FIGURE 63.4 Mole or junctional melanocytic nevus FST5.

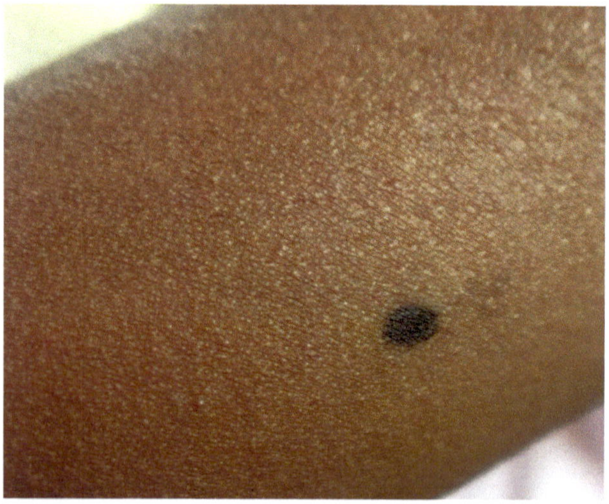

FIGURE 63.5 Mole or junctional melanocytic nevus FST5.

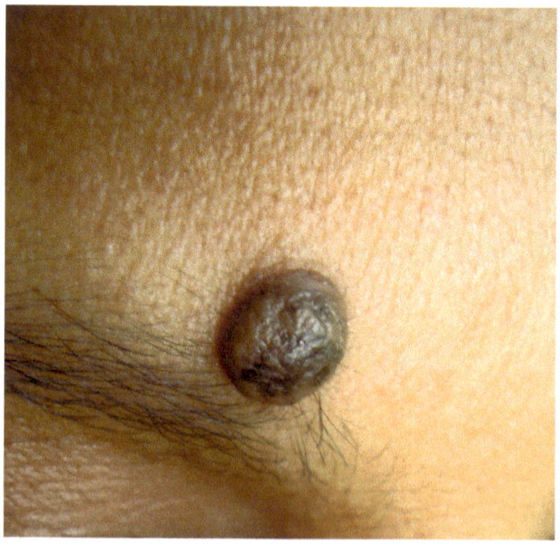

FIGURE 63.6 Compound nevus FST5.

64
MONGOLIAN SPOTS

Introduction

Mongolian spots are congenital macular areas of blue-gray pigmentation of varying size and shape located on the sacral area in normal infants. This is a state of dermal melanocytosis where there is a proliferation of dermal melanocytes in the dermis. These lesions have a bluish color owing to the Tyndall effect.

Usually presents as a single lesion, but multiple Mongolian spots may occasionally occur. The most common location is the lumbosacral region, but they can appear on the buttocks, flanks, shoulders, and lower legs in generalized lesions. This typically resolves during childhood but may occasionally persist into adult life.

Epidemiology

The Mongolian spot is uncommon in white skin. It is common in darker-skinned babies, increases in depth for a period during infancy, and then diminishes.

Associated diseases

Extensive Mongolian spots have been associated with Hurler syndrome, GM1 gangliosidosis type 1, and mucolipidosis II, as well as with bilateral Ota nevus.

Clinical characteristics in light skin (Fitzpatrick skin types I–III)

All the different types of dermal melanocytosis – Mongolian spot, Ota nevus in the zygomatico-maxillary region, nevus of Ito in the shoulder region, and some other rare forms – are extremely common in East Asians and Africans; however, the prevalence in fair-skinned newborns is below 1%. Clinically, the slate gray to bluish spots are easily seen in light skin although they are much less common than in skin of color. They usually fade between the ages of 2 to 6 years.

Histopathology shows an increased number of spindle-shaped melanocytes in the upper to mid-dermis. This may be slightly more marked in the Ota and Ito nevi.

As the classical Mongolian spots remain benign and tend to disappear spontaneously, no specific treatment is needed. Ota nevus may be treated with a pigment laser.

Clinical characteristics in dark skin (Fitzpatrick skin types IV–V)

Mongolian spots are very common in newborn babies in our setting (Figures 64.1 and 64.2). The lesion is a diffuse macule with a rather uniform, relatively faint blue to gray color. It has a round or oval shape, with a diameter of a few – usually up to 10 cm. The most common location is the lumbosacral region.

Investigations

This is a clinical diagnosis.

Treatments

No treatment is required; it typically resolves during childhood but may occasionally persist into adult life. Q-switched lasers, intense pulsed light, and bleaching creams have been used in persistent cases.

Further reading

Abdel-Naser MB (2019). The Color of Skin: Gray Diseases of the Skin, Nails, and Mucosa. *Clin Dermatol*;37(5):507–515.

Franceschini D, Dinulos JG (2015). Dermal Melanocytosis and Associated Disorders. *Curr Opin Pediatr*;27(4):480–485.

Jacobs AH, Walton RG (1976). The Incidence of Birthmarks in the Neonate. *Pediatrics*;58(2):218–222.

Shin JO, Roh D, Shin K, et al. (2023). High-Fluence 1064nm Q-Switched Nd:YAG Laser Treatment for Ectopic Mongolian Spot. *J Dermatolog Treat*;34(1):2255057.

Zhang Z, Ma M, Zhang W, et al. (2023). Phenotypic and Genetic Characteristics of 130 Patients with Mucopolysaccharidosis Type II: A Single-Center Retrospective Study in China. *Front Genet*;14:1103620.

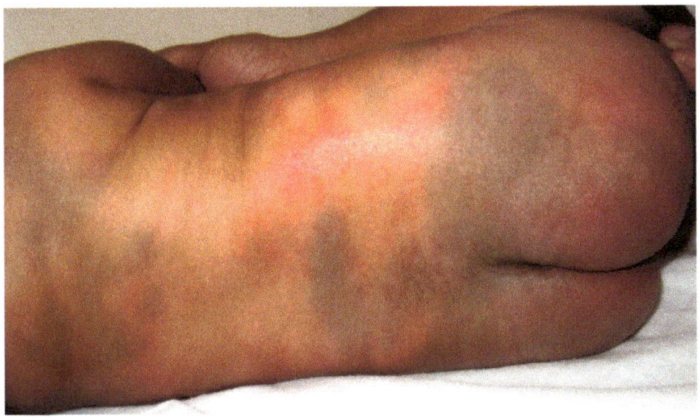

FIGURE 64.1 Multiple Mongolian spots are very common in dark-skinned newborn babies FST5.

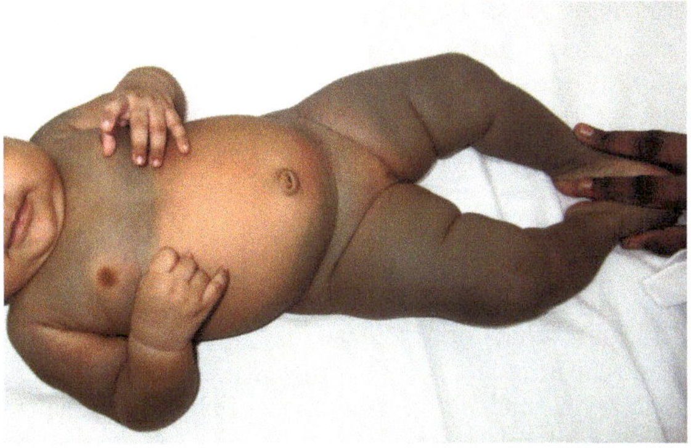

FIGURE 64.2 Multiple extensive Mongolian spots in a 5-month-old baby girl FST5. These spots on the upper trunk disappeared spontaneously over months.

DOI: 10.1201/9781003479512-64

65
MORPHEA

Introduction

Morphea is the term used in preference to 'localized scleroderma.' It comprises a group of related diseases that share a common underlying pathophysiology of increased collagen deposition in an autoimmune setting. They are largely confined to the skin and subcutaneous tissues. Overall, plaque morphea was the most common subtype (56%), followed in order of frequency by linear (20%), generalized (13%), and deep (11%) morphea.

Epidemiology

Morphea can occur at any age; it is more common in women, with a female to male ratio of 7:1.

Associated diseases

Since morphea is an autoimmune disease, generalized morphea associated with other autoimmune diseases is known. Cases of lichen sclerosus occurring in conjunction with morphea are now well documented.

Clinical characteristics in light skin (Fitzpatrick skin types I–III)

Circumscribed or localized scleroderma (morphea) is rare, though not uncommon (Figures 65.1 and 65.2). More than 20% of the cases begin in children and have a slightly higher involvement of the head. Four different clinical types are distinguished: *limited, linear, generalized,* and *mixed.* The skin is indurated, usually slightly depressed, with a lilac ring at the margin; this is usually seen as a sign of activity. There may be one or several lesions that are commonly asymptomatic. Linear morphea is a potentially crippling form with involvement of deep cutaneous structures, often also fascia and muscle; localization in the face may cause hemiatrophia faciei of Parry–Romberg or 'coup de sabre' when it affects the forehead and scalp. Generalized morphea is very rare but may be extremely severe.

Particularly histopathologically, there may be changes of lichen sclerosus et atrophicans in association with typical morphea.

Treatment is difficult, with superficial morphea responding to topical steroids and calcineurin inhibitors. Extensive forms and recalcitrant morphea usually respond well to methotrexate alone or in combination with systemic steroid pulses.

Clinical characteristics in dark skin (Fitzpatrick skin types IV–V)

Circumscribed or localized scleroderma (morphea) is the most common scleroderma presentation in our settings (Figures 65.3 to 65.6). However, the erythematous, edematous, inflammatory phase, which may be subtle and 'bruise-like' in appearance, is never observed in darker-skinned patients. The sclerotic phase, with central sclerotic area surrounded by an erythematous to violaceous so-called 'lilac ring,' is almost never observed in darker-skinned patients.

Most of the patients the author has observed presented with atrophic, hyperpigmented macules. Early presentation before atrophy has a very good prognosis, where lesions disappear completely with potent topical steroids.

Investigations

Histopathology is similar in all subtypes of morphea but varies in relation to the depth of involvement. For example, in plaque morphea, they may be limited to the dermis, whereas in linear and deep types, they may extend beyond the skin and into the underlying fascia, muscle, and bone. In the sclerotic stage, there are few recognizable fibroblasts and little inflammation. Collagen bundles are closely packed, highly eosinophilic, and oriented horizontally. The dermal appendages and subcutaneous fat are progressively lost.

Treatments

Treatment can then be based on the subtype, activity, extent, and depth of the disease, and patient symptoms.

- Limited superficial forms of morphea can generally be treated topically with topical corticosteroids or topical tacrolimus 0.1%.
- In extensive and generalized morphea, phototherapy, systemic corticosteroids, methotrexate, and intralesional platelet-rich plasma (PRP) had been tried with variable success.
- Recently, JAK inhibitors have had promising effects on the management of morphea and cutaneous fibrosis in systemic sclerosis.

Further reading

Al-Gburi S, Kreuter A, Moinzadeh P (2024). Lokalisierte Sklerodermie [Localized Scleroderma]. *Dermatologie (Heidelb)*; Mar;75(3):197–207.

McGaugh S, Kallis P, De Benedetto A, et al. (2022). Janus Kinase Inhibitors for Treatment of Morphea and Systemic Sclerosis: A Literature Review. *Dermatol Ther*;35(6):e15437.

Orteu CH (2024). Morphoea and Allied Scarring and Sclerosing Inflammatory Dermatoses. In: Griffiths C, et al. (eds). *Rook's Textbook of Dermatology*, 10th ed. John Wiley & Sons Ltd., UK; 55.1.

Rijal H, Bouadi N, Piguet V, et al. (2024). Treatment Outcomes of Scleroderma with Janus Kinase Inhibitors: A Systematic Review. *J Cutan Med Surg*;Sep–Oct;28(5):489–490.

Romanowska-Próchnicka K, Dziewit M, Lesiak A, et al. (2024). Scleroderma and Scleroderma-Like Syndromes. *Front Immunol*;Jun 3;15:1351675.

DOI: 10.1201/9781003479512-65

FIGURE 65.1 Localized morphea FST1. Sclerotic phase with central sclerotic area surrounded by an erythematous to violaceous so-called 'lilac ring.' (Courtesy Prof. Ian Coulson, UK.)

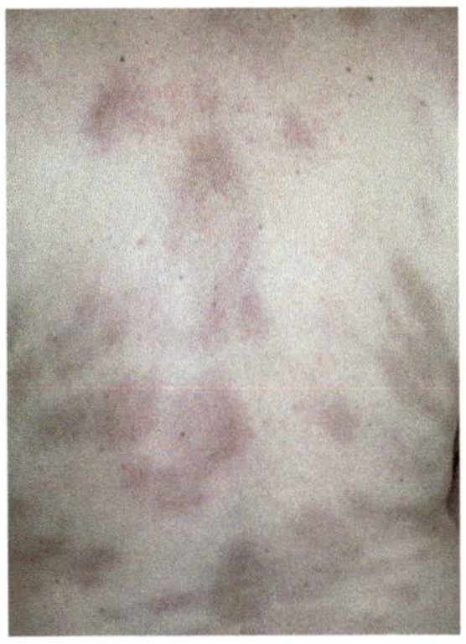

FIGURE 65.2 Generalized morphea FST1. (Courtesy Prof. Ian Coulson, UK.)

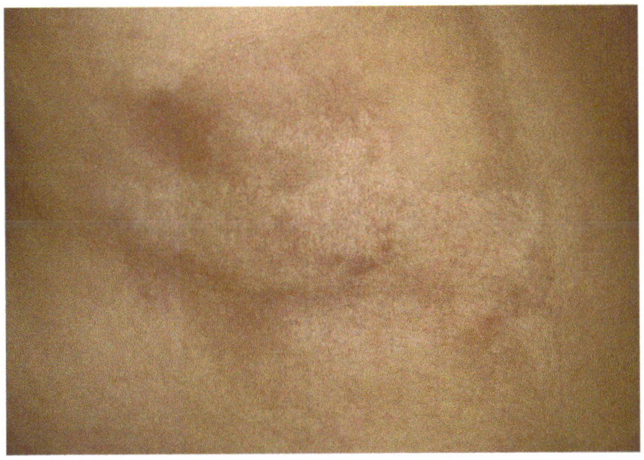

FIGURE 65.3 Localized morphea in early stage FST5. This early stage is reversible with potent topical steroids such as clobetasol ointments, or with 1% tacrolimus ointment.

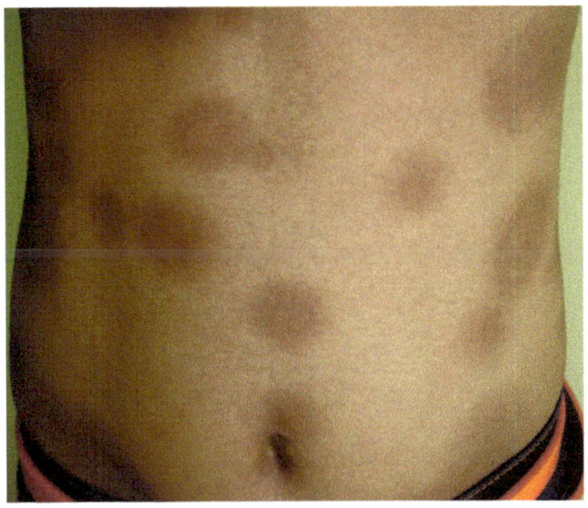

FIGURE 65.4 Generalized circumscribed morphea in early stage FST5. Even though the lesions are hyperpigmented, atrophy is minimal in early stages. Early, inflammatory morphea with erythema and bruise-like appearance is never observed in darker-skinned individuals.

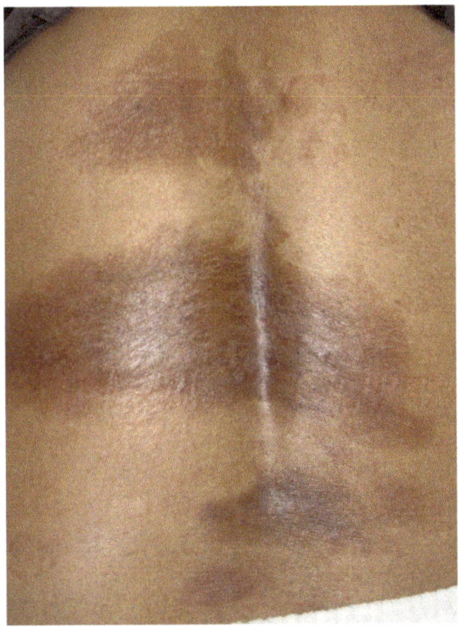

FIGURE 65.5 Circumscribed localized morphea in hyperpigmented atrophic stage which has lasted untreated for more than 4 years FST5.

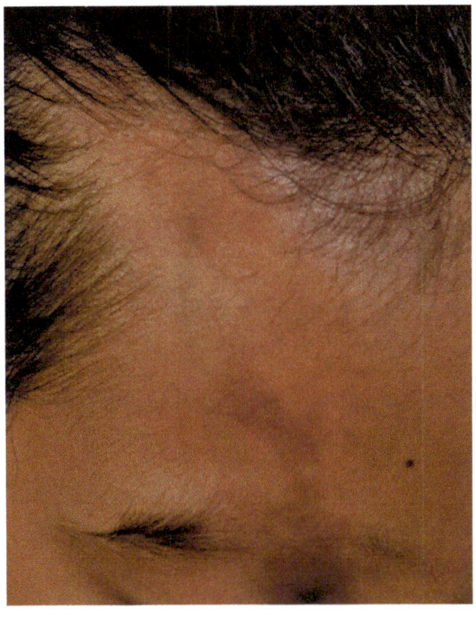

FIGURE 65.6 Linear localized morphea in the scalp (en coup de sabre) FST5.

66
MUCINOSES, SCLEREDEMA ADULTORUM, AND SCLEREDEMA DIABETICORUM

Introduction

Scleredema is a rare condition characterized by non-pitting swelling and induration of the upper part of the body caused by a thickened dermis and deposition of mucin. Scleredema can be divided into diabetic and non-diabetic types. The diabetic type is considered the most common, accounting for 25–50% of cases. It occurs mainly in obese middle-aged men with poorly controlled insulin-dependent diabetes. The non-diabetic form includes an idiopathic type (a post-infective type), and a monoclonal gammopathy-associated type (a type associated with anecdotal miscellaneous conditions such as autoimmune disorders, internal malignancies, exposure to organic solvents, and HIV infection).

In scleredema, mucin is deposited in the dermis and subcutaneous tissues, and also accumulates in skeletal muscle and the heart. Scleredema typically begins on the posterior neck and spreads to the upper back, shoulders, and scalp. The hands and feet are characteristically spared.

Epidemiology

Scleredema occurs in patients of all ages and is more prevalent in men 10:1.

Associated diseases

The post-infective type usually follows a streptococcal upper respiratory infection but also influenza, measles, mumps, chickenpox, cytomegalovirus, diphtheria, encephalitis, and dental abscesses.

A monoclonal gammopathy-associated type is associated with autoimmune disorders (e.g., rheumatoid arthritis, primary biliary cirrhosis, Sjögren syndrome, dermatomyositis, anaphylactoid purpura) and internal malignancies (malignant insulinoma, gallbladder carcinoma, carcinoid tumor, pituitary–adrenocortical neoplasms).

Clinical characteristics in light skin (Fitzpatrick skin types I–III)

The upper back, nape of the neck, lateral proximal extremities, and face with characteristic sparing of the hands and feet, develop an indolent swelling with a distinct hard feeling (Figures 66.1 and 66.2). The skin is like hard rubber and cannot be raised in folds. There is no hyperpigmentation; the skin may rather be slightly lighter. The disease remains stable over the years but may regress spontaneously depending on the possible etiologic associated diseases.

Histopathology shows massive deposition of acid mucopolysaccharides in the dermis and subcutaneous tissue.

Clinical characteristics in dark skin (Fitzpatrick skin types IV–V)

Patients present with feelings of tightness in the area affected, a movement restriction comprising limited body mobility and facial expressions, or difficulties in mastication and articulation (Figures 66.3 and 66.4). Erythema is not seen in dark skin, but one can feel the firm, indurated skin. *Peau d'orange* appearance of the skin is seen with careful observation and is accentuated when squeezing the area of the skin.

Investigations

Skin biopsy for histopathology to confirm the clinical diagnosis.

The epidermis is normal. The dermis is 3–4 times thicker than normal. The collagen fibers appear swollen and are separated by wide spaces. Mucin is found in the fenestrated spaces with special stains, such as Alcian blue stain at pH 2.5 or an iron colloidal stain. Subcutaneous tissue fat is replaced by coarse collagen fibers. Fibroblast proliferation is absent.

Investigations to detect the underlying disorder: FBS, HbA1C, serum protein electrophoresis.

Ultrasonography or magnetic resonance imaging (MRI) to evaluate skin thickness at baseline and after treatment.

Treatments

- Post-infective scleredema is benign, is self-limiting and resolves spontaneously within 6 months to 2 years.
- Scleredema associated with diabetes or monoclonal gammopathy is chronic and disabling, with little tendency to remission. In patients with associated conditions, the skin disorder can resolve or improve if the treatment of the primary disease is successful.
- At present, no effective treatment is known; however, phototherapy (UVA1, PUVA, and narrow-band UVB) is the first choice.
- Electron-beam radiotherapy, photopheresis, intravenous immunoglobulin, immunosuppressive agents (ciclosporin A, methotrexate), high-dose penicillin, corticosteroids (local, intralesional, and systemic), tamoxifen, and allopurinol have been used with variable success.

Further reading

Kreuter A (2018). Scleroedema adultorum: Klinik, Diagnostik, Differenzialdiagnose, therapeutisches Vorgehen [Scleredema adultorum: Clinical presentation, diagnostic workup, differential diagnosis, treatment option]. *Hautarzt*;69(11):908–915.

Pournazari M, Mohamadzadeh D, Assar S, et al. (2024). Treatment of Scleredema Adultorum of Buschke with Intravenous Immunoglobulin and Mycophenolate Mofetil in a 14-Year-Old Girl: A Case Report. *J Med Case Rep*;18(1):93.

Rongioletti F (2024). Cutaneous Mucinoses. In: Griffiths C, et al. (eds). *Rook's Textbook of Dermatology*, 10th ed. John Wiley & Sons Ltd., UK: 57.9.

DOI: 10.1201/9781003479512-66

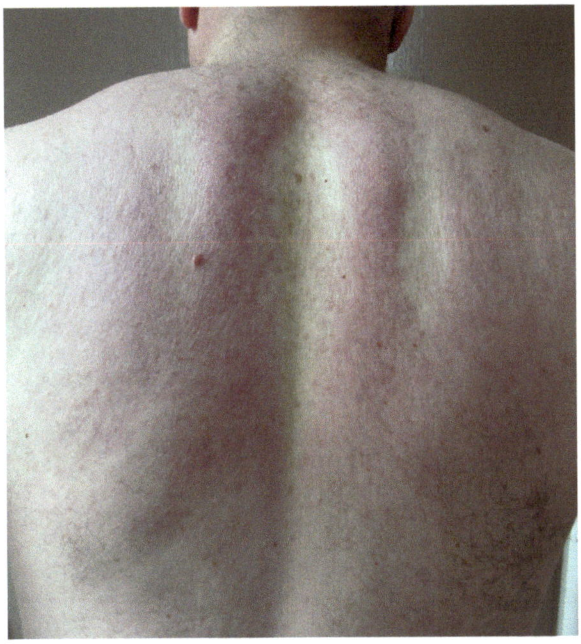

FIGURE 66.1 Scleredema in a diabetic patient with firm, non-pitting edema and induration on the upper back, neck, and shoulders on a red background FST1. (Courtesy Prof. Ian Coulson, UK.)

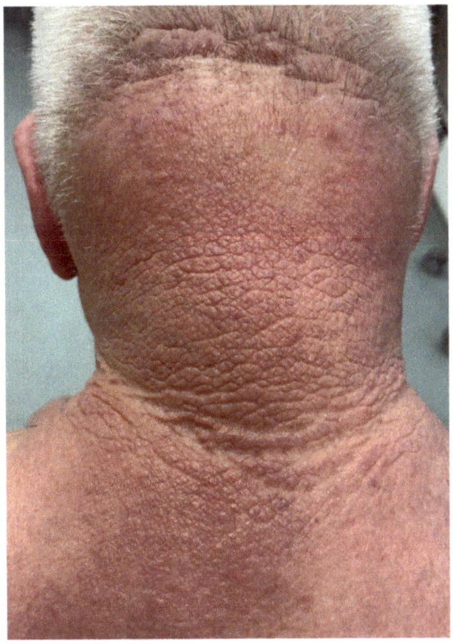

FIGURE 66.2 Scleredema adultorum of Buschke in a diabetic man FST1. Firm, non-pitting edema and induration on the upper back, neck, and shoulders on a red background. (Courtesy Dr. Richard Ashton, UK.)

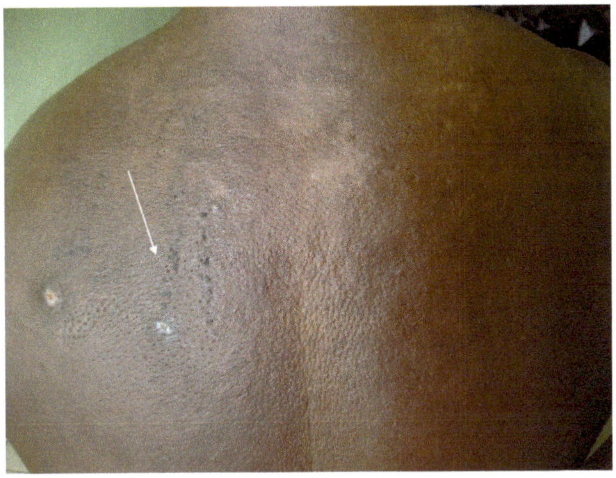

FIGURE 66.3 Scleredema in FST5. This 45-year-old diabetic man's complaint was tightening and feeling heaviness of the back of the upper chest and neck. Note erythema is not a feature in dark skin. The skin looks odematous, shiny and indurated. *Peau d'orange* appearance of the skin is seen in careful observation (arrow).

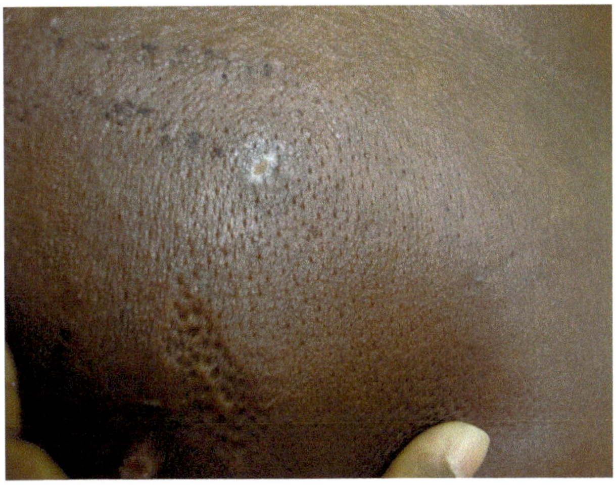

FIGURE 66.4 Scleredema in a diabetic man FST5. *Peau d'orange* appearance of the skin is accentuated when this area of the skin is squeezed.

67
MUCINOSES, SCLEROMYXEDEMA

Introduction

The main characteristic of cutaneous mucinoses is abnormal mucin deposition in the skin. Mucin is a normal component of the dermal extracellular matrix produced in small amounts by fibroblasts. Mucin is capable of absorbing 1000 times its own weight in water, thus playing a major role in maintaining the salt and water balance of the dermis. However, in disease conditions, mucin is increased, and since it holds water (hygroscopic), the dermal connective tissue is edematous.

The cutaneous mucinoses are divided into two groups: Primary (idiopathic) and secondary. Primary mucinoses can be divided into dermal and follicular mucinoses. Scleromyxedema, scleredema, and myxedema in thyroid disease (both localized [pretibial] and generalized myxedema) are primary dermal mucinoses.

Scleromyxedema is characterized by a generalized papular eruption on a sclerodermoid background, mucin deposition, increased fibroblast proliferation, fibrosis, and monoclonal gammopathy. It has systemic implications due to mucin deposition in the endocardium, the walls of myocardial blood vessels, interstitium of the kidneys, lungs, pancreas, adrenal glands, and nerves.

Epidemiology

Scleromyxedema is a rare disease that affects adults between the ages of 30 and 80 years (mean 59 years). It is rare in infants and young children.

Associated diseases

Systemic manifestations associated with mucinoses include monoclonal gammopathies (in scleromyxedema and scleredema), diabetes (in scleredema), hyperthyroidism (in pretibial myxedema), hypothyroidism (in generalized myxedema), or scleroderma (in papular and nodular mucinosis).

Clinical characteristics in light skin (Fitzpatrick skin types I–III)

Scleromyxedema is a rare chronic and progressive fibrosis of the dermis with mucin deposition without thyroid dysfunction (Figures 67.1 and 67.2). Most patients have paraproteinemia, which is probably etiological. There are several clinical variants despite the rarity of this condition. Most patients present the generalized form, which, however, may start as localized mucin deposition in the skin. Numerous tiny papules may be scattered on the trunk and extremities and coalesce to form large areas of induration. In particular, the face and hands may be erythematous. On the trunk, the thickened skin shows coarse bound-down folds. Other signs of mucin deposition are stiffness, muscle weakness, esophageal motility disturbances similar to scleroderma, and pulmonary dysfunction.

Clinical characteristics in dark skin (Fitzpatrick skin types IV–V)

This is a very rare condition (Figures 67.3 to 67.6). The typical skin features are a widespread eruption of 2–3 mm, firm, waxy, closely spaced, dome-shaped or flat-topped papules involving the dorsal aspect of the upper limbs, head and neck region, upper trunk, and thighs. Papules are arranged in a linear pattern; the surrounding skin is shiny and thick (i.e., sclerodermoid). Deep furrowing on the trunk, shoulders, limbs, and glabella. Edema and a brownish discoloration may be seen in the involved areas. Erythema is not a prominent feature in dark skin.

Investigations

In histopathology, scleromyxedema is characterized by a triad of microscopic features: (i) a diffuse deposit of mucin in the upper and mid-reticular dermis; (ii) an increase in collagen; (iii) a proliferation of irregularly arranged fibroblasts.

Mucin is seen on hematoxylin and eosin stains as a light blue-stained material between collagen bundles. Special stains are Alcian blue at pH 2.5 (blue color), colloidal iron, and toluidine blue at pH 4.0 (blue color).

Serum electrophoresis with immunofixation.

Thyroid function test results are normal.

Internal organ evaluation if clinically warranted.

Treatments

- There is no specific definitive treatment for scleromyxedema.
- Intravenous immunoglobulin therapy (alone or in combination with other drugs) is the first-line therapy for both skin involvement and extracutaneous manifestation. The dose is 2 g/kg for 5 days per month for at least 6 months. The response is not permanent, and maintenance infusions are spaced out to every 6–8 weeks.
- Thalidomide or lenalidomide (100–400 mg daily) and/or systemic steroids are the second line of treatment, more often in combination with intravenous immunoglobulins.
- Autologous peripheral blood stem cell transplantation can be considered a third line of treatment.

Further reading

Fasano G, Valenti G, D'Amico D, et al. (2023). Combination of Intravenous Immunoglobulin, Oral Prednisone, and Methotrexate for Managing Scleromyxedema: Case Report and Literature Discussion. *Dermatol Reports*;16(2):9803.

Guarneri A, Cioni M, Rongioletti F (2017). High-Dose Intravenous Immunoglobulin Therapy for Scleromyxoedema: A Prospective Open-Label Clinical Trial Using an Objective Score of Clinical Evaluation System. *J Eur Acad Dermatol Venereol*;31(7):1157–1160.

Rongioletti F (2024). Cutaneous Mucinoses. In: Griffiths C, et al. (eds). *Rook's Textbook of Dermatology*, 10th ed. John Wiley & Sons Ltd., UK: 57.2.

DOI: 10.1201/9781003479512-67

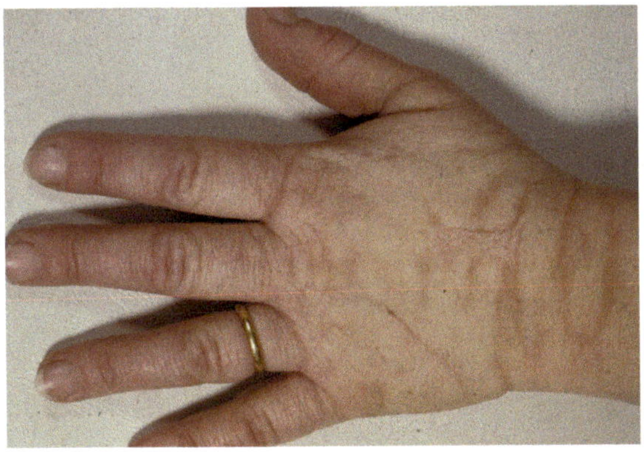

FIGURE 67.1 Scleromyxedema FST1. (Courtesy Dr. Richard Ashton, UK.)

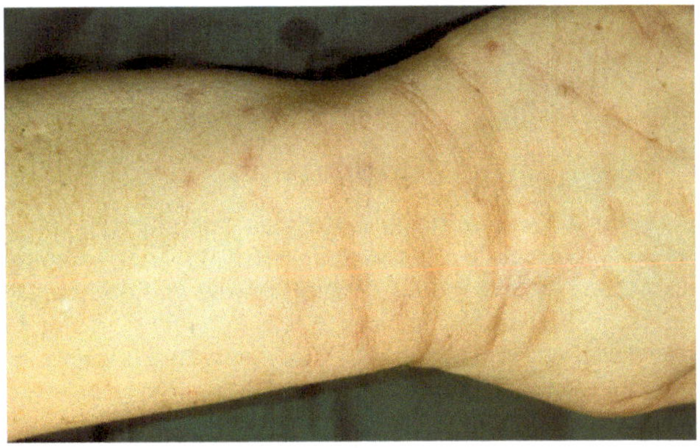

FIGURE 67.2 Scleromyxedema FST1. (Courtesy Dr. Richard Ashton, UK.)

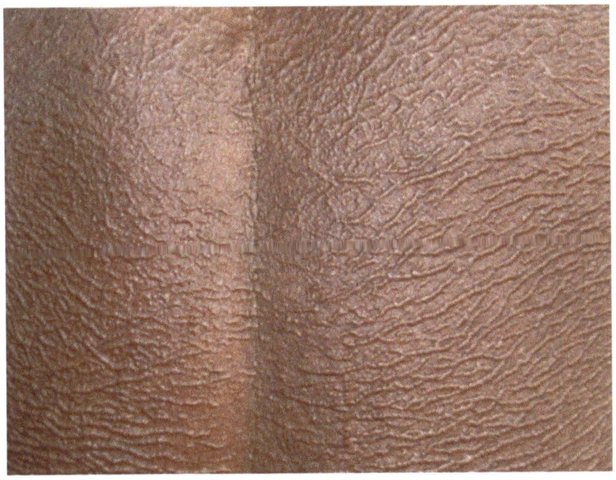

FIGURE 67.3 Scleromyxedema: Papules are arranged in a linear pattern in the back of the trunk FST5.

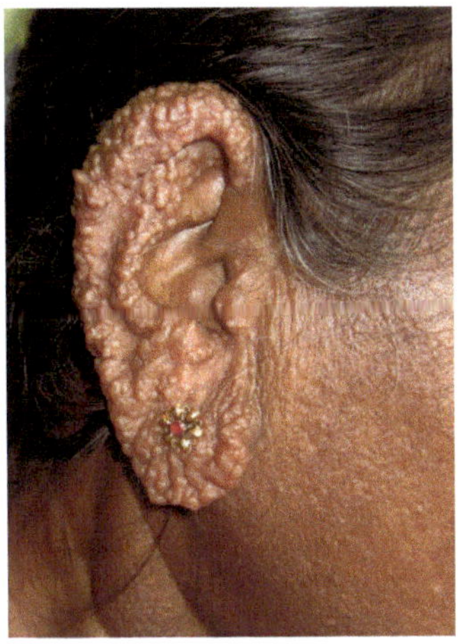

FIGURE 67.4 Scleromyxedema: Papules in the ear FST5.

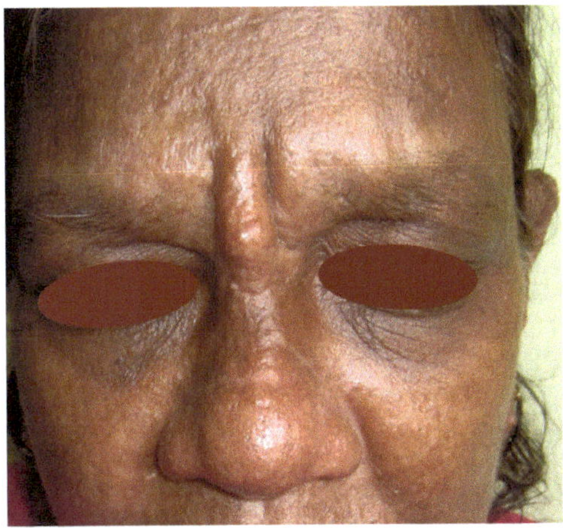

FIGURE 67.5 The glabella typically is involved with deep longitudinal folding that gives the appearance of a leonine face; skin is shiny and thick FST5.

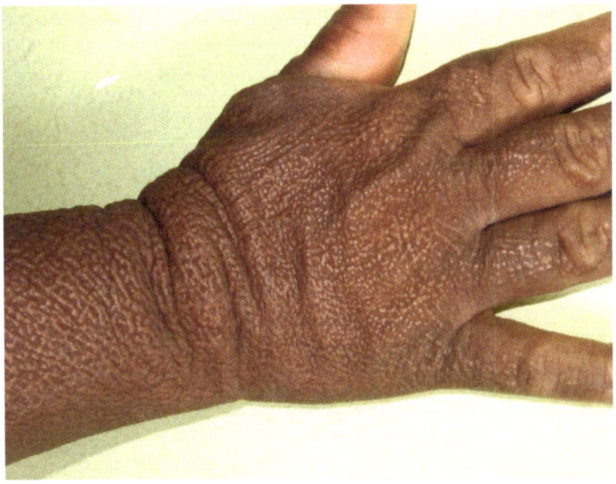

FIGURE 67.6 Scleromyxedema: Widespread eruption of closely spaced papules on the back of the hand FST5. Papules are arranged in a linear pattern. The surrounding skin is shiny and thick (i.e., sclerodermoid), and deep furrowing is evident on the dorsum of the hand. Note 'doughnut sign' over the proximal interphalangeal joints.

68
MYCOSIS FUNGOIDES

Introduction

Mycosis fungoides (MF) is the most common type of primary cutaneous T-cell lymphoma (CTCL). It is commonly associated with an indolent clinical course. Peripheral epidermotropic T-cells, the memory T-cells (CD45RO+) expressing the T-cell receptor (TCR) and CD4+ immunophenotype, are the main cell type. The etiology of MF is not yet established. It is suggested that UV radiation has a protective effect on MF and Sézary syndrome (SS).

MF may have many clinical forms: Hypopigmented asymptomatic patches with indistinct margins; scaly, slightly atrophic (wrinkled) erythematous patches; persistent, polymorphic, erythematous plaques; ulcers; tumors; or erythroderma. These are mostly asymptomatic but may become pruritic. There are many clinical variants of MF: Folliculotropic, poikiloderma, hypopigmented, capillaritis-like, verrucous/hyperkeratotic, psoriasiform, ichthyosiform, or bullous.

Epidemiology

The incidence of MF (0.64/100,000) is increasing possibly due to improved diagnosis as well as a genuine increase in disease incidence.

Clinical characteristics in light skin (Fitzpatrick skin types I–III)

The earliest lesions in light-skinned individuals are pink-to-slightly reddish patches with fine, dry scaling called parapsoriasis of Brocq (Figures 68.1 and 68.2). If the patches are under 6 cm in diameter, the condition is called small plaque parapsoriasis; if over 6 cm large plaque parapsoriasis, with the latter usually being seen as early MF. The patches may develop digitiform extensions, hence the term digitate dermatitis. They may persist for years until they coalesce, characteristically leaving spots of normal skin in them, which are called *nappes claires* or Leredde's sign. Over time, the patches may turn into palpable plaques, often with a bizarre outline like rings or horseshoes. The face and scalp, as well as palms and soles, may become involved. In the third stage, the fungus-like tumors, which gave the disease its historical name, develop. These have a tendency to ulcerate. However, there are also cases that begin with fungating tumors (MF d'emblée). Pruritus is characteristic, although not always present. The course of MF is often protracted, with years or decades being common. Depending on the skin structures primarily involved, many variants may be observed: follicular MF often appears with a goosebump-like eruption, purpuric and telangiectatic lesions may be seen, and hypopigmented MF is mainly a disease of children and is particularly obvious in late summer when light-skinned persons have a suntan. Syringotropic MF may be associated histopathologically with epithelial islands. MF palmaris and plantaris is rare, with only few cases reported. Nail involvement has been observed with generally uncharacteristic alterations. It may appear as eczematous, dyshidrotic, hyperkeratotic, verrucous, or ulcerated lesions, as dry pulpitis or pustulosis. Bullous MF is very rare. Pagetoid reticulosis of Woringer–Kolopp is a single plaque that is extremely chronic. Granulomatous slack skin is a rare variant with the localized loss of elastic fibers.

Histopathology is typical for MF with a positive T-cell receptor gene rearrangement in the majority of cases. However, a French study has shown that up to 16 biopsies were needed to establish the diagnosis in difficult cases. The prognosis is good in stages I and II. Resistance to topical steroids is common. The classical treatment consists of chlormethine gel and radiotherapy.

Sézary syndrome is a primarily erythrodermic and leukemic form with generalized lymph node swelling and circulating Sézary (Lutzner) cells characterized by convoluted nuclei.

Clinical characteristics in dark skin (Fitzpatrick skin types IV–V)

Hypopigmented MF (HMF) is the most common clinical presentation in darker-skinned individuals (Figure 68.3). HMF is characterized by striking hypopigmented patches often involving the trunk and limbs, especially the sunlight-covered areas such as buttocks, medial aspects of the upper arms, and upper thighs. The lesions are hypopigmented, dry, and finely scaly with ill-defined borders. They are clinically mistaken for pityriasis versicolor, leprosy, and early vitiligo, and in most patients, the diagnosis and treatment are delayed for many years (Ranawaka 2010, 2021). Presentation with erythematous plaques, poikilodermatous lesions, or papules and nodules has also been occasionally observed.

Investigations

The histological features of MF vary according to the clinical stage. The earliest pathological features of MF are the presence of a moderate lymphocytic infiltrate in the papillary dermis. As the disease progresses with the development of thicker plaques, prominent epidermotropism develops (i.e., selective colonization of the epidermis by atypical T-cells with cerebriform nuclei), often with Pautrier microabscesses (i.e., clusters of atypical lymphocytes in the non-spongiotic epidermis).

The histopathological diagnosis of early MF can be subjective and is best made in collaboration with the clinician (clinico-pathological correlation). It is often wise to take several elliptical biopsies from lesions that do not show secondary changes such as excoriation or impetiginization, and to repeat biopsies as the clinical picture evolves over a period of months or even years. Usually, clinical suspicion precedes histopathological confirmation by many years.

Modern diagnostics require immunophenotyping of the epidermotropic peripheral T-lymphocytes that are CD2+, CD3+, CD4+, and CD5+; a minority have a CD4− and CD8+, CD4− and CD8−, or CD4+ and CD8+ phenotype.

Immunostaining for multiple myeloma oncogene (MUM-1) may be useful for the differentiation of Sézary syndrome (positive) from mycosis fungoides (negative).

DOI: 10.1201/9781003479512-68

Treatments

- The choice of initial treatment for the MF patient will depend on the stage of the disease as well as the patient's performance status. A wide range of possible treatments exists, including topical steroids, topical chemotherapy (mechlorethamine [nitrogen mustard] and carmustine [BCNU]), and phototherapy – both UVB and psoralen with UVA (PUVA) and UVA-1 – that are mostly used by dermatologists. Other advanced therapies are decided by the oncologist.
- The prognosis of HMF is excellent, with overall survival rates at 5 and 10 years being 100%. There are several case reports where complete remission has been reported with treatment using topical potent steroids, topical tacrolimus, and phototherapy (NB-UVB, PUVA, or natural sunlight) in combination or as individual therapies (Ranawaka et al. 2011, Ranawaka 2021).

Further reading

André R (2024). Mycosis Fungoides Palmaris and Plantaris. *It J Dermatol Venereol*;159(1):1–3.

Fränken J, Haneke E (1995). Mycosis Fungoides Bullosa. *Hautarzt*;46(3):186–189.

Haneke E, Tulusan AH, Weidner F (1977). Histological Features of "Pagetoid Reticulosis" (Woringer-Kolopp) in Pre-Mycosis Fungoides. *Arch Dermatol Res*;258:265–273.

Lebowitz E, Geller S, Flores E, et al. (2019). Survival, Disease Progression and Prognostic Factors in Elderly Patients with Mycosis Fungoides and Sézary Syndrome: A Retrospective Analysis of 174 Patients. *J Eur Acad Dermatol Venereol*;33(1):108–114.

Ranawaka RR (2021). Hypopigmented Mycosis Fungoides. In Ranawaka RR, et al. (eds). *Atlas of Dermatoses in Pigmented Skin*. Springer, Singapore: 921.

Ranawaka RR, Abeygunasekara PH, de Silva MV (2011). Hypopigmented Mycosis Fungoides in Type V Skin: A Report of 5 Cases. *Case Rep Dermatol Med*;2011:190572.

Wilsch L, Schmidt G, Haneke E (1977). Spätmanifeste Dermatochalasis [Late-onset cutis laxa (generalized elastolysis)]. *Dtsch med Wschr*;102:1451–1454.

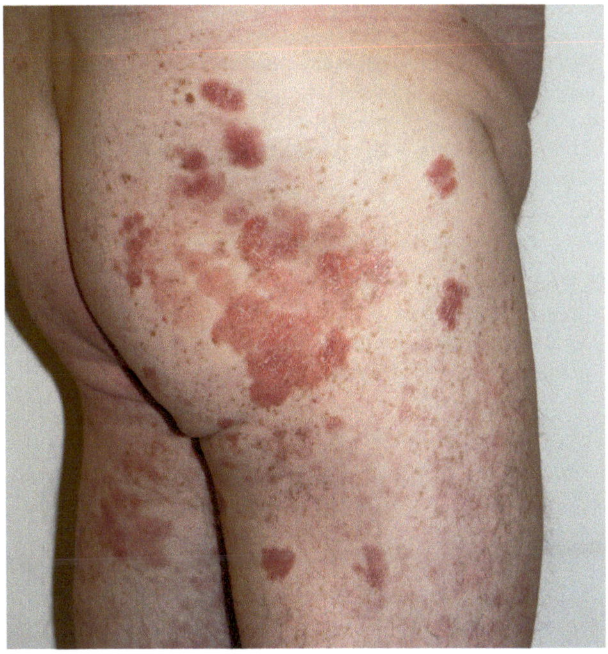

FIGURE 68.1 Cutaneous T-cell lymphoma present as psoriasiform plaques in a man FST1. (Courtesy Prof. Ian Coulson, UK.)

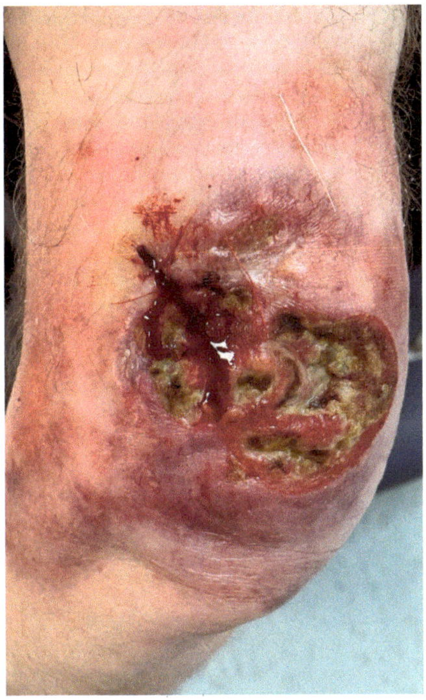

FIGURE 68.2 Ulcerated cutaneous T-cell lymphoma FST1. (Courtesy Prof. Ian Coulson, UK.)

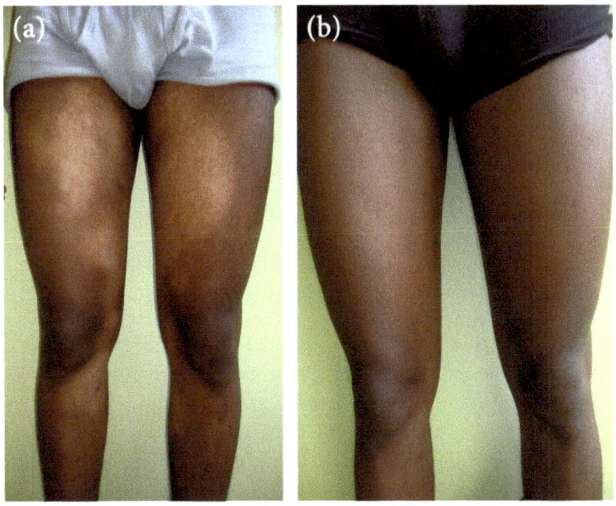

FIGURE 68.3 Hypopigmented mycosis fungoides in an 18-year-old boy. He was treated for vitiligo for more than 3 years. Note these patches are limited to medial aspect of limbs. He was treated with psoralen plus ultraviolet A (PUVA) (a) before treatments, (b) after 51 sessions of PUVA lesions have completely disappeared.

69
PRETIBIAL MYXEDEMA

Introduction

An infiltrative dermopathy due to mucin deposition, usually arising on the shins, is one of the signs of hyperthyroidism, especially of Graves' (Basedow) disease. Patients present with bilateral thickening and induration of the skin on the shins and dorsa of the feet. There are four main clinical variants: *Diffuse non-pitting edema* (43%); *plaque type* (27%); *nodular* (18%); and *elephantiasis* (5%).

Epidemiology

Pretibial myxedema is found in 1–5% of patients with Graves' disease, but in up to 25% of patients who have exophthalmos. Women are affected more often than men (3:1) with a peak of incidence at age 50–60 years.

Associated diseases

Pretibial myxedema is one of the signs of Graves' disease (along with goiter, exophthalmos, thyroid acropathy, and high circulating levels of long-acting thyroid-stimulating hormone).

Less commonly, it has been described in patients with Hashimoto thyroiditis and in those with no past or present history of thyroid dysfunction.

Clinical characteristics in light skin (Fitzpatrick skin types I–III)

Pretibial myxedema is an extrathyroidal manifestation of autoimmune thyroid disease. It is almost always associated with thyroid exophthalmus. It may cause a non-pitting edema on the shins or develop into large areas of hard waxy brownish swelling with a *peau d'orange* aspect (Figure 69.1). It is probably due to insulin-like growth factor 1 (IGF-1R) whose receptor colocalizes with the thyroid-stimulating hormone receptor in human orbital and possibly shin fibroblasts. Thus, treatment with teprotumumab, an inhibitor of IGF-1R, has successfully been used for its treatment.

Clinical characteristics in dark skin (Fitzpatrick skin types IV–V)

This is characterized by bilateral thickening and induration of the skin on the shins and dorsa of the feet (Figure 69.2). Plaques or nodules on the shins are skin-colored and may exhibit a characteristic orange peel appearance.

Investigations

Thyroid-stimulating hormone (TSH) is abnormally low and long-acting thyroid stimulator antibodies (free T4 and/or T3) are elevated in 50% of patients with Graves' disease.

Histopathology may show a diffuse deposit of mucin composed mostly of hyaluronic acid in the upper and mid-reticular dermis, confirmed with an Alcian blue stain at pH 2.5.

Treatments

- Normalizing thyroid function does not improve the cutaneous lesions.
- Localized myxedema may clear spontaneously in 3–5 years.
- The first line of pharmacological therapy is medium to high potency topical corticosteroids applied under occlusive dressings or delivered by intralesional injection.
- For the severe elephantiasis form, rituximab, plasmapheresis, intravenous immunoglobulins, and octreotide with and without surgical shave removal have been tried with some benefit.
- The use of compression stockings and gradient pneumatic compression is useful as they improve lymphedema.

Further reading

Bowens BK, Chou E, LaChance DP, et al. (2022). Graves' Disease Complicated by Concurrent Thyroid Eye Disease and Pretibial Myxedema Successfully Treated with Teprotumumab. *Clin Case Rep*;10(11):e6621.

Nguyen VB, Nguyen VVH, Van Le C, et al. (2024). Pretibial Myxedema in Graves' Disease: A Case Report and Treatment Review of the Literature. *Clin Case Rep*;12(2):e8478.

Rongioletti F (2024). Cutaneous Mucinoses. In: Griffiths C, et al. (eds). *Rook's Textbook of Dermatology*, 10th ed. John Wiley & Sons Ltd., UK: 57.11.

Wang S, Chen X, Bai J, et al. (2024). Tofacitinib Treatment for Pretibial Myxedema. *JAMA Dermatol*;160(5):578–580.

DOI: 10.1201/9781003479512-69

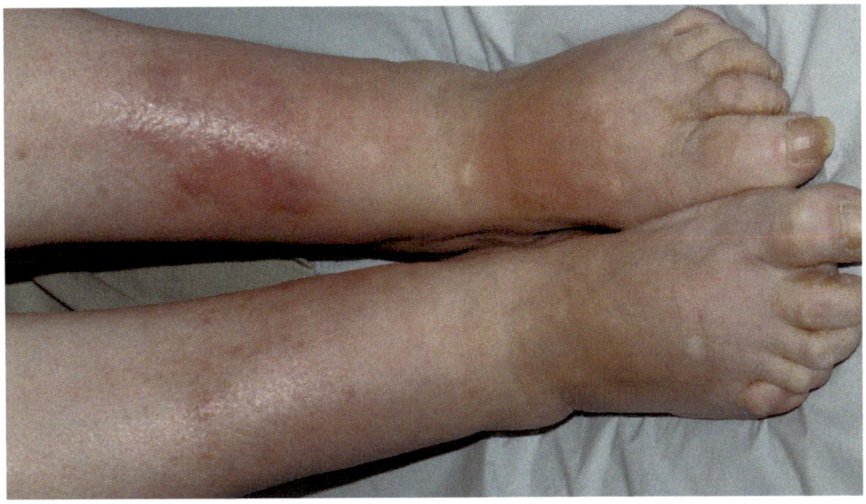

FIGURE 69.1 Pretibial myxedema, diffuse non-pitting edema type FST1. (Courtesy Prof. Ian Coulson, UK.)

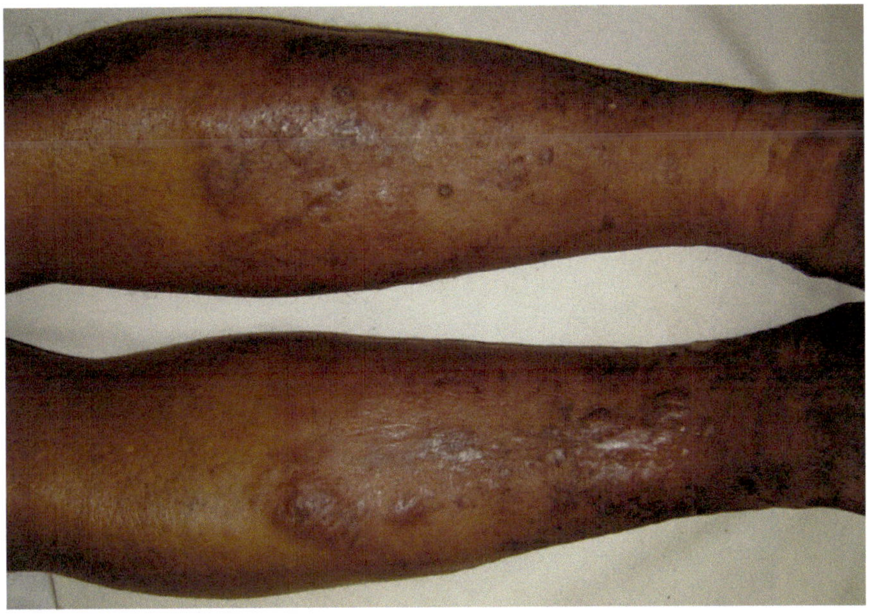

FIGURE 69.2 Pretibial myxedema, nodular type in a 76-year-old man with Graves' disease FST5.

70
EPIDERMAL NEVUS (KERATINOCYTIC NEVUS)

Introduction

Congenital hamartomas of epidermal structures can occur as isolated cutaneous lesions or in association with syndromes. These comprise a wide range of clinical and histological phenotypes. Congenital epidermal nevi (CEN) are usually present at birth, although some types can appear in the first few years of life. Single CEN lesions can be either round or linear, but larger or multiple lesions are often Blaschko linear in distribution. Epidermal nevi are very superficial and are therefore raised and can have the appearance of being 'stuck on' to the surface of the skin. Trichilemmal cyst nevus is deeper than the common epidermal nevi.

The term 'epidermal nevus syndrome' should be avoided as it is imprecise and comprises hard, soft, epidermolytic, comedonic, and sebaceous nevi with different prognoses and associations.

Associated diseases

CEN syndromes have a predilection for neurological, ophthalmological, skeletal, and endocrinological abnormalities. Examples are HRAS mosaicism, Proteus syndrome, PENS syndrome, CHILD syndrome, Becker nevus syndrome, and nevus comedonicus syndrome.

Clinical characteristics in light skin (Fitzpatrick skin types I–III)

There are different epidermal nevi that must be distinguished as they may be associated with different systemic alterations (Figure 70.1): Epidermal nevi with granular degeneration, or so-called epidermolytic nevi, have virtually no risk of association with neurocutaneous and other systemic manifestations, whereas 'soft epidermal nevi,' particularly those of sebaceous and basocellular types, may be part of a neurocutaneous syndrome (phacomatosis). This is important as it allows estimation of the risk at an early age when it is not yet clear whether there might be neurological and other symptoms.

Epidermolytic epidermal nevi are distributed in a Blaschko-linear pattern. The surface is rough, hard, verrucous, and often gray to brown. A parent with an epidermolytic nevus may have a child with epidermolytic ichthyosis, formerly called congenital bullous ichthyosiform erythroderma, a disease due to mutations of the genes for keratin 1 and 10.

Inflammatory linear verrucous epidermal nevus encompasses diverse inflammatory mosaic lesions that are characteristically pruritic. Its relationship to psoriasis is not yet entirely clear. The cases seen by the author were in girls and demonstrated a striking resemblance to linear psoriasis.

Munro's nevus is an acantholytic dyskeratotic epidermal nevus and probably represents a mosaic of Darier's dyskeratosis follicularis.

Blaschko-linear lesions may appear later in life. They are usually reddish lines and are called (adult) blaschkitis. Their histopathology varies from dyskeratosis follicularis to lichen planus, lichen striatus, eczema, psoriasis, etc.

Soft epidermal nevi may involve large areas and be linear or whorled in appearance. They are grayish brown to dark brown, sometimes covered with keratin masses. Biopsies may have a striking resemblance to so-called basal cell nevus or exophytic seborrheic keratosis.

Verrucous epidermal nevi may be clinically similar to soft epidermal nevi, but their histopathology is more wart-like, although without cytopathic HPV effects.

Linear sebaceous nevi are more yellowish-pink, often with a surface studded with large pore-like openings, sometimes with areas of hyperkeratosis.

A nevus comedonicus is a plaque or band-like lesion with many typical 'black-head' comedones.

As mentioned above, systematized non-epidermolytic epidermal nevi may be part of a neurocutaneous phacomatosis.

Clinical characteristics in dark skin (Fitzpatrick skin types IV–V)

Keratinocytic nevi in dark skin vary from pale brown to black with a soft velvety feel, verrucous or hyperkeratotic, and can have a prominent inflammatory component (inflammatory linear verrucous epidermal nevus – ILVEN) (Figures 70.2 and 70.3).

Investigations

Investigations are performed to assess neurological, ophthalmological, skeletal, and other organ system abnormalities, and should be assessed on an individual basis.

Biopsy of the epidermal nevus is required to make an exact diagnosis of the cellular origin type.

Investigation for extracutaneous abnormalities is individualized depending on the other system involvements.

Treatments

- Appropriate genetic counseling should be arranged as there is a possibility of transmitting the trait.
- Surgical excision can be suitable for small, single epidermal nevi.
- Ablative laser therapy is used to reduce thickness and/or hyperkeratosis of the lesion, and smaller verrucous lesions have been treated successfully with cryotherapy.

DOI: 10.1201/9781003479512-70

- Tangential (shave) excision is an easy alternative.
- ILVEN has been treated with CO_2 laser therapy with variable response.
- Topical calcipotriol, etanercept, and oral retinoids (acitretin) have been successful in some cases of ILVEN.

Further reading

Atzmony L, Ugwu N, Hamilton C, et al. (2022). Inflammatory Linear Verrucous Epidermal Nevus (ILVEN) Encompasses a Spectrum of Inflammatory Mosaic Disorders. *Pediatr Dermatol*;39(6):903–907.

Happle R (1991). How Many Epidermal Nevus Syndromes Exist? A Clinicogenetic Classification. *J Am Acad Dermatol*;25(3): 550–556.

Happle R, Haneke E (2021). More about Zlotnikov, the Man Who Explained Blaschko's Lines to Be a Mosaic. *Acta Derm Venereol*; 101(8):adv00521.

Morren MA, Fodstad H, Brems H, et al. (2024). Mosaic RASopathies Concept: Different Skin Lesions, Same Systemic Manifestations? *J Med Genet*;jmg-2023-109306.

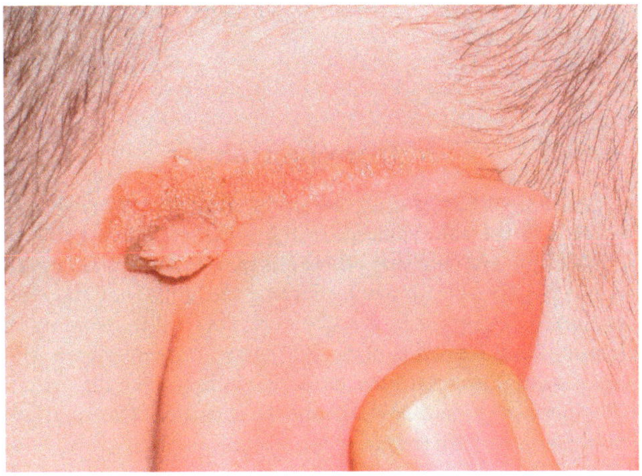

FIGURE 70.1 Linear epidermal nevus at the back of the ear FST1. (Courtesy Prof. Ian Coulson, UK.)

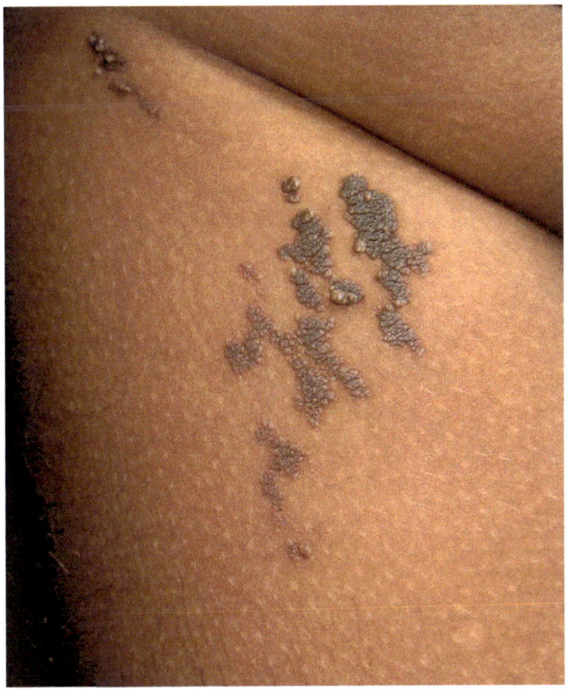

FIGURE 70.2 Congenital epidermal nevi in a 9-year-old girl FST5.

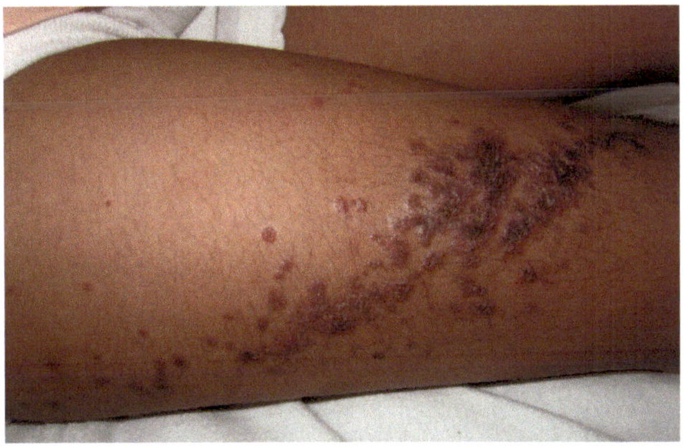

FIGURE 70.3 Inflammatory linear verrucous epidermal nevus FST5.

71
NEVUS OF OTA

Introduction

A nevus of Ota is a dermal melanocytosis that affects the sclera and the skin adjacent to the eye, distributed along the ophthalmic and maxillary divisions of the trigeminal nerve. It is an extensive, bluish patch affecting the bulbar and palpebral conjunctiva, the sclera, and the periorbital skin involving the temple, forehead, scalp, nose, ears, palate, and malar area. Most lesions are present at birth or develop during the first year of life, increasing in size and number in subsequent years. It does not disappear with time.

Epidemiology

Nevus of Ota usually presents in Asians and black people and is more common in women. It is especially common in the Japanese.

Associated diseases

It is rarely associated with nevus of Ito. Bilateral cases of nevus of Ota are sometimes associated with extensive Mongolian spots. Sturge–Weber and Klippel–Trenaunay syndromes have been infrequently associated with nevus of Ota. It may be associated with melanoma in the meninges or in the choroid, iris, or orbit.

Clinical characteristics in light skin (Fitzpatrick skin types I–III)

Nevus of Ota is a very rare condition in light-skinned persons (Figures 71.1 and 71.2). Usually, the extent is less than in skin of color.

Around the eye, with more lateral accentuation, a bluish-gray spot is found that may also affect the conjunctiva and bulbus oculi. It is cosmetically embarrassing but otherwise symptomless, except for ocular involvement where glaucoma was observed.

Clinical characteristics in dark skin (Fitzpatrick skin types IV–V)

Blue-dark gray pigmentation distributed along the ophthalmic and maxillary divisions of the trigeminal nerve, involving the adjacent sclera and conjunctiva (Figure 71.3).

Investigations

This is a clinical diagnosis.

Treatments

- Cosmetic camouflage.
- Q-switched lasers are the first-line treatment. Post-treatment hypo- or hyperpigmentation, scarring, and recurrence of the lesion can occur.
- Rare occurrences of malignant transformation have been reported. Any new subcutaneous nodule arising on a nevus of Ota should be investigated to exclude the possibility of melanoma.
- Close ophthalmological monitoring is essential in cases where the eye is involved.

Further reading

Chan JC, Shek SY, Kono T, et al. (2016). A Retrospective Analysis on the Management of Pigmented Lesions Using a Picosecond 755-nm Alexandrite Laser in Asians. *Lasers Surg Med*;48(1):2–9.

Gowda Venkatesha RR, Rajaram Mohan K, Sridhar Rao V, et al. (2024). Concurrent Occurrence of Trichilemmal Cyst and Nevus of Ota: Case Series. *Cureus*;16(1):e52439.

Huang WH, Wang HW, Sun QN, et al. (2013). New Classification of Nevus of Ota. *Chin Med J*;126(20):3910–3914.

Zhao W, Yang Y, Shi H, et al. (2024). Picosecond Alexandrite Laser Treatment of Nevus of Ota in Children. *Lasers Surg Med*;56(5):437–445.

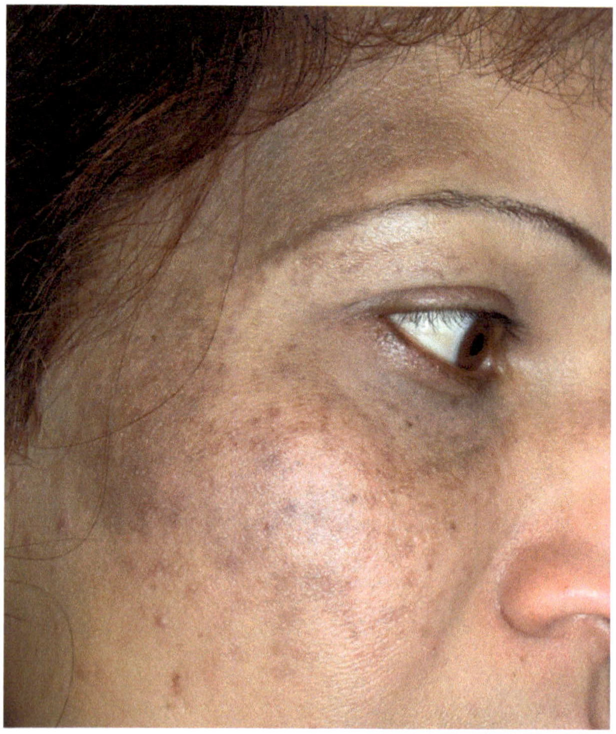

FIGURE 71.1 Nevus of Ota FST3. (Courtesy Prof. Ian Coulson, UK.)

DOI: 10.1201/9781003479512-71

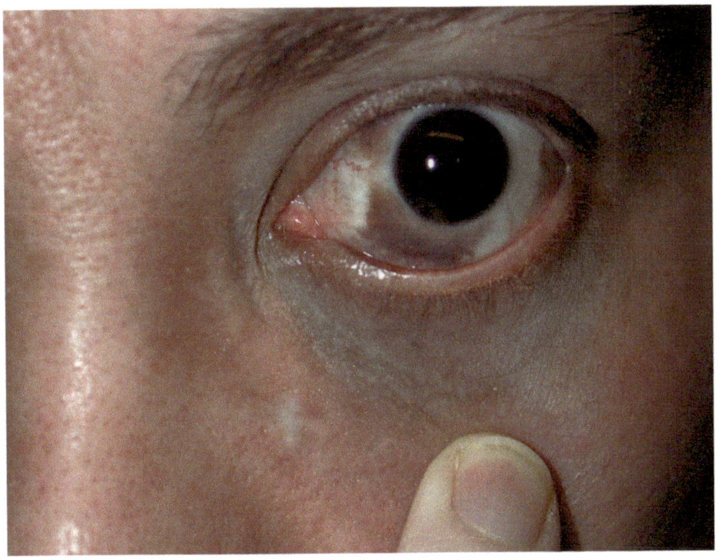

FIGURE 71.2 Nevus of Ota involving the sclera FST1. (Courtesy Dr. Richard Ashton, UK.)

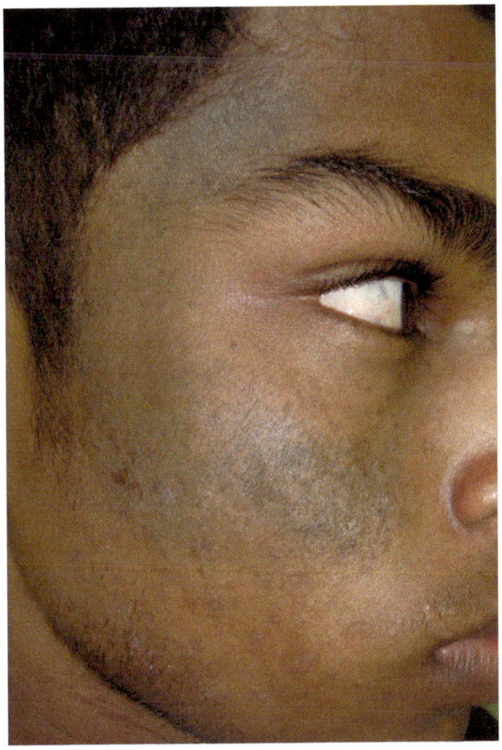

FIGURE 71.3 Nevus of Ota FST5.

72
SEBACEOUS NEVUS

Introduction

This is a congenital epidermal nevus where the predominant cells develop into sebaceous glands. Epidermal nevi are by their nature very superficial and are therefore raised, and can have the appearance of being 'stuck on' to the surface.

For single isolated sebaceous nevi, the evidence suggests that they are benign tumors with a risk of malignant transformation. Syringocystadenoma papilliferum occurs in sebaceous nevi in approximately 1%, whereas basal cell carcinoma occurs in less than 1%, and squamous cell carcinoma is rare.

Epidemiology

Nevus sebaceous, by definition of congenital epidermal nevi, is present at birth or becomes apparent in the first years of life. Its appearance develops over time and becomes hyperkeratotic.

Associated diseases

Linear sebaceous nevus syndrome may be associated with central nervous system, ocular, skeletal, and cardiovascular anomalies, as well as cognitive developmental delay; the nevus sebaceous is often on the face, neck, and scalp.

Clinical characteristics in light skin (Fitzpatrick skin types I–III)

Isolated sebaceous nevus is a circumscribed yellowish lesion with a cobblestone surface. Its color may take on a pink tone (Figure 72.1). The lesion may increase during puberty due to the effect of androgenic hormones. It is often localized on the face, particularly on the forehead and scalp. With time, secondary skin tumors may develop, most commonly syringocystadenoma papilliferum, trichoblastoma, basal cell carcinoma, and squamous cell carcinoma. This is seen as a nodular growth which may show oozing in syringocystadenoma papilliferum and ulceration in basal cell carcinoma.

Clinical characteristics in dark skin (Fitzpatrick skin types IV–V)

Sebaceous nevi have a greasy feel and appearance, and are often yellowish or pink at birth. Later, they become more verrucous and deeply pigmented to brown or black (Figures 72.2 and 72.3).

Investigations

Histopathology is performed to confirm the clinical diagnosis of the nevus and any potential secondary tumors.

Treatments

- Sebaceous nevus is permanent if not surgically removed. Surgical excision can be suitable for small, single, epidermal nevi.
- Ablative laser therapy is used to reduce thickness and/or hyperkeratosis of the lesion, and smaller verrucous lesions have been treated successfully with cryotherapy.
- Trametinib interferes downstream of KRAS and HRAS in the MAPK signaling pathway and was shown to improve sebaceous nevus.

Further reading

Dartaha R, Jobran AWM (2023). Therapeutic Effects of CO_2 Laser Therapy for Congenital Sebaceous Nevus. *J Surg Case Rep*;2023(8):rjad467.

Haller CN, Leszczynska MA, Brichta L, et al. (2024). Topical Trametinib for Epidermal and Sebaceous Nevi in a Child with Schimmelpenning-Feuerstein-Mims Syndrome. *Pediatr Dermatol*;May–Jun;41(3):523–525.

Pang S, Cevik J, Sreedharan S, et al. (2024). Rate of Benign and Malignant Secondary Tumors Associated with Nevus Sebaceous: A Systematic Review and Meta-Analysis. *Ann Plast Surg*;92(6):711–719.

Pelivani N, Houriet C, Haneke E (2010). Trichilemmal Cyst Nevus with a Sebaceous Nevus Component. *Dermatology*;221(4):289–291.

Ponomarev IV, Topchiy SB, Andrusenko YN, et al. (2023). Successful Treatment of Sebaceous Nevus with Copper Vapor Laser. *J Lasers Med Sci*;14:e20.

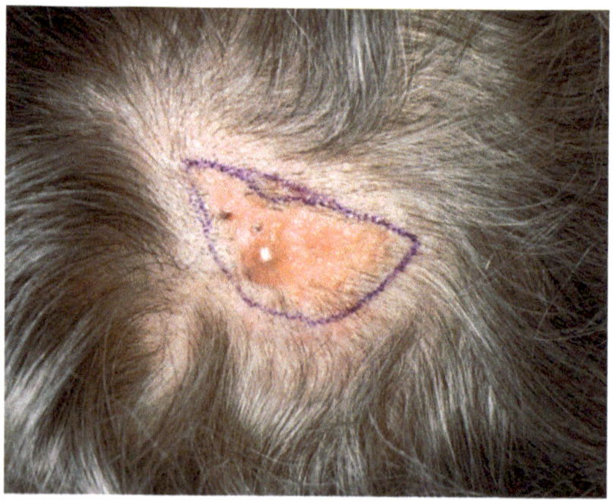

FIGURE 72.1 Sebaceous nevus on the scalp FST1. (Courtesy Prof. Ian Coulson, UK.)

DOI: 10.1201/9781003479512-72

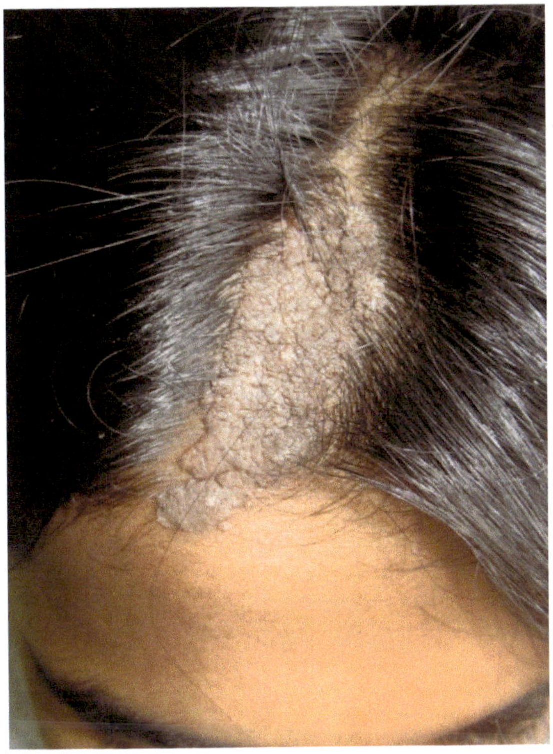

FIGURE 72.2 Sebaceous nevus on the scalp in a 15-year-old girl FST5.

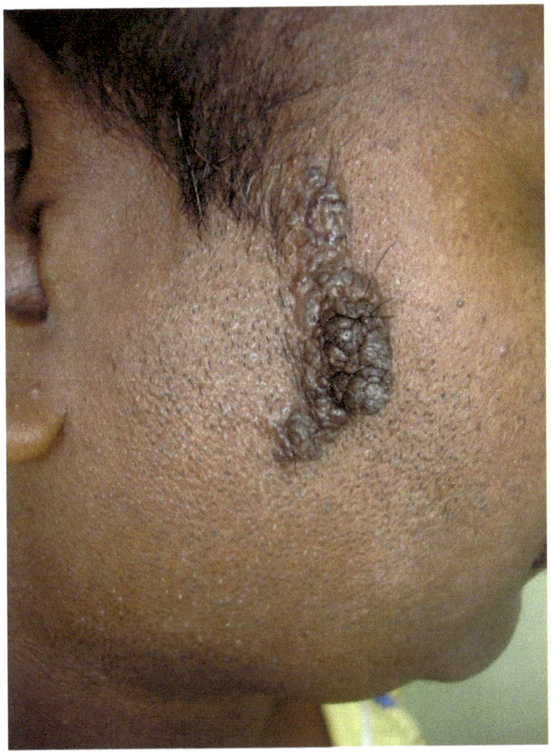

FIGURE 72.3 Sebaceous nevus on the face in a 45-year-old man FST5. With time this becomes more verrucous and deeply pigmented.

73
OCHRONOSIS

Introduction

Ochronosis is gray-brown or blue-black discoloration of the skin. This can be endogenous or exogenous. Endogenous ochronosis occurs in patients with alkaptonuria. Alkaptonuria is a rare, congenital, autosomal recessive inherited disorder. The patients present with lower back pain between 25 and 40 years of age, which later progresses to kyphosis and/or ankylosis. Darkening appears on the ear cartilages, sclerae, conjunctivae, and less often the axillae and groin. On the face, brown mottled pigmentation (sometimes in a butterfly distribution), dusky discoloration of the neck and trunk, and rarely, pigmentation of the palmar and plantar skin are seen.

Exogenous ochronosis is more common and is due to topical use of bleaching creams primarily containing hydroquinone, but it may also be caused by the use of phenol or resorcinol. This can occur in all skin phototypes, but it is more common in darker skin types (Fitzpatrick skin types IV, V–VI) who live in Western countries with white people.

Epidemiology

Exogenous ochronosis is common among women of darker skin types.

Alkaptonuria is very rare (1:250,000 to 1: 1,000,000).

Associated diseases

Alkaptonuria patients may have disabling arthritis mainly in the hip and knee joints. Older patients often develop calcification of the aortic or mitral valves or coronary arteries.

Clinical characteristics in light skin (Fitzpatrick skin types I–III)

Ochronosis, also called black urine disease, is a rare autosomal recessive metabolic disease due to the accumulation of homogentisic acid that undergoes a characteristic color change when deposited in the skin, predominantly on the zygoma, but extending to the entire face and other exposed areas, the skin takes on a dusky grayish-brown hue (Figure 73.1).

Exogenous ochronosis is due to the long-term topical application of phenolic compounds, particularly hydroquinone in skin-lightening creams, which are probably accumulated in elastic tissue and oxidized under the influence of sunlight in the skin to form a melanin-like agranular brown pigment. It is virtually not seen in light-skinned persons.

Clinical characteristics in dark skin (Fitzpatrick skin types IV–V)

Endogenous ochronosis or alkaptonuria is very rare in our setting.

Exogenous ochronosis has only recently been observed in Sri Lanka with the high trend of unsupervised use of whitening/ bleaching creams (Figure 73.2). This discoloration is either dark gray or blackish; blue-black discoloration is never observed in dark skin.

Investigations

Alkaptonuria diagnosis is established by urine organic acid analysis, which reveals homogentisic acid.

Exogenous ochronosis diagnosis is clinical.

Histopathological examination of both endogenous and exogenous ochronosis is similar and is characterized by comma- or banana-shaped ochronotic collagen bundles and ochre (brownish-yellow) pigment in the papillary dermis.

Treatment

Treatment of alkaptonuria: No definitive treatment exists; nitisinone, ascorbic acid 1 g/day in divided doses, and a low tyrosine and phenylalanine, protein-restricted diet (1.3 g/kg/ day) may be beneficial.

Treatment of exogenous ochronosis:

- Discontinuation of hydroquinone use; strict sun protection/avoidance. Treatment of discoloration is difficult.
- Some improvement may occur with the use of retinoic acid.
- Topical low-potency corticosteroids may be of benefit in combination with photoprotection.
- Exogenous ochronosis may improve with superficial dermabrasion using carbon dioxide laser, glycolic acid peels, or Q-switched laser.

Further reading

Bhattar PA, Zawar VP, Godse KV, et al. (2015). Exogenous Ochronosis. *Indian J Dermatol*;60(6):537–543.

Ishack S, Lipner SR (2022). Exogenous Ochronosis Associated with Hydroquinone: A Systematic Review. *Int J Dermatol*;61(6):675–684.

Lazar M, De La Garza H, Vashi NA (2023). Exogenous Ochronosis: Characterizing a Rare Disorder in Skin of Color. *J Clin Med*;12(13):4341.

Narayanan D, Tyring SK (2024). Hyperpigmented Macules and Patches on the Face: Exogenous Ochronosis or Lichen Planus Pigmentosus? *J Drugs Dermatol*;23(7):567–568.

Rajesh Gulwani P, Parekh AR, Shah HA (2024). Intradermal Vitamin C: A New Paradigm in the Treatment of Exogenous Ochronosis. *Indian J Dermatol Venereol Leprol*;March 14:1–3.

DOI: 10.1201/9781003479512-73

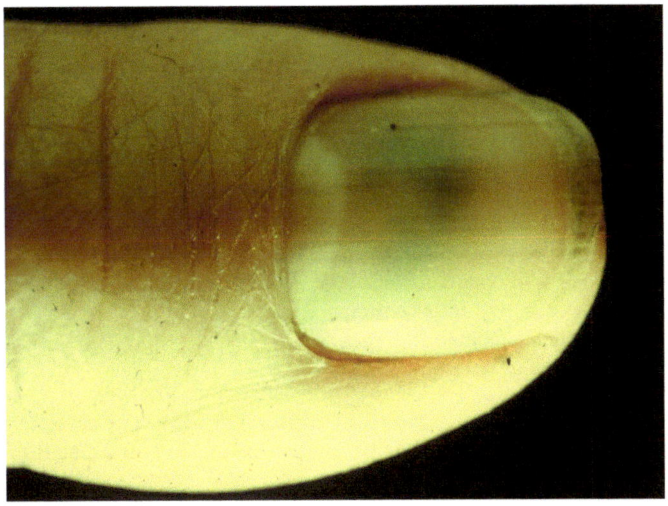

FIGURE 73.1 Ochronosis of the nail bed. (Courtesy of Jan Kejda, Czechia.)

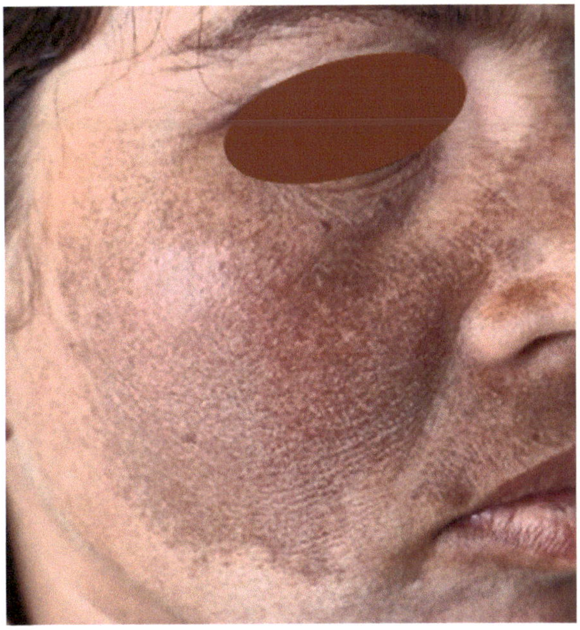

FIGURE 73.2 Worsening of melasma after initial response to hydroquinone-containing creams should alert the diagnosis of exogenous ochronosis. Blue-black discoloration is barely visible in dark skin. (Courtesy Dr. Daniel Henry, India.)

74
PAGET DISEASE OF THE BREAST

Introduction

Paget disease is an invasion of the epidermis of the nipple and areola by malignant cells, which commonly, but not always originate from an intraductal carcinoma of the breast. This is important as the underlying tumor is usually small and superficial, so early recognition may allow curative intervention. Patients present with scaling and erythema, sometimes with oozing and crusting, on or around the nipple.

Extramammary Paget disease is not uncommon.

Epidemiology

Paget disease of the nipple is uncommon, occurring in fewer than 3% of breast cancers. Most patients are over 60 years of age. It occurs mainly in women, although rare cases have been recorded in men.

Associated diseases

Eczema, psoriasis, hyperkeratosis, and erosive adenomatosis are in the clinical differential diagnosis of mammary Paget disease.

Clinical characteristics in light skin (Fitzpatrick skin types I–III)

Mammary Paget disease usually presents as a one-sided nipple 'eczema' with a red, slightly raised plaque that tends to desquamate and later ooze (Figures 74.1 to 74.3).

Extramammary Paget's may involve the genito-inguinal, perineal, and perianal skin, rarely the axillae and exceptionally other skin regions. It is thought to derive from apocrine glands. It may form large red plaques with scaling and later erosive oozing areas. Areas with increased friction may develop papillomatous lesions covered with macerated keratin, finally giving a cauliflower aspect. Any such lesion in a person – male or female – should be biopsied and submitted for histopathology, which shows the characteristic large round intraepidermal cells that are PAS and mucin positive and can be stained for keratin 7. It is important to look for the hair follicles as they may also be populated by Paget cells, a reason why superficial excision may lead to recurrence. Further, extramammary Paget may be associated with urogenital carcinoma.

Clinical characteristics in dark skin (Fitzpatrick skin types IV–V)

Early lesion clinically resembles nipple eczema; a small, crusted and intermittently moist area on the nipple gives a brownish stain on clothing, or produces itching, pricking, or burning sensations (Figures 74.4 and 74.5).

The nipple, areola, and, at a later stage, the skin of the breast are erythematous and moist or crusted. The change is sharply marginated. The nipple is retracted or completely destroyed.

Investigations

Histologically, there may be diagnostic problems from other disorders with Pagetoid spread, such as some melanomas or Bowen's disease, and also from a benign proliferation of Toker cells termed clear cell papulosis.

Mammogram or ultrasound to establish whether or not there is deeper pathology in the underlying breast, as this will help determine the extent of surgery required.

Treatments

Surgery should be carried out as for carcinoma of the breast.

Further reading

Ranawaka RR, Madarasinghe NP, Kannangara AP, et al. (2020) Cutaneous Disorders of Breast. In: Smoller B, et al. (eds). *Atlas of Dermatology, Dermatopathology and Venereology.* Springer, Cham; 991–1038.

Swarnkar B, Anand GRP, Ramam M, et al. (2023). Two Cases of Vulval Extramammary Paget's Disease Treated with Topical Imiquimod Cream. *Indian Dermatol Online J*;15(1):129–131.

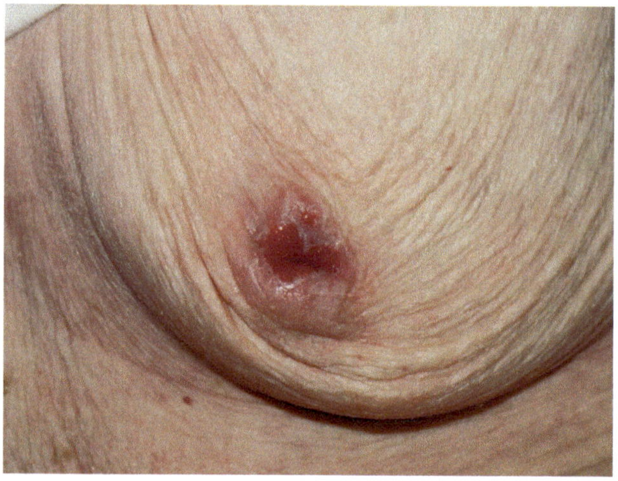

FIGURE 74.1 Paget disease of the nipple FST1. (Courtesy Prof. Ian Coulson, UK.)

DOI: 10.1201/9781003479512-74

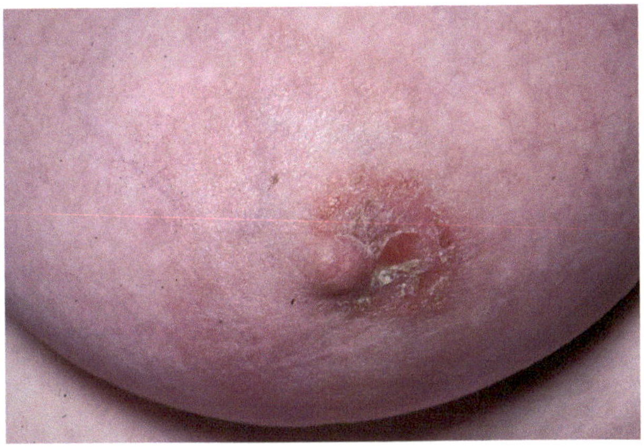

FIGURE 74.2 Paget disease of the nipple.

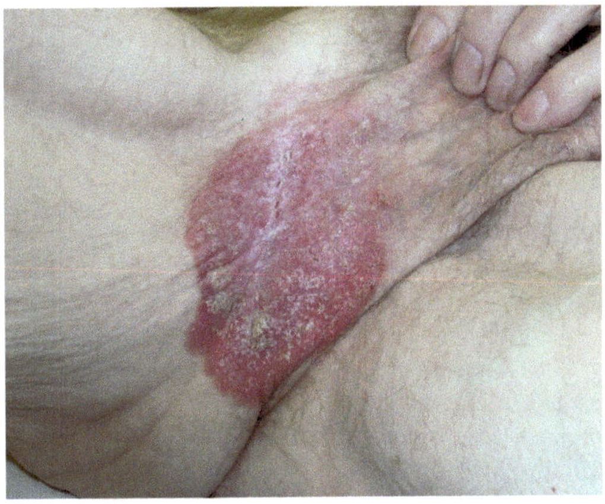

FIGURE 74.3 Extramammary Paget disease FST1. (Courtesy Prof. Ian Coulson, UK.)

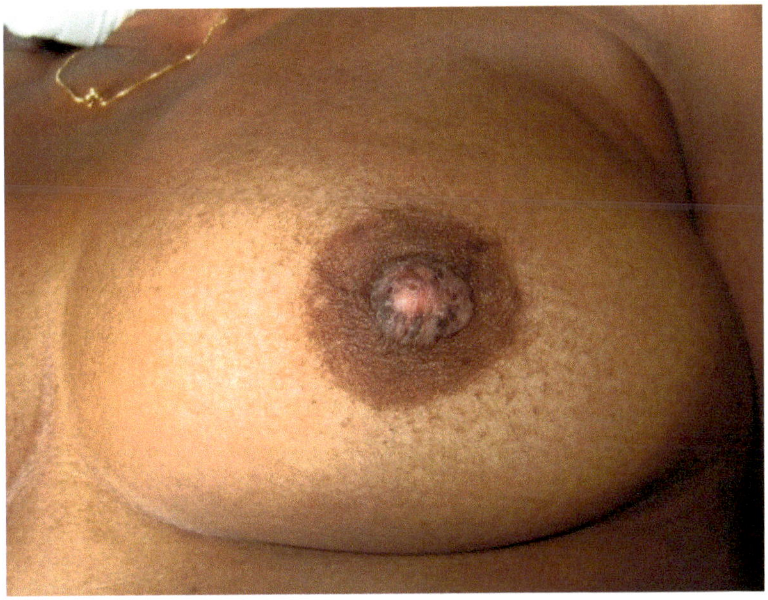

FIGURE 74.4 Paget disease of the nipple, early stage, in a 65-year-old woman FST5; note unilateral nipple destruction, sharply marginated lesion.

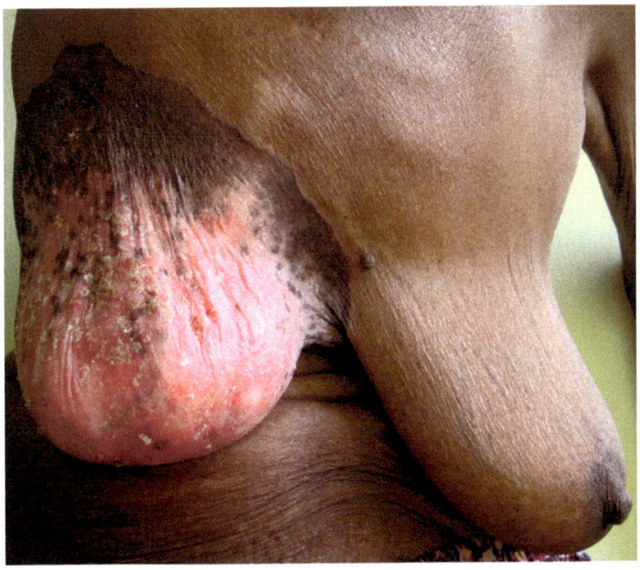

FIGURE 74.5 Paget disease of the breast, advanced disease, in an 85-year-old woman FST5.

75
PANNICULITIS

Introduction

Panniculitis is an inflammatory disease of the subcutaneous fat. Histopathologically, this is classified as either predominantly septal or predominantly lobular panniculitis. The next diagnostic step requires assessment of whether vasculitis is or is not present and, when it is present, of the size and nature of the involved blood vessels. The final diagnostic step requires the microscopic identification of the composition of the inflammatory infiltrate involving the septa and/or the fat lobule, and the type of adipocyte necrosis.

Associated diseases

There are many causes for panniculitis: Predominantly septal panniculitides including superficial migratory thrombophlebitis, cutaneous polyarteritis nodosa, necrobiosis lipoidica, deep morphea, subcutaneous granuloma annulare, rheumatoid nodule, necrobiotic xanthogranuloma, and erythema nodosum.

Predominantly lobular panniculitides include erythema nodosum leprosum, erythema induratum of Bazin, sclerosing panniculitis, calciphylaxis, cold panniculitis, lupus panniculitis, pancreatic panniculitis, α1-antitrypsin deficiency panniculitis, infective panniculitis, factitious panniculitis, subcutaneous Sweet syndrome, and subcutaneous sarcoidosis, etc.

Clinical characteristics in light skin (Fitzpatrick skin types I–III)

Clinically, the diagnoses of erythema induratum and erythema nodosum are usually obvious. The lesions in erythema nodosum are bright red, warm, tender nodules with a smooth surface, painful to touch and pressure, and mostly distributed on the anterior side of the lower legs, rarely on the thighs, and exceptionally other skin areas (Figures 75.1 to 75.3).

Erythema induratum of Bazin, in contrast, is mainly localized on the posterior side of the lower legs, is neither warm nor painful, and tends to ulcerate after some weeks to months. The legs are often slightly edematous and livid. The overlying skin takes on an orange peel aspect when it is gently moved together from the sides.

Calciphylaxis is a rare disease involving the necrosis of affected vessels. It is often a sign of a very serious underlying condition.

Most other panniculitides require an in-depth examination to define the exact diagnosis; see above.

Clinical characteristics in dark skin (Fitzpatrick skin types IV–V)

Induration of a localized area of the skin with features of acute inflammation (erythema, warmth, and tenderness). The overlying skin is warm and an orange peel appearance is marked when pinching or squeezing the skin (Figure 75.4).

Investigations

Histopathology to differentiate the type of panniculitis, and further investigations are performed depending on the cause.

Treatments

Identify the cause and the specific treatment that is prescribed for that condition.

Further reading

Baskaran N, Bharti P, Arava S, et al. (2023). Linear and Annular Lupus Panniculitis of the Scalp with Annular Lupus Panniculitis of the Face in a Child. *Indian Dermatol Online J*;15(4):634–636.

Requena L, Cerroni L (2024). Panniculitis. In: Griffiths C, et al. (eds). *Rook's Textbook of Dermatology*, 10th ed. John Wiley & Sons Ltd., UK: 97.1.

DOI: 10.1201/9781003479512-75

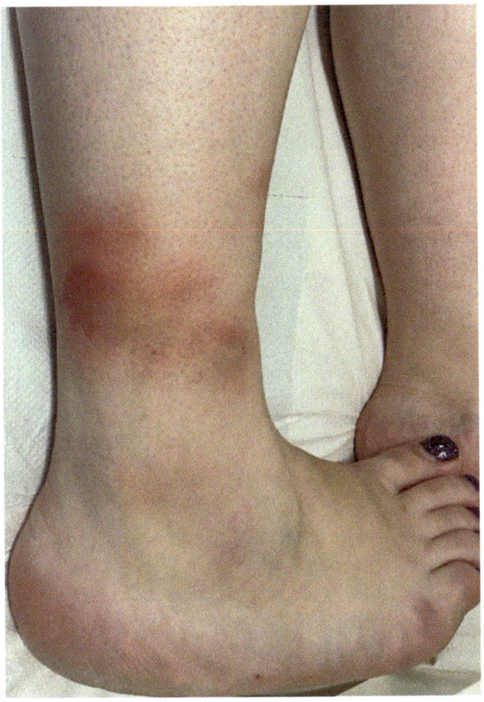

FIGURE 75.1 Panniculitis FST1. (Courtesy Dr. Richard Ashton, UK.)

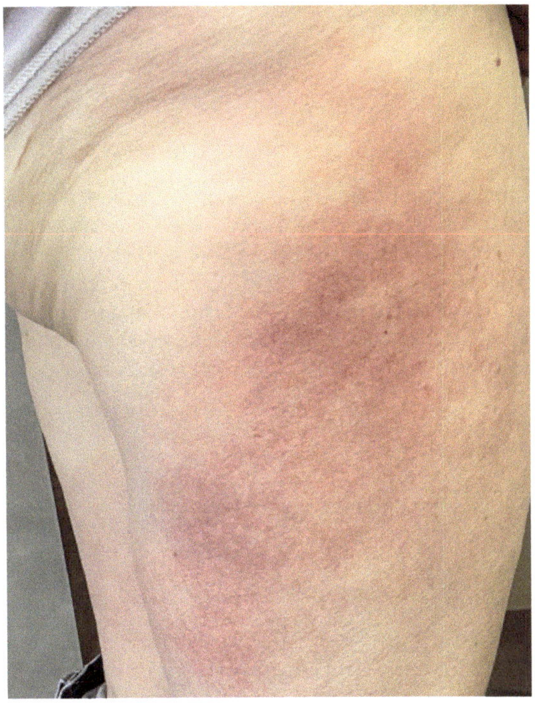

FIGURE 75.2 Panniculitis (cold panniculitis) FST1. (Courtesy Dr. Richard Ashton, UK.)

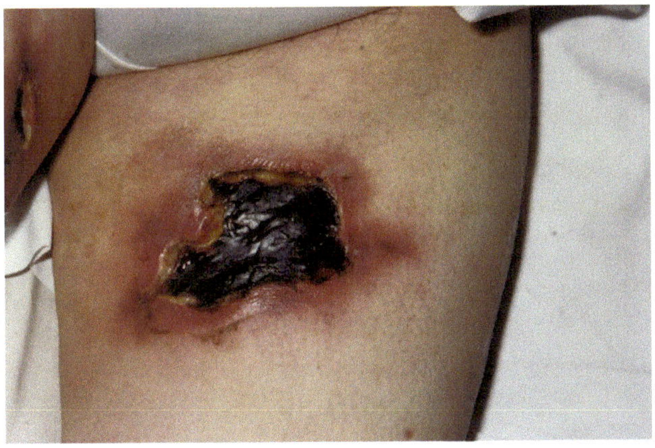

FIGURE 75.3 Calciphylaxis FST1. (Courtesy Prof. Ian Coulson, UK.)

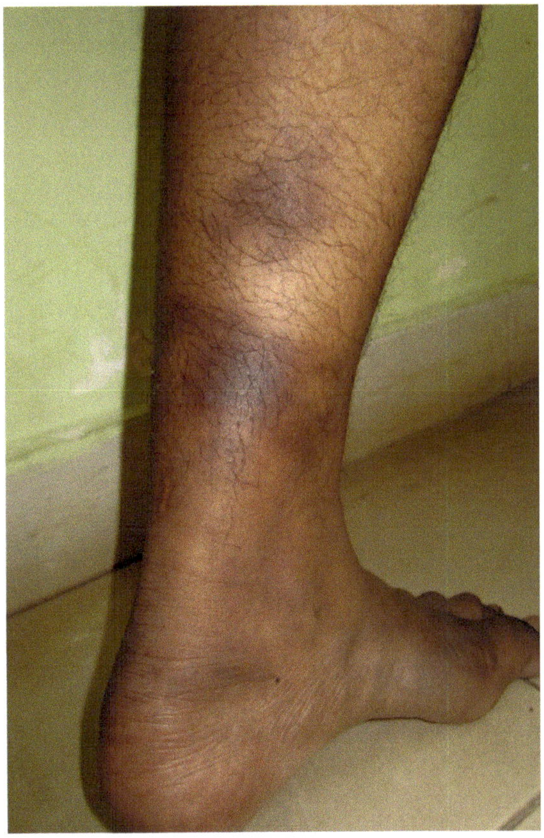

FIGURE 75.4 Erythema induratum of Bazin in a 37-year-old woman FST5. This woman presented with panniculitis and histopathology confirmed cutaneous tuberculosis.

76
PEMPHIGOID BULLOUS

Introduction

Bullous pemphigoid (BP) is the most frequent autoimmune blistering disease in white skin. It often starts with pruritus and urticated and erythematous lesions. Later, tense blisters are characteristic both on erythematous and on normal skin. Mucosal involvement only develops in a minority of patients and is not predominant. There are identified clinical variants: Localized BP, childhood BP, mucous membrane pemphigoid, etc.

Epidemiology

It mainly affects elderly people (formerly known as pemphigus of the aged).

Associated diseases

In older patients, neurological and psychiatric disorders, including cognitive impairment, Parkinson's disease, stroke, epilepsy, multiple sclerosis, and uni- and bipolar disorders, have been associated with BP. Patients with BP have a three times higher risk of pulmonary infection and embolism.

Clinical characteristics in light skin (Fitzpatrick skin types I–III)

BP is a relatively common autoimmune blistering disease mainly observed in people over 50 years of age (Figure 76.1). Starting with itch and erythema, which is sometimes called the premonitory stage and can occasionally last longer, tense blisters develop that may be grouped but reach a much bigger size than the vesicles of dermatitis herpetiformis. Its pathogenesis involves autoantibodies against the hemidesmosomal proteins BP180 and BP230, which lead to detachment at the dermo-epidermal junction with blister formation. They can be used for diagnosis and control of therapy with immunoassays. BP is associated with coexisting co-morbidities and drug exposure.

There are a number of particular BP forms such as non-bullous itchy erythema, dyshidrosiform BP of the palms and soles, oral mucosal BP, paronychia-like lesions and pterygium due to nail involvement, localized BP, pemphigoid vegetans, pemphigoid nodularis, and drug-induced BP.

The differential diagnoses comprise cicatricial mucosal pemphigoid, epidermolysis bullosa acquisita, bullous lupus erythematosus, bullous lichen planus, pemphigoid gestationis, IgM BP, and orf-induced BP.

Clinical characteristics in dark skin (Fitzpatrick skin types IV–V)

In South Asian skin, BP is less common than pemphigus vulgaris and is a disease of the elderly (Figures 76.2 and 76.3). The prodromal phase may last weeks or months; pruritus, from mild to intractable, is typical in this phase and may even occur without skin lesions. The bullous stage is characterized by intense pruritus accompanied by widespread tense blisters and vesicles on apparently normal or erythematous skin. Mucosal involvement is rare. The Nikolsky sign is negative. These lesions heal without scarring.

Investigations

Histopathology of a lesional biopsy reveals a subepidermal blister with a dense eosinophil-rich infiltrate within the papillary dermis and along the dermo-epidermal junction (DEJ).

Direct immunofluorescence microscopy of a *perilesional* biopsy shows linear deposits of IgG (IgG4 and IgG1 are the predominant subclasses) and/or C3, and to a lesser extent of IgA and IgE, seen along the DEJ.

Specific serological tests to identify autoantibodies to BP180, BP230, laminin 332.

Treatments

- Topical and systemic steroids are the mainstay of treatment.
- Azathioprine, dapsone, doxycycline, methotrexate, and mycophenolate are second-line therapies with or without systemic prednisolone.
- Immunoadsorption, rituximab, or IVIG are the third-line therapies with systemic prednisolone. Promising options are rituximab, dupilumab, eosinophil-targeted molecules, omalizumab, complement inhibitors, interleukin (IL)-17 and IL-23 inhibitors, neonatal Fc receptor antagonists, topical therapies, and Janus kinase inhibitors.

Further reading

Altan Ferhatoglu Z, Yucesoy SN, Ak T, et al. (2024). Omalizumab in the Treatment of Bullous Pemphigoid: A Single-Center Series of 15 Cases. *Medicine*;103(30):e38684.

Geng RSQ, Wei E, Wilken B, et al. (2024). Serum Biomarkers in Bullous Pemphigoid: A Systematic Review. *J Cutan Med Surg*;Sep–Oct;28(5):463–467.

Haneke E, Borradori L (2020). Pterygium in Bullous Pemphigoid: An Unusual Complication. *JAAD Case Rep*;6(8):737–739.

Karakioulaki M, Eyerich K, Patsatsi A (2024). Advancements in Bullous Pemphigoid Treatment: A Comprehensive Pipeline Update. *Am J Clin Dermatol*;25(2):195–212.

Schmidt E, Groves R (2024). Immunobullous Diseases. In: Griffiths C, et al. (eds). *Rook's Textbook of Dermatology*, 10th ed. John Wiley & Sons Ltd., UK; 50.10.

DOI: 10.1201/9781003479512-76

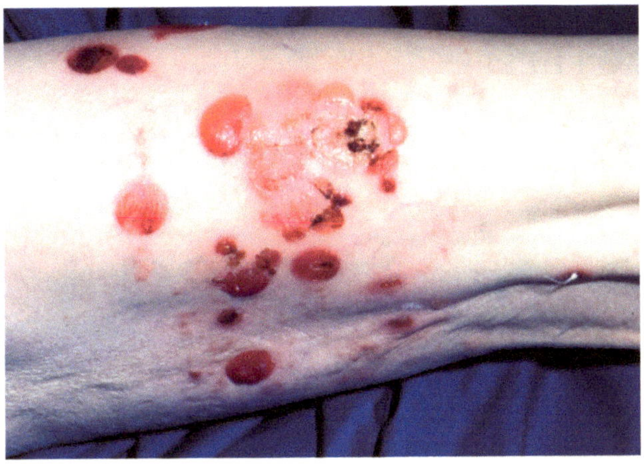

FIGURE 76.1 Bullous pemphigoid FST1. (Courtesy Prof. Ian Coulson, UK.)

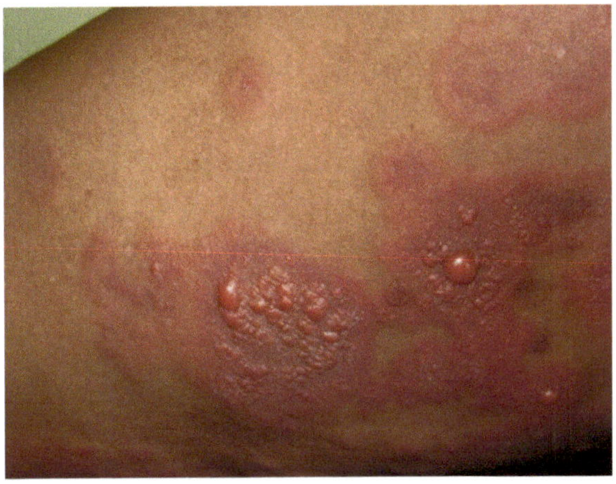

FIGURE 76.2 Bullous pemphigoid in a 65-year-old woman FST5. Note tense blisters on erythematous urticated skin.

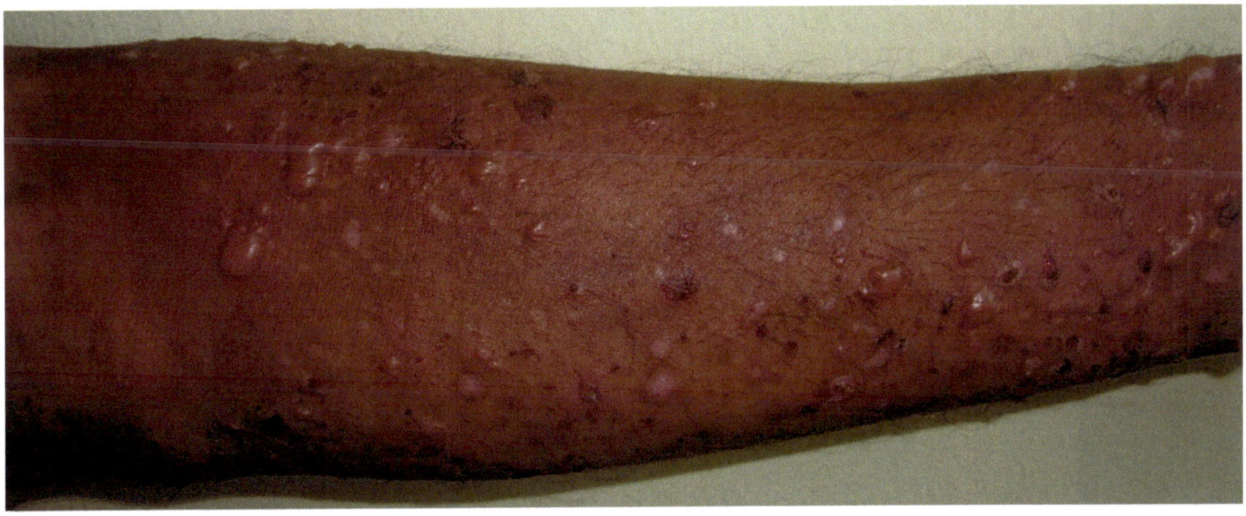

FIGURE 76.3 Tense bullae in bullous pemphigoid in a 67-year-old man FST5.

77
PEMPHIGOID GESTATIONIS OR HERPES GESTATIONIS

Introduction

Pemphigoid gestationis (PG) is a rare, autoimmune, bullous disorder that presents mainly in late pregnancy or the immediate postpartum period. It can also occur in association with trophoblastic tumors (choriocarcinoma, hydatidiform mole).

Initially, erythematous urticarial papules and plaques typically develop on the abdomen, characteristically involving the periumbilical region, then spreading to the entire skin surface. It then progresses to tense blisters that resemble those of bullous pemphigoid (BP). The face and mucous membranes are usually spared. The natural course of PG is characterized by exacerbations and remissions during pregnancy, with frequent improvement in late pregnancy followed by a flare-up at the time of delivery (75% of patients). After delivery, the lesions usually resolve within weeks to months but may recur with menstruation and hormonal contraception. There is an increase in fetal prematurity and small-for-date babies. Due to a passive transfer of antibodies from the mother to the fetus, about 10% of newborns may develop mild skin lesions (neonatal PG) that resolve spontaneously within days to weeks.

Epidemiology

PG can recur in subsequent pregnancies and with the use of oral contraceptive therapy. When PG recurs, it often presents at an earlier gestation and with increased severity.

Associated diseases

There is an increased risk of developing other organ-specific autoimmune diseases, in particular Graves' disease.

Clinical characteristics in light skin (Fitzpatrick skin types I–III)

PG, like BP, is due to autoantibodies against the BP antigens 180 and 230. It begins with an immune response within the placenta, stimulating maternal antibody production to abnormal placental antigens. These antibodies bind both to the placental antigen and the antigen in the epidermal basement membrane. Tense bullae form on the skin, often beginning on the abdomen and later spreading to other areas, but rarely the face (Figures 77.1 and 77.2). Pruritus may be intense. Inflammatory papules and plaques turn into blisters within a few days to weeks that characteristically resolve spontaneously after delivery. Recurrences are frequent with subsequent pregnancies.

Like BP, histopathology is characterized by intense eosinophilia, often eosinophil spongiosis, and subepidermal blisters.

Clinical characteristics in dark skin (Fitzpatrick skin types IV–V)

This entity is very rare in our setting (Figures 77.3 and 77.4).

Investigations

Histopathology of the bullous stage demonstrates subepidermal blistering.

Direct immunofluorescence of perilesional skin, the gold standard in the diagnosis of PG, shows linear C3 deposition along the dermo-epidermal junction in 100% of cases.

Circulating IgG antibodies in the patient's serum may be detected by indirect immunofluorescence in 30–100% of cases.

Antibody levels may also be monitored using ELISA and immunoblot techniques and show a good correlation with disease activity.

Treatments

- Topical corticosteroids with or without oral antihistamines may be sufficient in cases of mild pre-BP.
- Systemic corticosteroids (prednisolone, usually started at a dose of 0.5–1 mg/kg/day) are the mainstay of treatment.
- Cases unresponsive to systemic corticosteroid treatment may benefit from third-line treatments including azathioprine, intravenous immunoglobulins, and plasma exchange.

Further reading

Himeles JR, Pomeranz MK (2022). Recognizing, Diagnosing, and Managing Pregnancy Dermatoses. *Obstet Gynecol* ;140(4):679–695.

Sood S, Yeung J, Mufti A (2023). Biologic Therapy for Refractory Pemphigoid Gestationis: An Evidence-Based Systematic Review. *JAAD Int*;13:134–136.

Stanway A (2024). Dermatoses of Pregnancy. In: Griffiths C, et al. (eds). *Rook's Textbook of Dermatology*, 10th ed. John Wiley & Sons Ltd., UK; 113.17.

Xie F, Lehman JS, Baban F, et al. (2024). Pemphigoid Gestationis and Polymorphic Eruption of Pregnancy: Treatment and Outcomes in a Retrospective Cohort Study. *Int J Dermatol*;63(1):e29–e32.

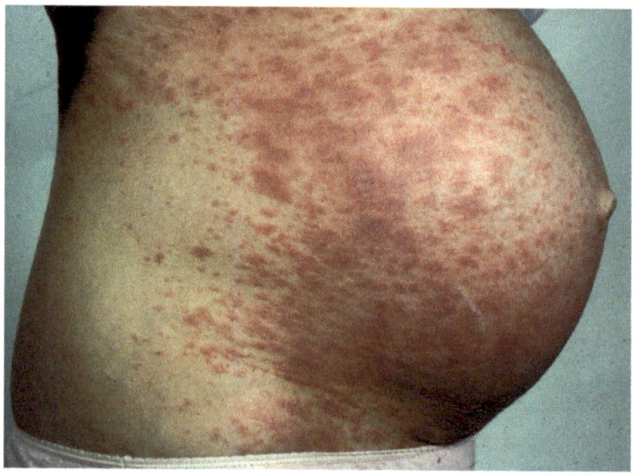

FIGURE 77.1 Pemphigoid gestationis FST1. (Courtesy Dr. Richard Ashton, UK.)

DOI: 10.1201/9781003479512-77

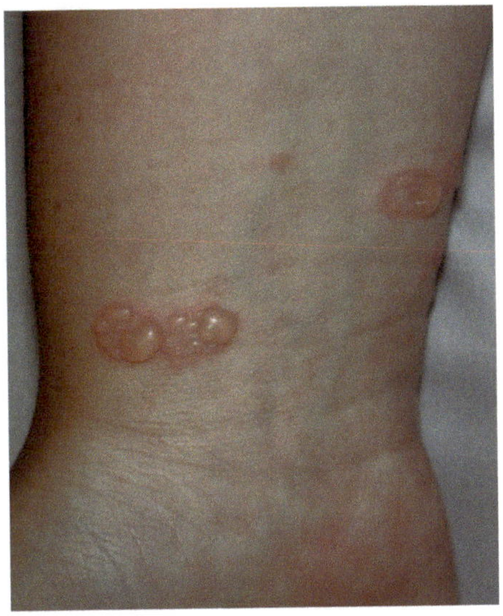

FIGURE 77.2 Pemphigoid gestationis FST1: A closer view showing blisters. (Courtesy Dr. Richard Ashton, UK.)

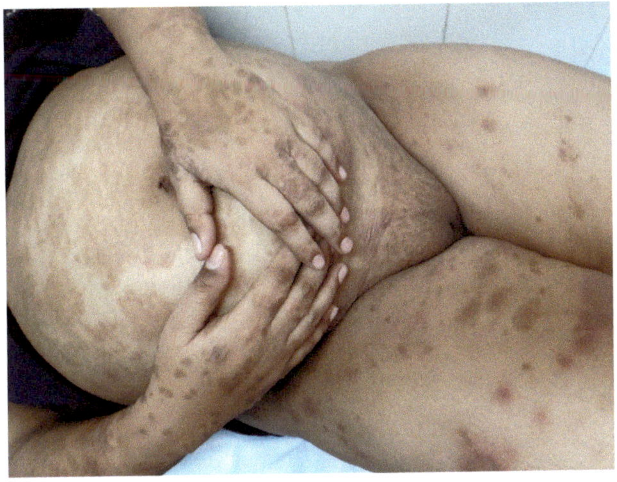

FIGURE 77.3 Pephigoid gestationis FST4. (Courtesy Prof. Archana Singal, India.)

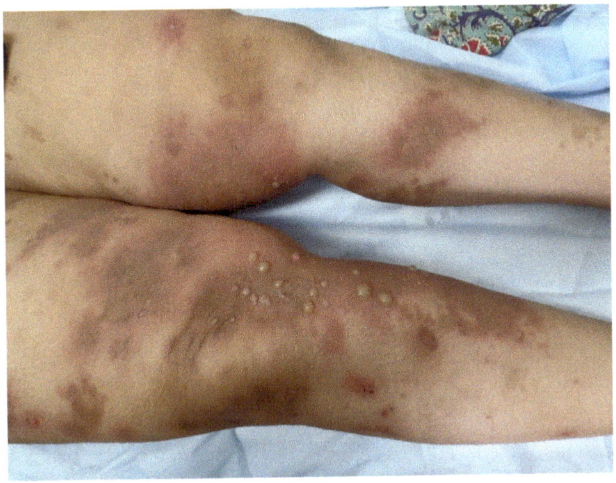

FIGURE 77.4 Pephigoid gestationis FST4. (Courtesy Prof. Archana Singal, India.)

78
PEMPHIGUS VULGARIS

Introduction

Pemphigus vulgaris (PV) is an immunobullous disorder that represents a group of conditions characterized by antibody-mediated autoimmune responses against structural elements of the epidermis, resulting in blistering of the skin and mucosae. In pemphigus, antibodies are present against desmosomal adhesion proteins, desmogleins (Dsg) 3 and sometimes Dsg 1, and desmocollins.

Nearly all patients have mucosal lesions (ill-defined irregularly shaped buccal or palatal erosions), and PV presents with oral lesions in 50–70% of patients. These may precede cutaneous lesions by months or be the only manifestation of the disease. Flaccid blisters filled with clear fluid either arise on normal skin or an erythematous base. A positive Nikolsky sign can be demonstrated on normal-looking skin adjacent to blisters or erosions. Healing occurs without scarring, but pigmentary change may occur in resolving lesions.

Epidemiology

PV is the more common form in South Asia, including India and Sri Lanka. PV can occur at any age but is usually seen between the fourth and sixth decades of life. Pemphigus is rare in childhood. It seems to affect men and women equally. PV has been reported in all ethnic groups but is more common in Ashkenazi Jews, and Mediterranean, Iranian, and Indian populations.

Associated diseases

PV has been associated with many other autoimmune diseases, particularly thyroid disease, rheumatoid arthritis, and type I diabetes. Paraneoplastic pemphigus occurs in association with hematological malignancy.

Clinical characteristics in light skin (Fitzpatrick skin types I–III)

PV is a classical immunobullous disease of squamous epithelia, thus including the epidermis, oral and genital mucosa, as well as hair follicles and nails. There are about eight distinct forms of pemphigus, with pemphigus vulgaris (PV) and pemphigus foliaceus (PF) being the most frequent. Generally, patients are between 50 and 70 years old. Flaccid blisters arise on normal or slightly erythematous skin (Figure 78.1). As they are due to acantholysis, i.e., the dissolution of the intercellular adhesions (the desmosomes), they are not resistant and erosions soon develop. This is particularly the case in the oral cavity where blisters are very rarely seen. However, the erosions have a red base in the beginning, as the basal cell layer is left intact by the disease process, in contrast to subepidermal blistering diseases which show shallow ulcers covered with fibrin. Nevertheless, PV may finally be fatal, with a one-year mortality rate of 4–8%, as the body loses proteins and electrolytes during the long course.

Endemic PF is probably induced, at least in part, by particular flies that occur in hot climates; Brazil and Tunisia have the highest incidence of PF, which is called fogo selvagem (fire of forest) in Brazilian Portuguese. Whereas PV has antibodies to desmoglein 3 and 1 splitting the spinous cells in the Malpighian layer, PF has only Dsg 1 antibodies that act on the granular layer, and thus there is a splitting of the epidermis in the subcorneal layer; the oral mucosa has virtually no Dsg 1 and is therefore not affected in PF. A PF variant with mainly facial involvement and skin redness is called pemphigus seborrhoeicus or pemphigus erythematosus.

Pemphigus vegetans is a rare variant with the same immunoserological profile as PV but with a vegetating/papillomatous proliferation of the blister base. It occurs mainly in the intertriginous areas and periorificially around the mouth and genitals.

IgA pemphigus should be considered in patients with vesiculopustular eruptions and circinate plaques with involvement of the trunk and extremities. Immunofluorescence and serology show IgA class intercellular antibodies.

As the term implies, pemphigus herpetiformis combines clinical features of PV with those of dermatitis herpetiformis; however, it is often severely inflammatory and pruritic, and acantholysis may be lacking. The mucosae remain free. The main histopathological feature is eosinophilic spongiosis; hence, it was also called eosinophilic pemphigus.

Immunoglobulin G (IgG)/immunoglobulin A (IgA) pemphigus is another very rare variant with a clinically benign course. It is mainly seen in middle-aged persons. Skin lesions are either like those of PV or may show annular and arciform erythemas with marginal blisters.

Paraneoplastic pemphigus (PNP) is also called paraneoplastic autoimmune multiorgan syndrome (PAMS). It occurs mainly in patients with lymphoproliferative disorders, but other malignant and less frequently benign tumors may be associated. Humoral and cell-mediated immunities contribute to the pathogenesis, with autoantibodies against the plakin family proteins being characteristic. Recalcitrant severe stomatitis and polymorphous skin lesions are typical. Bronchiolitis obliterans is a frequent complication contributing to the high PNP/PAMS mortality rate.

Finally, several drugs and lately both COVID-19 as well as COVID vaccinations were seen to elicit cases of various pemphigus forms.

The differential diagnosis comprises bullous pemphigoid (BP), erythema multiforme, excoriation disorders, familial benign pemphigus Hailey–Hailey, linear IgA dermatosis, papular urticaria, and bullous scabies, to mention just a few.

Clinical characteristics in dark skin (Fitzpatrick skin types IV–V)

PV is more common than BP in South Asian skin (Figures 78.2 and 78.3). PV is mostly seen in young men and women of the 20–40 age group. Flaccid blisters filled with clear fluid either arise on normal skin or an erythematous base. Nearly all patients have mucosal lesions. This has an excellent response to dexamethasone-cyclophosphamide pulse (DCP) therapy introduced by Pasricha et al. from India in 1981. After the initiation of DCP therapy in Sri Lanka in 2000, the author has

DOI: 10.1201/9781003479512-78

not encountered any fatality or extensive PV, as DCP is started early in our patients. Recurrences are almost unseen with a fully completed DCP regime.

Investigations

The diagnosis of pemphigus is confirmed by IgG, which can be demonstrated on direct and indirect immunofluorescence (IF) testing. Direct IF shows IgG and often C3 deposited on the surface of keratinocytes throughout the epidermis in perilesional skin. Circulating pemphigus autoantibodies are detected by indirect IF in over 80% of patients.

Treatments

- If left untreated, immunobullous disorders may be associated with significant morbidity and mortality, and thus prompt, accurate diagnosis and treatment are mandatory.
- Systemic corticosteroid therapy remains the mainstay of therapy, generally in combination with a steroid-sparing immunosuppressant: cyclophosphamide, azathioprine, mycophenolate mofetil.
- Advent of intravenous dexamethasone-cyclophosphamide pulse therapy (DCP) by Pasricha et al. in 1981 has revolutionized the therapy of pemphigus.
- Intravenous immunoglobulin, rituximab, immunoadsorption, and plasmapheresis are considered in resistant cases.

Further reading

Anderson HJ, Huang S, Lee JB (2023). Paraneoplastic Pemphigus/Paraneoplastic Autoimmune Multiorgan Syndrome: Part I. Clinical Overview and Pathophysiology. *J Am Acad Dermatol*; S0190-9622(23)02512-4.

Kridin K, Patel PM, Jones VA, et al. (2020). IgA Pemphigus: A Systematic Review. *J Am Acad Dermatol*;82(6):1386–1392.

Montagnon CM, Tolkachjov SN, Murrell DF, et al. (2021). Intraepithelial Autoimmune Blistering Dermatoses: Clinical Features and Diagnosis. *J Am Acad Dermatol*;84:1507–1519.

Pasricha JS, Srivastava G (1986). Cure in Pemphigus a Possibility. *Indian J Dermatol Venereol Leprol*;52:185–186.

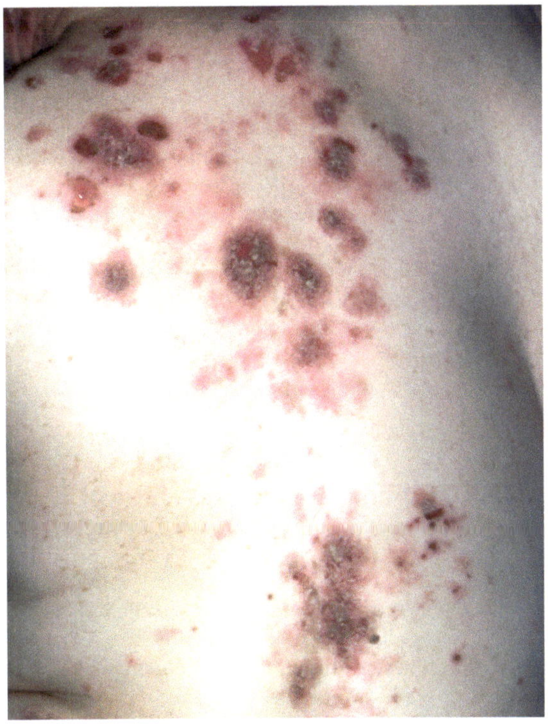

FIGURE 78.1 Pemphigus vulgaris in a 67-year-old woman FST1. (Courtesy Prof. Ian Coulson, UK.)

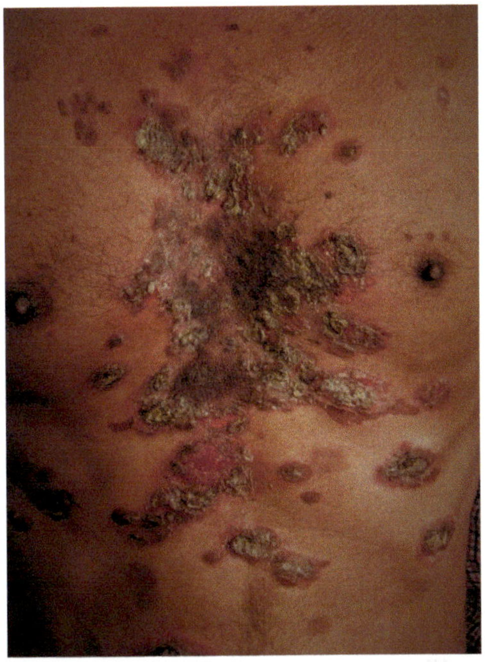

FIGURE 78.2 Pemphigus vulgaris; crusted erosions in a 37-year-old man FST5.

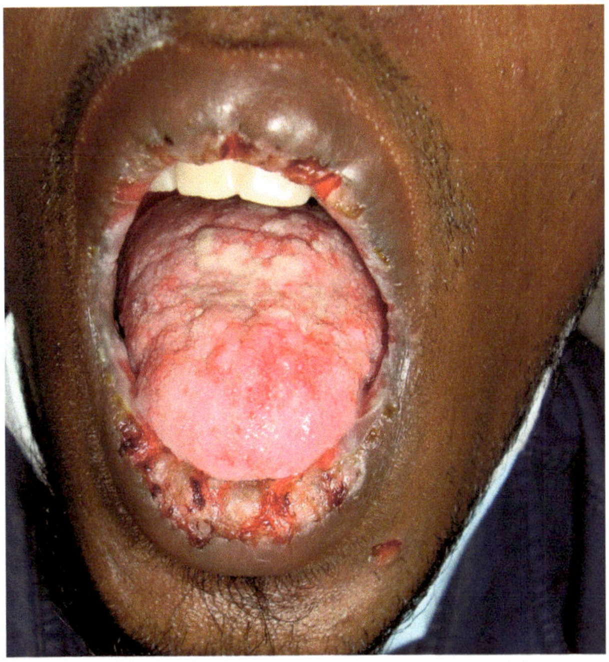

FIGURE 78.3 Pemphigus vulgaris; painful oral erosions and ulcers in a 29-year-old man.

79
PHOTOTOXIC DRUG ERUPTIONS

Introduction

Phototoxic drug eruptions are an abnormal photosensitivity induced by drugs. A phototoxic reaction is the most common reaction pattern with chemotherapeutic agents; it is non-immunologically mediated and is characterized by an exaggerated sunburn reaction. It is characterized by a burning sensation occurring within 12–24 hours of culprit drug exposure in light-exposed sites over the face, neck, anterior 'V' of the chest, and forearms. It can present with painful, well-demarcated erythema and edema progressing to blistering and desquamation.

Photo-onycholysis is a form of phototoxicity that involves the distal one-third of the nail and can be associated with tenderness.

Associated diseases

This is common with cancer chemotherapy agents.

Clinical characteristics in light skin (Fitzpatrick skin types I–III)

The most common type of acute phototoxic reaction seen in fair-skinned persons in Europe is probably phytophotodermatitis, historically also called dermatitis bullosa pratensis (Figure 79.1). It is seen in summer when uncovered skin comes into contact with plants that contain furocoumarins, e.g., giant hogweed (*Heracleum mantegazzianum*) sap. Therefore, the pattern is often characteristic with flagellate, fiercely red lesions that develop small blisters with a tendency to enlarge and merge. A great number of drugs may cause phototoxic dermatitis, such as antibiotics, anticancer drugs, modern antifungals, antihypertensives, diuretics, some non-steroidal anti-inflammatory drugs, and many more. Also, fruits and vegetables such as limes, figs, celery, parsnip, and more may cause phototoxic reactions.

Apparently, an 'odd' distribution of lesions should be searched for, as particular professional and hobby activities may encompass handling phototoxic substances.

Intense questioning often reveals the culprit. The diagnosis is limited to the area of contact with the phototoxin and sun exposure and has no tendency to spread like photoallergic reactions.

Phytophotodermatitis characteristically leaves hyperpigmentation in light-skinned individuals as it is usually due to furocoumarins. However, in contrast to dark skin, this hyperpigmentation soon resolves in skin types I–III.

Clinical characteristics in dark skin (Fitzpatrick skin types IV–V)

Erythema may not be marked in dark skin (Figure 79.2). However, a well-demarcated area of edema and tenderness with mild erythema confined to sun-exposed areas is noted, progressing to blistering and desquamation.

Investigations

This is a clinical diagnosis.

Treatments

Symptomatic treatments include discontinuing the culprit chemotherapeutic agent and dose reduction can sometimes be helpful. The use of topical steroids, broad-spectrum sunscreens, and UV light-protective clothing is also recommended.

Further reading

Fearfield L, Edwards C (2024). Cutaneous Side Effects of Chemotherapy and Radiotherapy. In: Griffiths C, et al. (eds). *Rook's Textbook of Dermatology*, 10th ed. John Wiley & Sons Ltd., UK; 119.10.

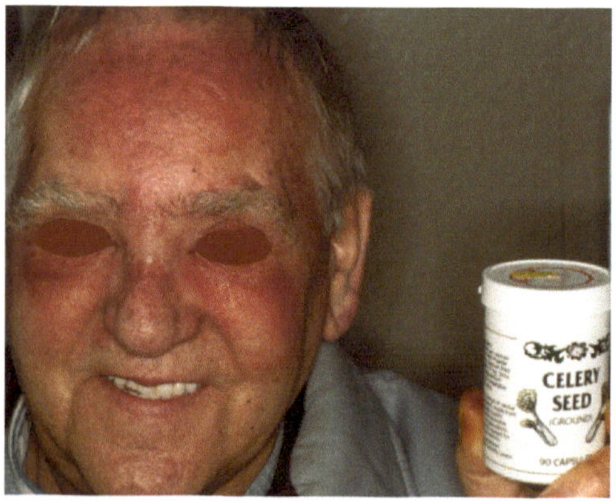

FIGURE 79.1 Phytophotodermatitis due to celery FST1. (Courtesy Prof. Ian Coulson, UK.)

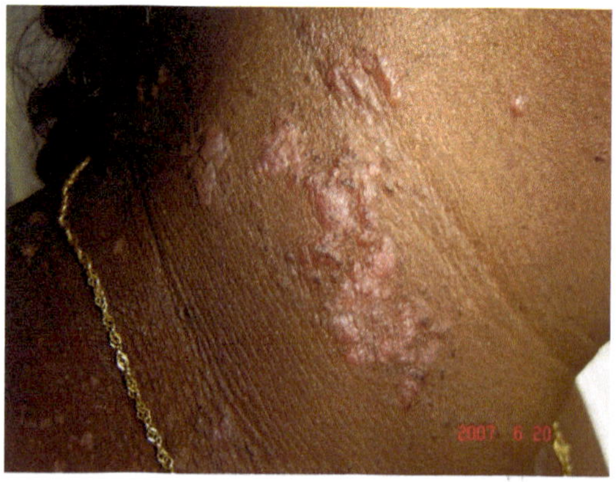

FIGURE 79.2 Phototoxic drug eruption in a 67-year-old vendor woman FST5 who was on thiazides.

DOI: 10.1201/9781003479512-79

80
PIEBALDISM

Introduction

Piebaldism is a rare autosomal dominant trait characterized by well-demarcated irregular hypopigmented macules. Histology has shown the absence of melanocytes and melanosomes in the hypomelanotic areas or sometimes reduced numbers of abnormally large melanocytes.

The extent of the areas of depigmentation is variable. The most typical and common clinical feature of the disease is a white forelock, often associated with a V-shaped area of leukoderma on the mid-forehead. The hypopigmented lesions of piebaldism have a predilection for the anterior part of the body and the mid-portion of the limbs. Often, white patches occur on the upper chest, abdomen, and limbs, bilaterally but not symmetrically.

Piebaldism is usually not associated with extracutaneous manifestations.

Epidemiology

Incidence is less than 1 in 20,000. Both sexes are affected equally and no population is spared.

Associated diseases

If the interpupillary distance is increased or the patient is deaf (sensorineural deafness), the diagnosis of Waardenburg syndrome (WS) must be considered.

Clinical characteristics in light skin (Fitzpatrick skin types I–III)

Piebaldism is a rare anomaly of the cutaneous melanocyte system (Figure 80.1). The name derives from the magpie, which is black and white. The most characteristic sign is the white forelock, often associated with a triangular white spot on the upper forehead. Furthermore, there may be white triangular areas pretibially and white spots on the trunk.

This is a genetic condition with no treatment available. The spots are already present at birth and do not grow.

Clinical characteristics in dark skin (Fitzpatrick skin types IV–V)

Depigmentation is marked and easily visible in dark skin. Therefore, this is diagnosed at birth and is a great cosmetic concern in dark skin (Figures 80.2A and 80.2B).

Investigations

This is a clinical diagnosis.
If WS is suspected, further investigations are performed.

Treatments

- Sun protection is recommended to protect the amelanotic areas from burning.
- Epidermal cell or skin grafting has been successful in piebaldism.
- Autologous cultured melanocyte transplantation may provide better repigmentation in piebaldism patients than non-cultured epidermal cell suspension transplantation with no significant side effects (Jin et al. 2024).
- Phototherapy and topical corticosteroids are ineffective for piebaldism.

Further reading

Bertolotti A, Leone G, Taïeb A, et al. (2021). Assessment of Non-cultured Autologous Epidermal Cell Grafting Resuspended in Hyaluronic Acid for Repigmenting Vitiligo and Piebaldism Lesions: A Randomized Clinical Trial. *Acta Derm Venereol*;101(7):adv00506.

Jin R, Hong W, Ye Z, et al. (2024). Comparative Outcomes of Autologous Cultured Melanocytes Transplantation and Non-Cultured Epidermal Cell Suspension Transplantation in Piebaldism Patients: A Retrospective Study. *Skin Res Technol*;30(1):e13580.

Morice-Picard F, Taieb A (2024). Genetic Disorders of Pigmentation. In: Griffiths C, et al. (eds). *Rook's Textbook of Dermatology*, 10th ed. John Wiley & Sons Ltd., UK; 68.3.

Yamaguchi Y, Peeva E, Duca ED, et al. (2024). Ritlecitinib, a JAK3/TEC Family Kinase Inhibitor, Stabilizes Active Lesions and Repigments Stable Lesions in Vitiligo. *Arch Dermatol Res*; 316(7):478.

Wang Y, Lin M, Huang F, et al. (2024). Efficacy and Safety of Fire Needle Therapy in Treating Non-Segmental Stable Vitiligo: A Randomized Self-Controlled Clinical Trial. *J Cosmet Dermatol*; Oct;23(10):3335–3334.

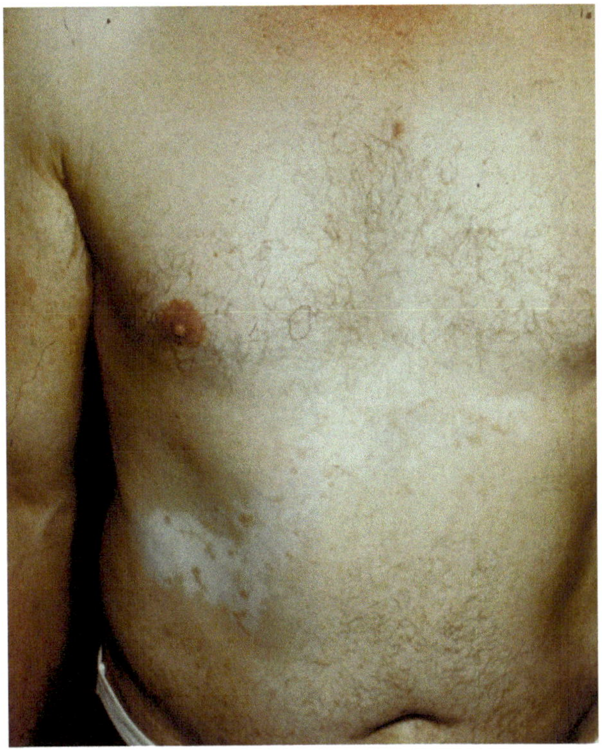

FIGURE 80.1 Piebaldism FST2. (Courtesy Dr. Richard Ashton, UK.)

DOI: 10.1201/9781003479512-80

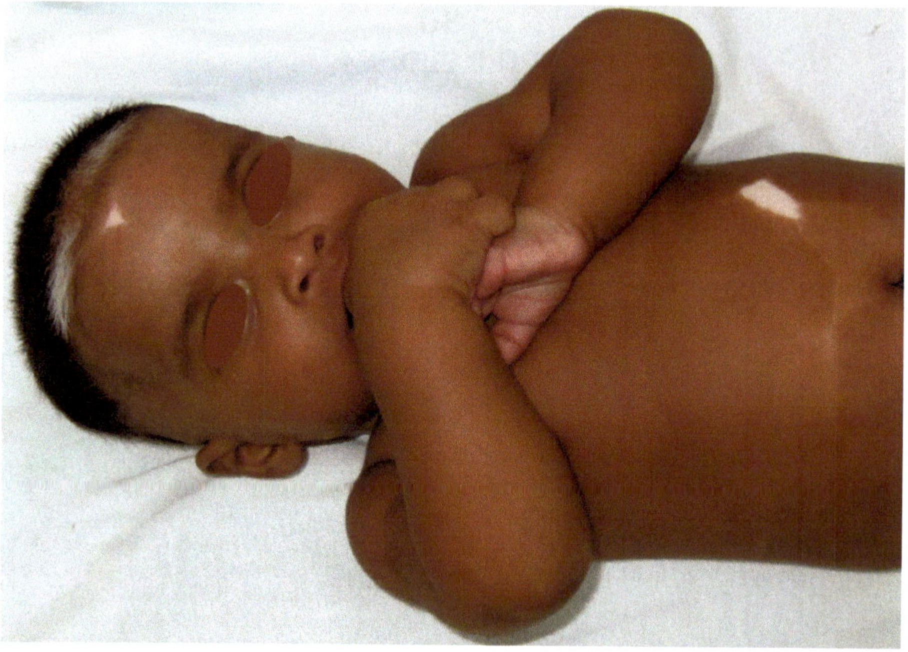

FIGURE 80.2A Piebaldism in a 7-month-old baby boy FST5. White forelock, often associated with a V-shaped area of leukoderma on the mid-forehead and hypopigmented macules on the anterior abdomen.

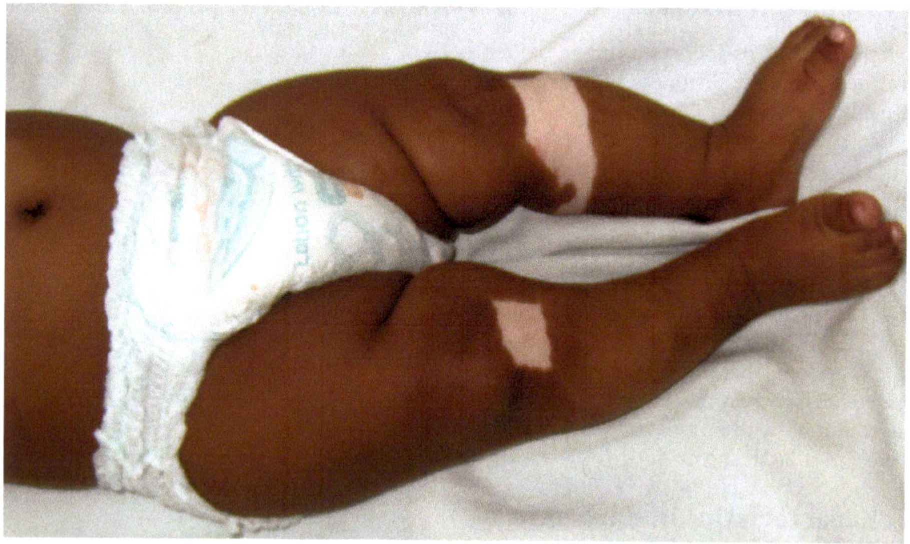

FIGURE 80.2B Piebaldism in the same baby boy FST5. The hypopigmented macules on mid-portion of the limbs are bilateral but not symmetrical.

81
PIGMENTED PURPURIC DERMATOSES

Introduction

The pigmented purpuric dermatoses (Schamberg's purpura pigmentosa progressive and Gougerot–Blum's dermatitis lichenoides purpurica et pigmentosa, as well as many other very similar purpuras) are a set of diseases of unknown etiology, which may be secondary to capillaritis. These are found to be distinctive purpuric lesions that are characterized by petechial hemorrhage (or extravasation of erythrocytes in the skin with marked hemosiderin deposition). Gravity and increased venous pressure are important localizing factors in many cases. Exercise may be a provoking factor.

Epidemiology

Common in middle-aged to older men.

Associated diseases

Obesity is a risk factor, but it is common in non-obese individuals too.

Clinical characteristics in light skin (Fitzpatrick skin types I–III)

This is a chronic progressive purpuric disease of unknown etiology in most cases, although drug-induced cases are not rare, particularly carbamides used as sedatives. Starting with red points on both lower legs, they may coalesce and form large areas (Figures 81.1 to 81.3). With time, the legs and buttocks as well as the forearms may be involved. The extravasated erythrocytes are degraded, leaving hemosiderin that is only slowly removed by tissue macrophages that become siderophages.

Although this is a clinical diagnosis, patch tests in the affected skin are occasionally positive.

If the disease is associated with tiny lichenoid papules, it is called lichenoid purpuric and pigmented dermatitis (Gougerot–Blum).

Clinical characteristics in dark skin (Fitzpatrick skin types IV–V)

Early purpuric lesions or petechial hemorrhages are not seen in dark skin. Dark-skinned individuals present with asymptomatic, discrete, pinpoint hyperpigmented macules, which later coalesce into larger macular areas (Figure 81.4). This starts around the ankles and slowly spreads upward along the lower legs to the dorsum of the feet, and is limited to the lower legs.

Investigations

This is diagnosed clinically.

Treatments

- Reassurance only.
- Withdrawal of the potentially etiological drugs. Abstain from drinks containing quinine.

Further reading

Levell NJ (2024). Purpura. In: Griffiths C, et al. (eds). *Rook's Textbook of Dermatology*, 10th ed. John Wiley & Sons Ltd., UK; 99.7.

Zaldivar Fujigaki JL, Anjum F (2023). Schamberg Disease. In: *StatPearls* [Internet]. StatPearls Publishing, Treasure Island, FL; 2024.

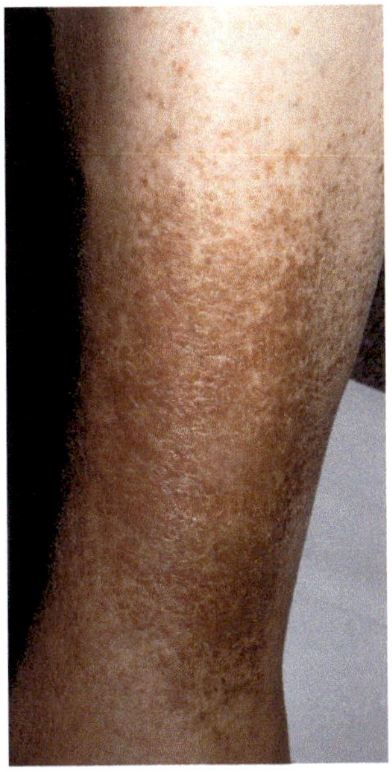

FIGURE 81.1 Pigmented purpuric eruption FST1. (Courtesy Dr. Richard Ashton, UK.)

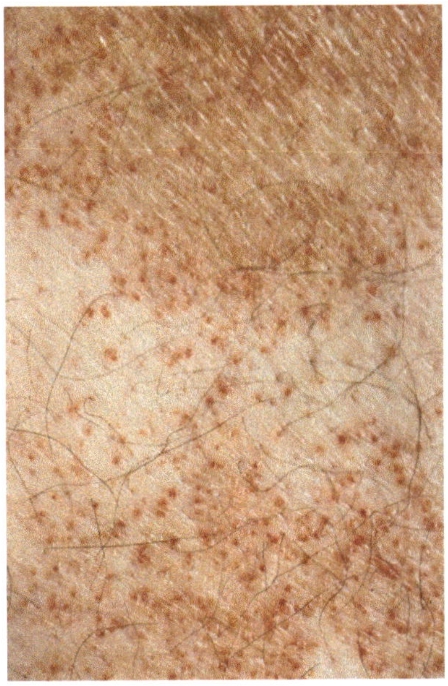

FIGURE 81.2 Pigmented purpuric eruption FST1: A closer view. (Courtesy Dr. Richard Ashton, UK.)

DOI: 10.1201/9781003479512-81

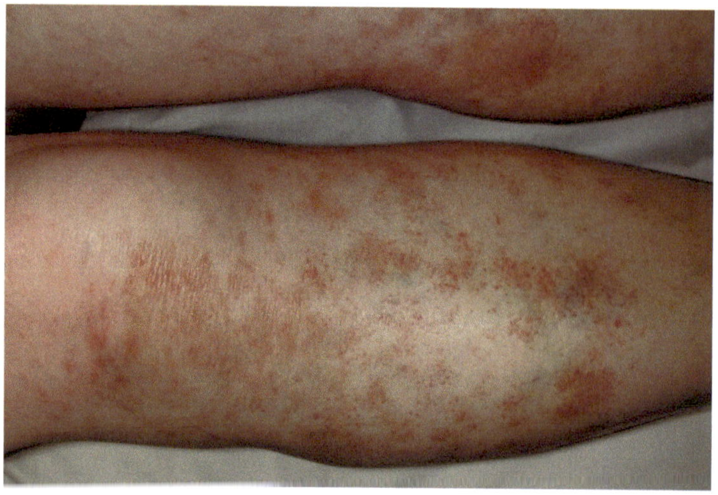

FIGURE 81.3 Schamberg disease showing pigmented purpura FST1. (Courtesy. Prof Ian Coulson, UK.)

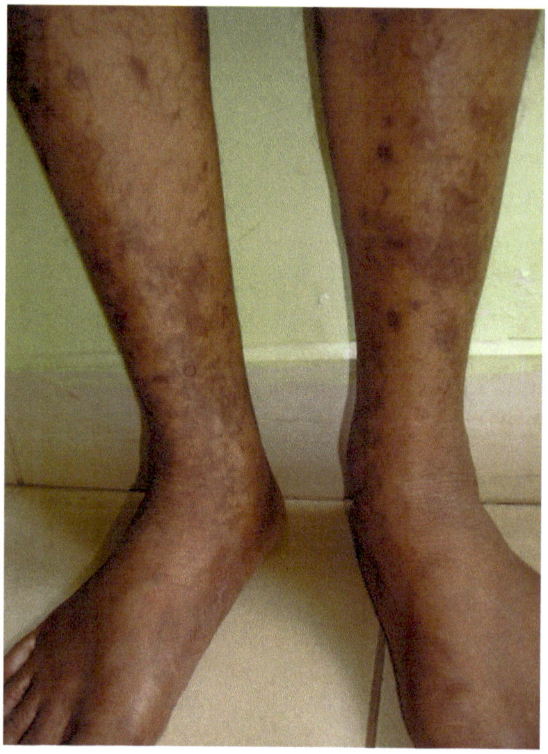

FIGURE 81.4 Pigmented purpuric dermatoses in a 37-year-old non-obese man FST5.

82
PIGMENTED TRANSVERSE NASAL BAND

Introduction

Pigmented transverse nasal band/groove is an asymptomatic benign condition characterized by the development of a hyperpigmented, well-demarcated, transverse groove at the junction of the middle and lower two-thirds of the nasal dorsum. This condition is often associated with facial seborrhea. The exact etiology of this condition is still unclear; a developmental defect of nasal cartilage, genetic predisposition, and embryological origin have been suggested to account for the transverse nasal crease. The cause of pigmentation is not yet clear.

Differentiation from the crease of allergic rhinitis (allergic salute) and wrinkles of photoaging/chronological aging is easy as the former is always associated with allergic rhinitis, has short creases that do not extend the full width of the nose, and the creases disappear when stretching the skin. Wrinkles due to photoaging or old age occur in elderly women and are associated with other signs of photoaging and old age.

Epidemiology

Female preponderance is common in adolescents and young adults and peak in the third decade.

Associated diseases

Associated with seborrhea or seborrheic dermatitis.

Clinical characteristics in light skin (Fitzpatrick skin types I–III)

This is entirely dependent on the intensity of the individual's pigmentation. The author has not seen this in fair-skinned persons, although transverse nasal grooves do exist. It demarcates the border between the bony and the cartilaginous portions of the nose and is mainly seen in patients with chronic allergic rhinitis, particularly in atopic individuals (allergic salute). However, some authors interpret it as an embryological error of development.

Clinical characteristics in dark skin (Fitzpatrick skin types IV–V)

Clinically, this presents as a 1–2 mm hyperpigmented transverse band or groove on the dorsum of the nose which extends from end to end (Figure 82.1). This is asymptomatic and cosmetically disturbing. Concomitant development of milia, pseudocomedones, and cysts within the groove causes distress. Most patients who have this condition have seborrhea or seborrheic dermatitis, even though acne is not a frequent association.

Investigations

This is diagnosed clinically.

Treatments

- Reassurance.
- Topical retinoids have been effective in lightening pigmentation, and especially when associated with milia and comedones.
- Mild-to-moderate topical steroids may show some improvement if associated with seborrheic dermatitis.

Further reading

Agarwal K, Podder I, Sarkar R (2022). Pigmented Transverse Nasal Band: A Review. *Indian J Dermatol Venereol Leprol*;88(2):144–147.

Panasia S, Paradisi M (2004). Transverse Nasal Groove. *Eur J Pediat Dermatol*;14(2):91.

Wimmershoff MB, Hohenleutner U, Landthaler M (2001). Transverse Nasal Groove. A Rare Embryological Error in Nature. *Hautarzt*;52:828–830.

Zawar V, Daga S, Pawar M, et al. (2019). Pigmented Transverse Nasal Band: A Distinct Presentation. *J Cosmet Dermatol*;18(1):301–302.

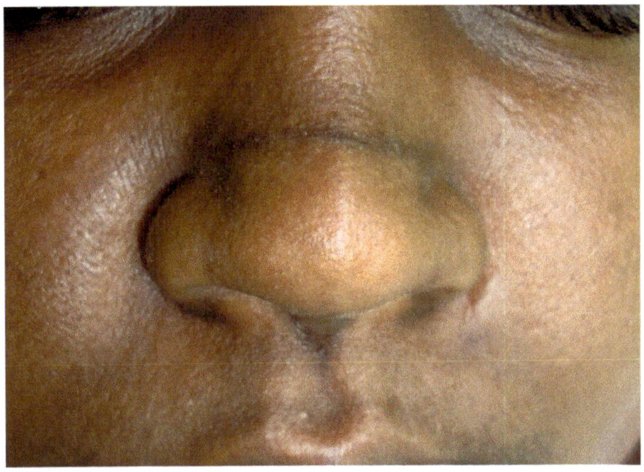

FIGURE 82.1 Pigmented transverse nasal band in a 29-year-old woman FST5. Note seborrhea and associated seborrheic melanosis around the mouth.

DOI: 10.1201/9781003479512-82

83
PITYRIASIS ALBA

Introduction

This is a pattern of dermatitis in which hypopigmentation is the most conspicuous feature. Transient, hypopigmented areas on the face are associated in some cases with fine scaling. It is most frequent on the lower cheeks. The lesions are ovoid in shape with indistinct margins, and size ranging from 0.5 to 2 cm in diameter. This is entirely asymptomatic. The lesions are often confined to the face but can appear on the neck, arms, and shoulders, or as scattered lesions on the trunk and limbs. The hypopigmentation is most conspicuous in pigmented skin, and in lighter skin may become more evident after sun tanning. Nevus depigmentosus, vitiligo, nummular dermatitis in an atopic child, hypopigmented mycosis fungoides (HMF), pityriasis versicolor, and photodermatitis are to be differentiated.

Epidemiology

Pityriasis alba occurs predominantly in older children and is more marked in darker skin. It is uncommon in infants.

Associated diseases

Pityriasis alba is often a manifestation of atopic eczema, but it is not confined to atopic individuals. Hypopigmented mycosis fungoides is difficult to distinguish clinically and histologically, so follow up and repeated biopsies are sometimes required if HMF is clinically suspected.

Clinical characteristics in light skin (Fitzpatrick skin types I–III)

Pityriasis alba (simplex) is a very common condition in children and young adolescents, mostly atopics (Figure 83.1). Predominantly on the face, often also on the extremities where the skin is dry, white patches develop that show fine scaling. They are otherwise asymptomatic; however, vigorous treatment by a parent may cause irritation with erythema. Treatment is either just bland emollients or a mild hydrocortisone cream or calcineurin inhibitor cream. The parents have to be informed that hypopigmentation remains for some time even after successful therapy.

Clinical characteristics in dark skin (Fitzpatrick skin types IV–V)

Transient, hypopigmented areas on the face, sometimes associated with fine scales, mostly appear on the lower cheeks (Figure 83.2). The lesions are ovoid in shape with indistinct margins. Even though this condition is entirely asymptomatic, it may be a source of great concern to parents.

Investigations

This is a clinical diagnosis. Histopathology will help to differentiate it from mimics.

Treatments

- Emollients can help reduce the scale.
- Topical steroids should be avoided.

Further reading

Lv Y, Gao Y, Lan N, Sun M, Zhang C, Gao J, Wang N, Yang X (2022). Analysis of Epidemic Characteristics and Related Pathogenic Factors of 2726 Cases of Pityriasis Alba. *Clin Cosmet Investig Dermatol*;15:203–209.

Maymone MBC, Watchmaker JD, Dubiel M, Wirya SA, Shen LY, Vashi NA (2019). Common Skin Disorders in Pediatric Skin of Color. *J Pediatr Health Care*;33(6):727–737.

Mughal AA, Ingram JR (2024). Eczematous Disorders. In: Griffiths C, Barker J, Bleiker T, Hussain W and Simpson R (eds). *Rook's Textbook of Dermatology*, 10th ed. John Wiley & Sons Ltd., UK; 39.26.

Shahin MM, Quach HT, Marathe KS (2024). Pediatric Dermatology for People of Color. *Pediatr Ann*;53(4):e146–e151.

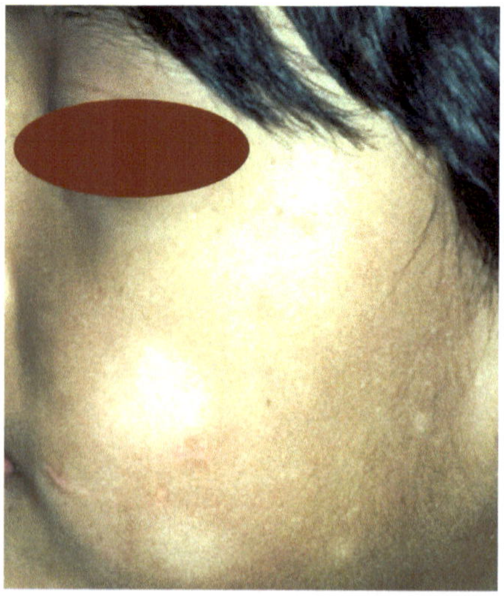

FIGURE 83.1 Pityriaisis alba in a 7-year-old boy FST3. (Courtesy Prof. Ian Coulson, UK.)

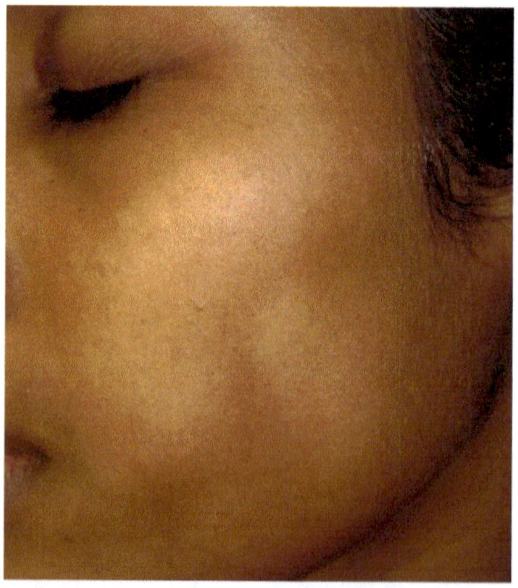

FIGURE 83.2 Pityriaisis alba in a 14-year-old girl FST5.

DOI: 10.1201/9781003479512-83

84
PITYRIASIS LICHENOIDES ACUTA

Introduction

The cause of pityriasis lichenoides is unknown. Clinically, pityriasis lichenoides is divided into two main conditions: Pityriasis lichenoides chronica (PLC) and pityriasis lichenoides et varioliformis acuta (PLEVA). However, it is not clear whether they are really a chronic and an acute variant of the same condition. A third, much rarer and aggressive form, febrile ulceronecrotic Mucha–Habermann disease (FUMHD), is also described.

Clinical characteristics in light skin (Fitzpatrick skin types I–III)

PLEVA is also called Mucha–Habermann disease. It is an acute to subacute condition with hemorrhagic papules that tend to become necrotic and leave pox-like scars (Figure 84.1). Its etiology is still not exactly known.

Often occurring after a febrile infection or spontaneously, crops of hemorrhagic or even papulo-necrotic lesions develop that have a characteristic brownish-red color and are of variable size. They may persist and enlarge for weeks or even longer, may recur or disappear spontaneously. Papules with pronounced necrosis heal with a fine varioliform scar.

Clinical characteristics in dark skin (Fitzpatrick skin types IV–V)

This is very rare in our setting. A high degree of clinical suspicion is needed to diagnose PLEVA or FUMHD in an ill patient who does not respond to systemic varicella treatments. They resemble ulcerative and/or hemorrhagic generalized varicella infection (chickenpox) (Figure 84.2).

Investigations

A skin biopsy is needed for histology, immunohistochemistry, and T-cell receptor (TCR) and immunoglobulin gene rearrangement analysis.

In cases of FUMHD, a causative infectious agent may be implicated, and investigations should be tailored to each patient's presentation: Antistreptolysin (ASO) titre, throat swab, hepatitis, Epstein–Barr virus (EBV), and human immunodifficiency virus (HIV) serology, monospot, and investigations for *Toxoplasma* infection.

Treatments

- Depending on the causal disease, broad-spectrum antibiotics (tetracyclines or erythromycin) may be given, sometimes in combination with medium-dose systemic steroids.
- Topically, mild steroids or topical tacrolimus ointment may be given to improve symptoms.
- In adults, phototherapy is usually the first-line treatment of choice: Natural sunlight, UVB, narrow-band UVB, UVA-1, and psoralen and UVA (PUVA).
- In more aggressive or refractory disease of PLEVA or FUMHD pattern, immunosuppressive agents including methotrexate, ciclosporin, and dapsone and intravenous immunoglobulin may prove successful.

Further reading

Chen Y, Zhao M, Xiang X, et al. (2020). Oral Erythromycin in Pityriasis Lichenoides Chronica and Pityriasis Lichenoides et Varioliformis Acuta. *Dermatol Ther*;33(3):e13311.

Child F, Whittaker SJ (2024). Lymphocytic Infiltrates. In: Griffiths C, et al. (eds). *Rook's Textbook of Dermatology*, 10th ed. John Wiley & Sons Ltd., UK; 134.3.

Jiao L, Liu Y, Xiang X, et al. (2019). A Case of Pityriasis Lichenoides et Varioliformis Acuta Pemphigoides Successfully Treated with Methotrexate and Corticosteroids. *Dermatol Ther*;32(4):e12833.

Ogrum A, Takci Z, Seckin HY, et al. (2018). A Case of Pityriasis Lichenoides: Rapid Resolution with Azithromycin Monotherapy in 3 Weeks. *Dermatol Ther*;31(5):e12681.

Somasundaram A, Gupta A, Sathishkumar D, et al. (2024). Rapid Recovery in a Child with Febrile Ulceronecrotic Mucha-Habermann Disease Following Intravenous Immunoglobulin Administration. *Pediatr Dermatol*; 41(3):518–522.

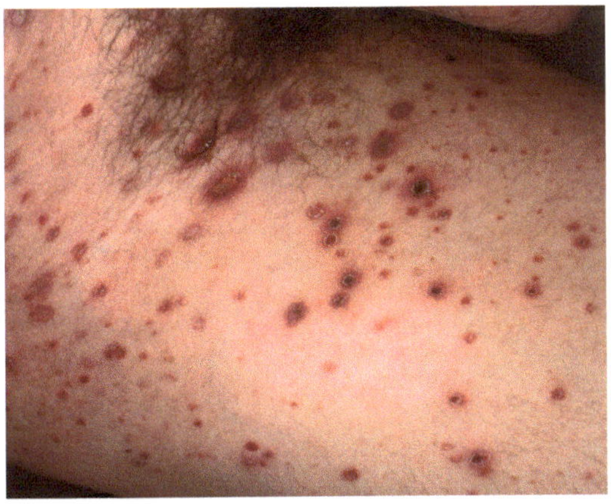

FIGURE 84.1 Pityriasis lichenoides et varioliformis acuta (PLEVA) FST2. (Courtesy Prof. Ian Coulson, UK.)

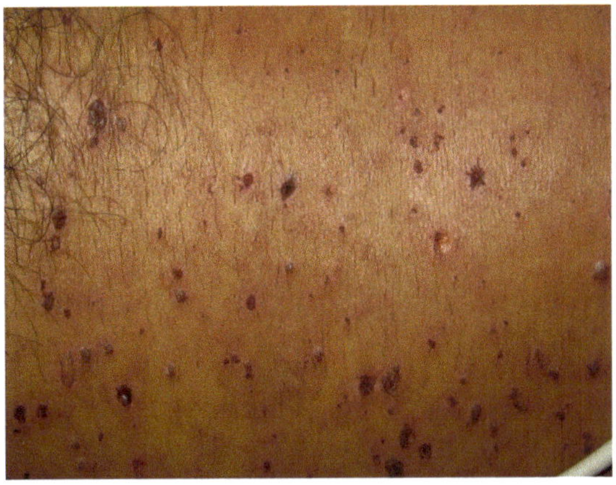

FIGURE 84.2 Pityriasis lichenoides et varioliformis acuta (PLEVA) in a 40-year-old man FST5. This man died in spite of intensive management.

DOI: 10.1201/9781003479512-84

85
PITYRIASIS LICHENOIDES CHRONICA

Introduction

The cause of pityriasis lichenoides is unknown. Clinically, pityriasis lichenoides is divided into two main conditions: Pityriasis lichenoides chronica (PLC) and pityriasis lichenoides et varioliformis acuta (PLEVA). PLC can closely resemble guttate psoriasis, but the lesions are usually less evenly scattered, have a brownish-red or orange-brown color and are capped by a 'mica-like' or watch-glass scale. PLC lasts for an average 18 months with an episodic course.

Epidemiology

It occurs most frequently in children and young adults.

Associated diseases

PLC-like lesions have been described in patients with typical features of mycosis fungoides.

PLC overlap with 'parapsoriasis' is described. In the older literature, PLC was grouped into the parapsoriasis conditions.

Clinical characteristics in light skin (Fitzpatrick skin types I–III)

In patients with light skin, dark-red papules with a brownish tint develop that are surprisingly asymptomatic (Figure 85.1). With time, they develop a single scale that can be gently lifted and removed as a whole from the lesional surface. The course of the disease is chronic progressive in most cases, although there may be periods of improvement and exacerbation.

The etiopathogenesis is not yet clear. Whereas some believe it to be an infection-allergic reaction as there is often a history of a previous infection, others dismiss this as narrow-band UVB is at least as effective as antibiotics.

Clinical characteristics in dark skin (Fitzpatrick skin types IV–V)

The characteristic lesion is a small, firm, lichenoid papule 3–10 mm in diameter, and reddish brown in color (Figure 85.2). An adherent 'mica-like' scale can be detached by gentle scraping to reveal a shining brown surface – a distinctive diagnostic feature. Over the course of 3 or 4 weeks, the papule flattens and the scale separates spontaneously to leave a pigmented macule, which gradually fades. Post-inflammatory hypopigmentation is common, and may persist.

Investigations

This is a clinical diagnosis. Histopathology helps to diagnose doubtful cases.

Treatments

- Topical corticosteroids may improve symptoms and healing of lesions but do not alter the course of the disease.
- Antibiotics such as tetracyclines or erythromycin are second-line therapies in children and adults.
- When systemic therapy is indicated, we propose that oral erythromycin and narrow-band ultraviolet B phototherapy should be first-line treatment options for children with PL since they have been shown to be effective and well-tolerated (Geller et al. 2015).
- In adults, phototherapy is usually the first-line treatment of choice and includes natural sunlight, UVB, narrow-band UVB, UVA-1, and psoralen and UVA (PUVA).
- Methotrexate, ciclosporin, and dapsone are third-line therapies in both, while acitretin and acitretin plus PUVA can be used in adults.

Further reading

Child F, Whittaker SJ (2024). Lymphocytic Infiltrates. In: Griffiths C, et al. (eds). *Rook's Textbook of Dermatology*, 10th ed. John Wiley & Sons Ltd., UK; 134.3.

Geller L, Antonov NK, Lauren CT, et al. (2015). Pityriasis Lichenoides in Childhood: Review of Clinical Presentation and Treatment Options. *Pediatr Dermatol*;32(5):579–592.

Zang JB, Coates SJ, Huang J, et al. (2018). Pityriasis Lichenoides: Long-Term Follow-Up Study. *Pediatr Dermatol*;35(2):213–219.

DOI: 10.1201/9781003479512-85

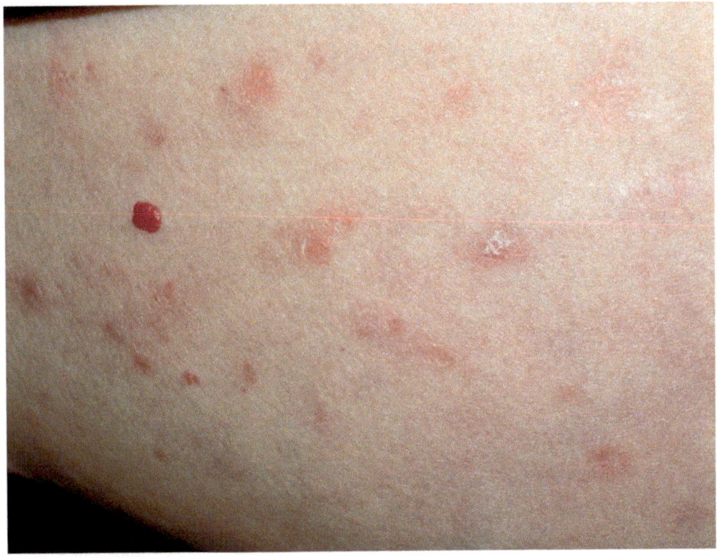

FIGURE 85.1 Pityriasis lichenoides chronica, a closer view showing adherent 'mica-like' scale FST1. (Courtesy Prof. Ian Coulson, UK.)

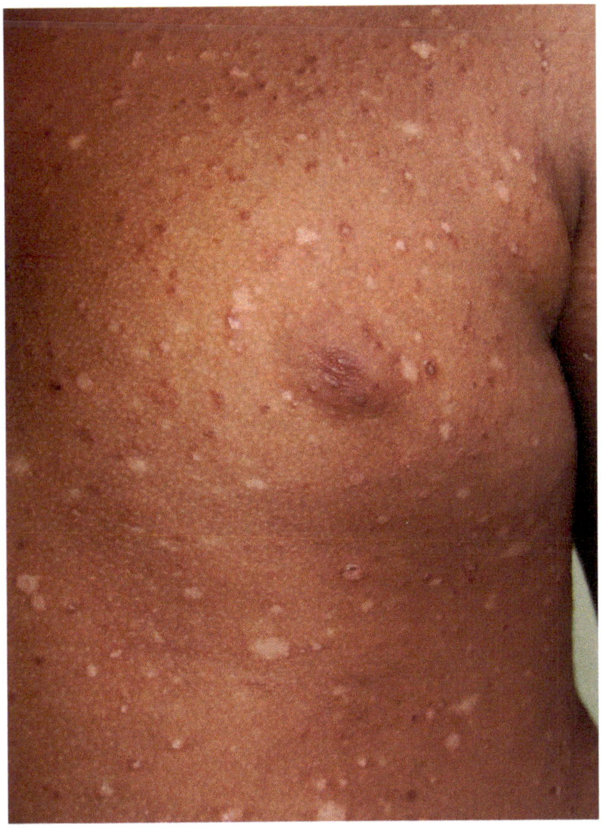

FIGURE 85.2 Pityriasis lichenoides chronica in a 12-year-old boy FST5. Note post-inflammatory hypopigmentation is common and striking. This hypopigmentation which last many months is the primary complaint in most affected children.

86
PITYRIASIS ROSEA

Introduction

Pityriasis rosea is an acute self-limiting disease, probably infective in origin, affecting mainly children and young adults. A drug-induced pityriasis rosea-like reaction has been reported with captopril, adalimumab, aspirin, allopurinol, barbiturates, beta-blockers, omeprazole, etc.

Epidemiology

Pityriasis rosea is a common eruption occurring throughout the world.

Associated diseases

Involvement of two herpes viruses, HHV-6 and HHV-7, has been suggested as the cause of the eruption.

Clinical characteristics in light skin (Fitzpatrick skin types I–III)

Often beginning with one patch, slightly scaling, mildly inflammatory lesions develop on the trunk and proximal extremities (Figure 86.1). They are usually slightly marginated and may itch. In most cases, the rash is rather embarrassing than really disturbing. New lesions develop from small papules to slightly raised plaques. The first lesion, the herald patch, remains the largest over the entire disease duration. Commonly, the rash takes 3–4 weeks to develop, remains another 3–4 weeks like this and slowly disappears over the course of 3–4 weeks. Treatment is symptomatic with zinc oxide lotion or a mild topical steroid; however, it is not certain that this really shortens the disease duration.

Clinical characteristics in dark skin (Fitzpatrick skin types IV–V)

The lesions are skin-colored with mild erythema or hypopigmented and covered by fine dry silvery-gray scales (Figures 86.2 and 86.3). The center tends to clear and assumes a wrinkled, atrophic appearance with a marginal collarette of scale attached peripherally, with the free edge of the scale internally.

Investigations

This is a clinical diagnosis. A skin biopsy may help in uncertain cases.

Treatments

- No treatment is needed in the common asymptomatic and self-limiting cases.
- If itch is troublesome, or the appearance distressing, a topical steroid (moderate potency) or UVB can be helpful.
- In resistant cases, aciclovir (400 mg five times a day for a week) or oral erythromycin antibiotic (1 g four times a day for 2 weeks for adults) may help to clear the lesions.

Further reading

Ashforth GM, Youssef S, Bhagavathi V, et al. (2023). What's Old Is New: Valacyclovir for the Treatment of Pityriasis Rosea, a Retrospective Case Series. *JAAD Case Rep*;37:98–102.

Harwood CA, Sterling JC (2024). Viral Infections. In: Griffiths C, et al. (eds). *Rook's Textbook of Dermatology*, 10th ed. John Wiley & Sons Ltd., UK; 25.123.

Wu H, Ji QJ, Xu YY, et al. (2024). A Case of Persistent Pityriasis Rosea Successfully Treated by a Short Course of Therapy with Abrocitinib. *Clin Cosmet Investig Dermatol*;17:843–846.

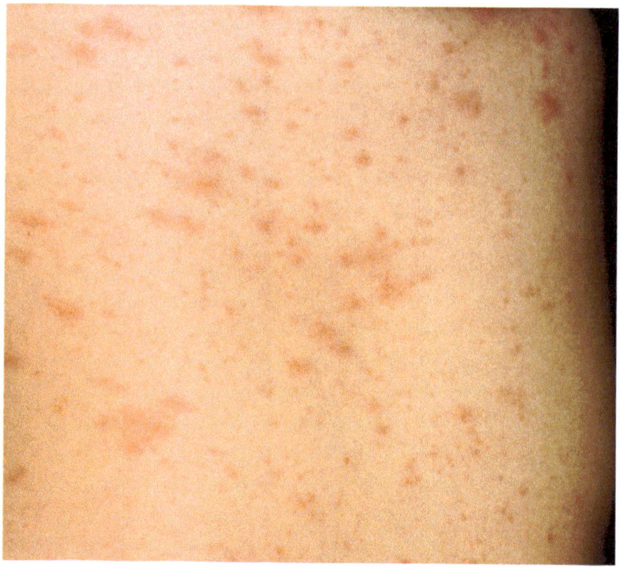

FIGURE 86.1 Pityriasis rosea FST2. (Courtesy Prof. Ian Coulson, UK.)

DOI: 10.1201/9781003479512-86

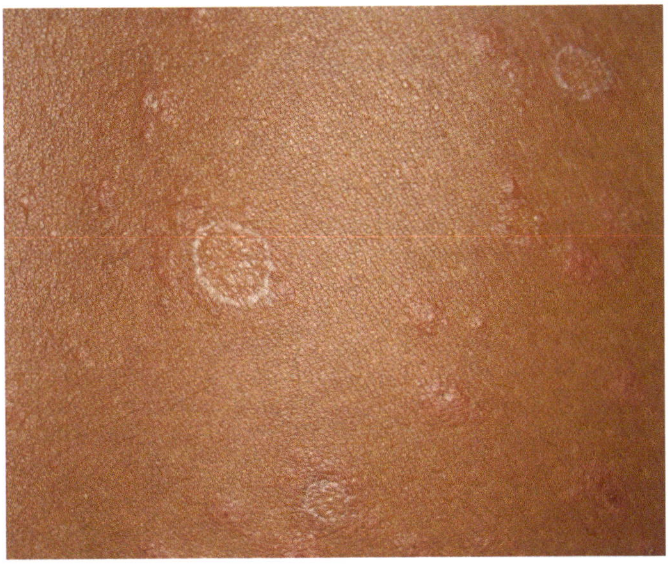

FIGURE 86.2 Pityriasis rosea, asymptomatic or mildly itchy lesions, showing a classical marginal collarette of scale attached peripherally FST5.

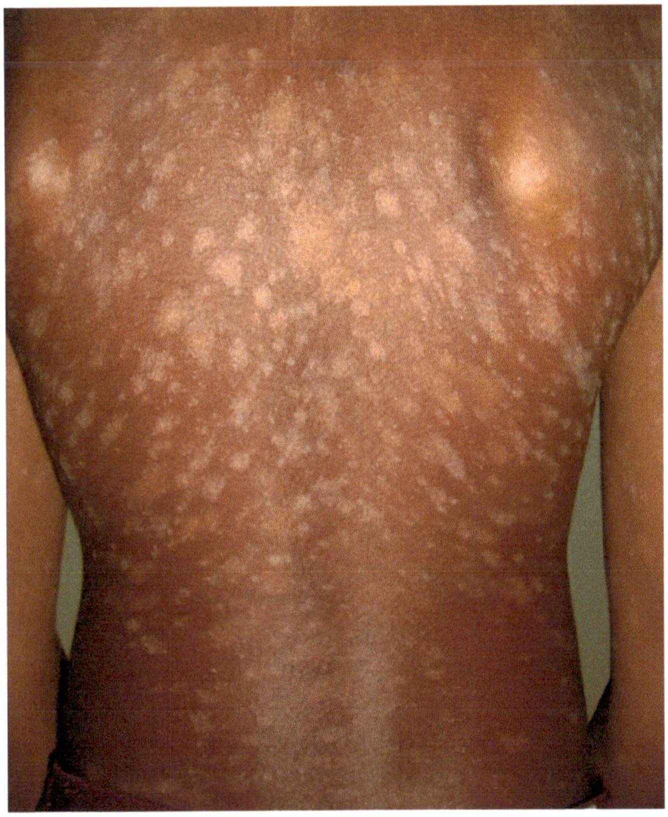

FIGURE 86.3 Pityriasis rosea FST5. Note these lesions are either skin colored or hypopigmented in dark skin.

87
PITYRIASIS RUBRA PILARIS

Introduction

Pityriasis rubra pilaris (PRP) is the name given to a group of clinically similar papulosquamous dermatoses. Its etiology is unknown. It has been divided into six clinical types depending on the distribution, age of onset, and the speed of onset. The familial form of PRP (type V) is inherited as an autosomal dominant trait and has a slow and gradual onset. The more common generalized sporadic forms (types I and III) tend to have an acute onset.

They initially present with erythematous hyperkeratotic perifollicular papules, which tend to coalesce into plaques but may progress to erythroderma. In most cases, sharply demarcated islands of unaffected skin 1 cm in diameter or larger remain as a helpful diagnostic sign ('island of sparing,' nappes claires, or Leredde's sign).

Epidemiology

PRP is an uncommon condition and has equal sex distribution. The familial type (type V) starts in early childhood, while the acquired forms of PRP have a bimodal age distribution with peaks in the first and fifth decades.

Associated diseases

PRP is not associated with an increased incidence of malignancy or with various autoimmune diseases such as systemic sclerosis and autoimmune thyroiditis.

Clinical characteristics in light skin (Fitzpatrick skin types I–III)

Fair-skinned individuals develop slightly infiltrated red areas with tiny follicular keratoses (Figures 87.1 to 87.3). They often display a characteristic yellowish to orange tint. Uninvolved clear spots (nappes claires or Leredde's sign) are very common. The palms may become diffusely hyperkeratotic with accentuated creases and a very characteristic yellowish-red color. Often, elbows, knees, and the trunk demonstrate more evolved lesions and may show white scaling.

The different clinical forms cannot be distinguished on clinical grounds alone but require a detailed personal and family history.

Single patches may be similar to psoriasis. Also, the biopsy of PRP and an old psoriasis lesion may be strikingly similar and require the experience of the dermatopathologist.

Clinical characteristics in dark skin (Fitzpatrick skin types IV–V)

Present with either skin-colored or hyperpigmented scaly plaques on trunks, knees, and elbows that do not respond to conventional treatments (Figures 87.4 to 87.6). Well-defined salmon-red or orange-red dry scaly plaques described in white skin are not a feature in dark-skinned individuals.

Investigations

Diagnosis is made based on clinical features and supported by histology. No other tests are indicated.

The histological features of PRP are not pathognomonic and change with the evolution of the disease, and allow differentiation from psoriasis and other causes of erythroderma.

Treatments

- Patients who are erythrodermic may need intensive supportive care to prevent hypothermia, electrolyte imbalance, protein loss, and sepsis.
- First-line treatments are emollients, topical corticosteroids, and acitretin or isotretinoin.
- Second-line therapies are topical calcipotriol, topical tazarotene, methotrexate, or ustekinumab.
- Third-line therapies are TNF-α antagonists, UVB phototherapy, or extracorporeal photochemotherapy.

Further reading

Boyd AH, Polcari IC (2018). Methotrexate Treatment in a Case of Juvenile Pityriasis Rubra Pilaris. *Pediatr Dermatol*;35(1):e62–e63.

Conrad C (2024). Pityriasis Rubra Pilaris. In: Griffiths C, et al. (eds). *Rook's Textbook of Dermatology*, 10th ed. John Wiley & Sons Ltd., UK; 36.1.

Kim EJ, Corey K, Damji Y (2024). Rapid Clearance of Extensive Juvenile Pityriasis Rubra Pilaris with Ixekizumab. *Pediatr Dermatol*;Nov–Dec;41(6):1235–1237.

Smyk J, Kamińska A, Borowy P, et al. (2024). Pityriasis Rubra Pilaris – A Difficult Path to Optimal Treatment: Case Report. *Pol Merkur Lekarski*;52(3):363–367.

DOI: 10.1201/9781003479512-87

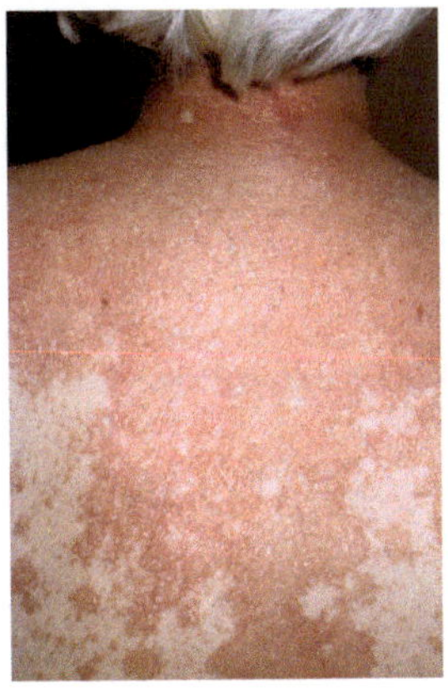

FIGURE 87.1 Pityriasis rubra pilaris FST1. (Courtesy Prof. Ian Coulson, UK.)

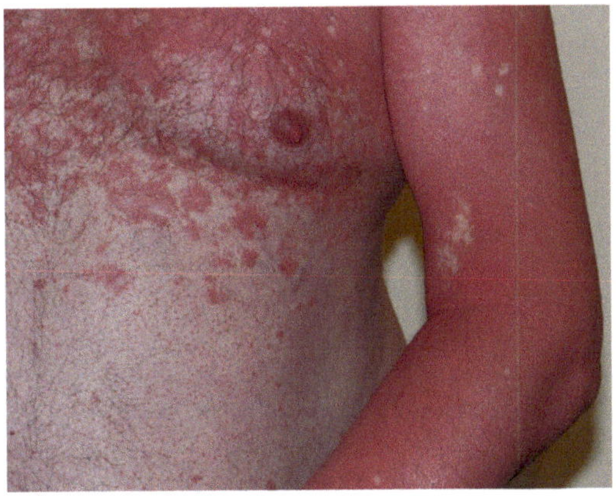

FIGURE 87.2 Pityriasis rubra pilaris FST1. (Courtesy Prof. Ian Coulson, UK.)

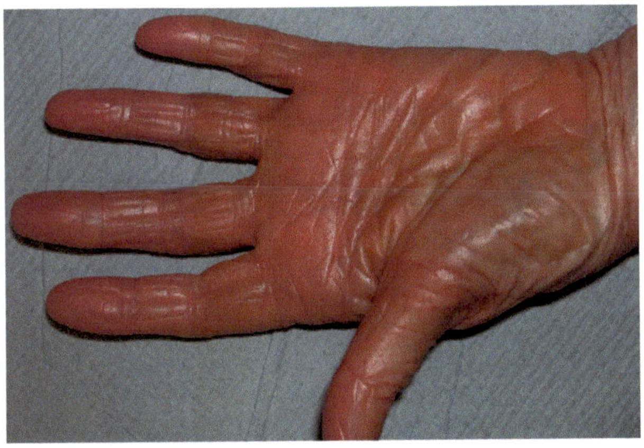

FIGURE 87.3 Pityriasis rubra pilaris palms FST1. (Courtesy Prof. Ian Coulson, UK.)

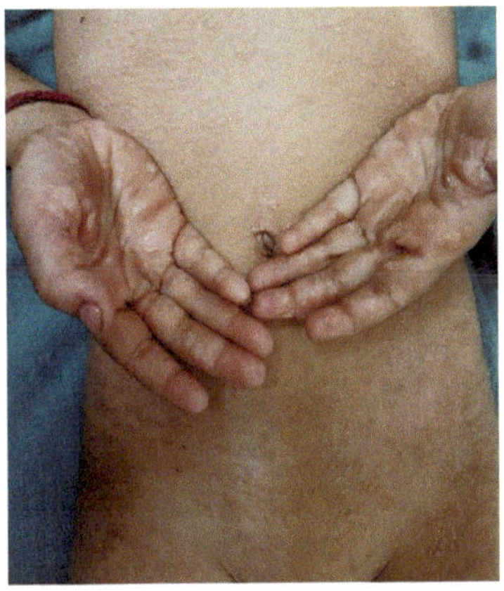

FIGURE 87.4 Pityriasis rubra pilaris palms and trunk FST5. Note well-defined salmon-red or orange-red dry scaly plaques described in white skin is not present in dark skin. (Courtesy Prof. Archana Singal, India.)

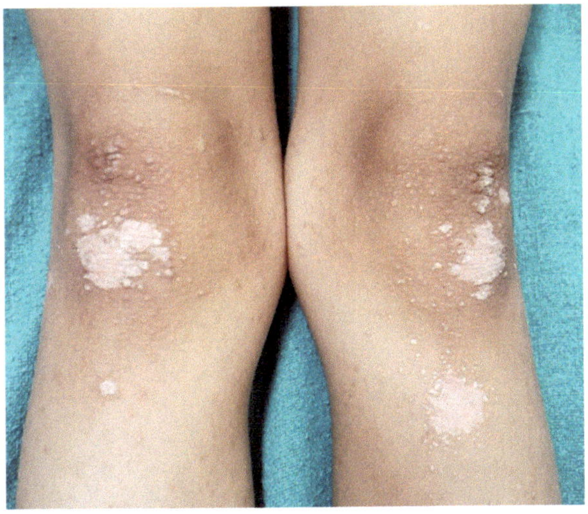

FIGURE 87.5 Pityriasis rubra pilaris FST5. (Courtesy Prof. Archana Singal, India.)

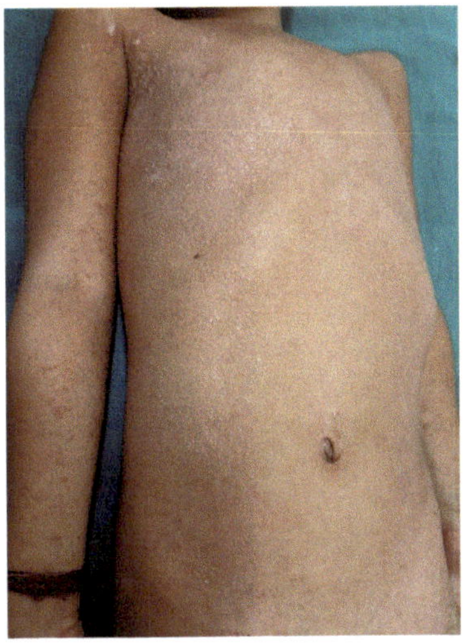

FIGURE 87.6 Pityriasis rubra pilaris in an 11-year-old boy FST5. Note erythema is not marked in dark skin. (Courtesy Prof. Archana Singal, India.)

88
PITYRIASIS VERSICOLOR

Introduction

Pityriasis versicolor (PV) is a mild, chronic, very common infection of the skin caused by lipophilic yeasts in the normal flora of the skin: *Malassezia* yeasts; *M. globosa* and possibly *M. sympodialis*, and *M. furfur.* Colonization by these species is especially dense in the scalp, the upper trunk, and flexures – areas rich in sebaceous glands and their secretions.

Epidemiology

More common in the late teens, with a peak in the early 20s.

Associated diseases

PV has been claimed to be more common in Cushing's syndrome, spontaneous and iatrogenic, and possibly in malnutrition. PV does not appear to be more common in acquired immune deficiency syndrome (AIDS) patients.

Clinical characteristics in light skin (Fitzpatrick skin types I–III)

This chronic and often relapsing infection by lipophilic yeasts of the genus *Malassezia* is very common. It is characterized by the development of asymptomatic or slightly itching macules that are light brown on fair skin and thus may cause cosmetic concern (Figure 88.1). When the patient first consults a dermatologist, the lesions may be just a few centimeters in diameter or already cover large areas of the trunk with a characteristic distribution over the midline. The skin itself is a bit velvety, and upon scraping with a wooden tongue depressor, fine scales can be made visible. This is also the means to take a specimen for direct microscopy: A transparent tape is pressed on the scaly skin and then put on a drop of methylene blue on a glass slide. Under 200–400-fold magnification, groups of yeast cells and short filaments are seen, the so-called spaghetti with meatballs picture.

A bothersome feature of PV for the patient is its long permanence and high recurrence rate. First, instead of the light brown patches, pale ones remain due to the depigmenting and melanocyte-inhibiting properties of *Malassezia* metabolic products; this may last several months (versicolor means color changing). Second, PV apparently involves persons with a (genetic? metabolic?) susceptibility to develop this disease, and this is not amenable to treatment. Third, as outlined above, *Malassezia* spp. are abundant on the scalp and trunk where many sebaceous glands are, and thus auto-infection is common. Therefore, the author recommends repeating a course of antifungal treatment, for instance with ketoconazole shampoo for the whole body first fortnightly, then once a month to suppress recurrences.

Clinical characteristics in dark skin (Fitzpatrick skin types IV–V)

A sharply demarcated macule characterized essentially by fine scaling and satellite lesions. The color of the scales may vary from pale ochre to medium brown (Figures 88.2 and 88.3). In ordinary cases that settle spontaneously or as a result of treatment, the residual hypopigmentation may remain for many months without any scaling.

Investigations

Direct microscopy shows oval yeasts. The characteristic appearance on microscopy has been likened to 'spaghetti and meatballs' or 'bananas and grapes.'

Wood's lamp examinations help to differentiate PV from erythrasma when it occurs on the flexures. Erythrasma and PV may occasionally coexist. PV lesions may show pale yellow fluorescence, while erythrasma shows pink fluorescence under the Wood's lamp.

Treatments

- Relapse is very common regardless of what primary treatment is used.
- Patients should be warned that repigmentation may take several months; otherwise, they will often report treatment failure.
- The first line of treatment is topical antifungal therapy.

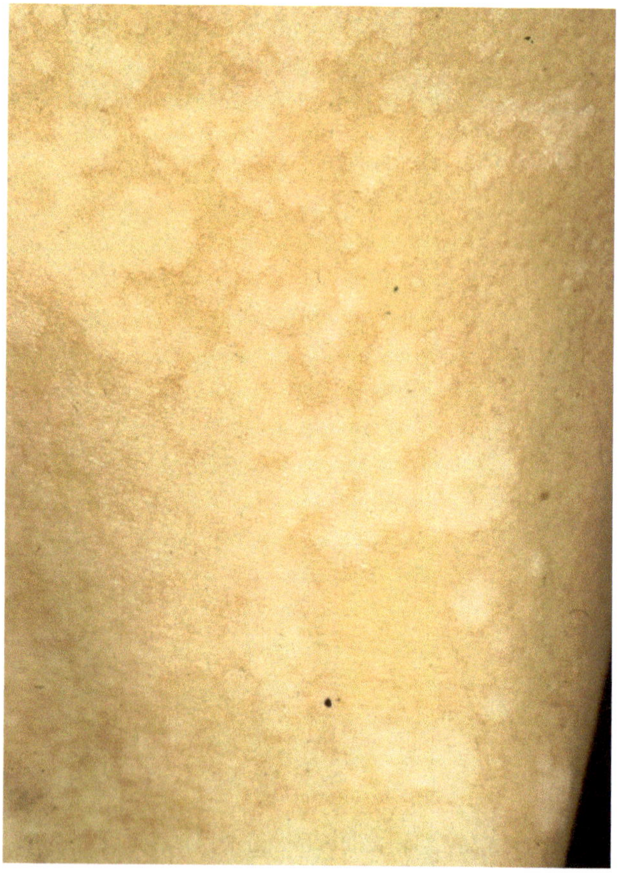

FIGURE 88.1 Hypopigmented pityriasis versicolor FST3. (Courtesy Prof. Ian Coulson, UK.)

DOI: 10.1201/9781003479512-88

- Topical azole creams (clotrimazole, ketoconazole, oxiconazole, econazole, miconazole) twice daily for 2–3 weeks.
- Terbinafine 1% cream twice daily for 2–3 weeks.
- Whitfield lotion (20% sodium hyposulphite solution and 50:50 propylene glycol in water) should be applied daily until clearance.
- Ketoconazole shampoo twice weekly for 2–3 weeks in a patient with extensive spread.
- 2.5% selenium shampoo on alternative days for 2–3 weeks is applied to all the affected areas and left overnight. This is an irritant if applied to the face or genitalia. It also stains clothes and bedding.
- Oral itraconazole 200 mg daily for 5 days for extensive or recalcitrant cases.
- In recurrent PV, long-term once-weekly application of ketoconazole shampoo.

Further reading

Chang CH, Stein SL (2024) Malassezia-Associated Skin Diseases in the Pediatric Population. *Pediatr Dermatol*;Sep–Oct;41(5):769–77.

Hay RJ (2024). Fungal Infections. In: Griffiths C, et al. (eds). *Rook's Textbook of Dermatology*, 10th ed. John Wiley & Sons Ltd., UK; 32.10.

Kallini JR, Riaz F, Khachemoune A (2014). Tinea Versicolor in Dark-Skinned Individuals. *Int J Dermatol*;53(2):137–41.

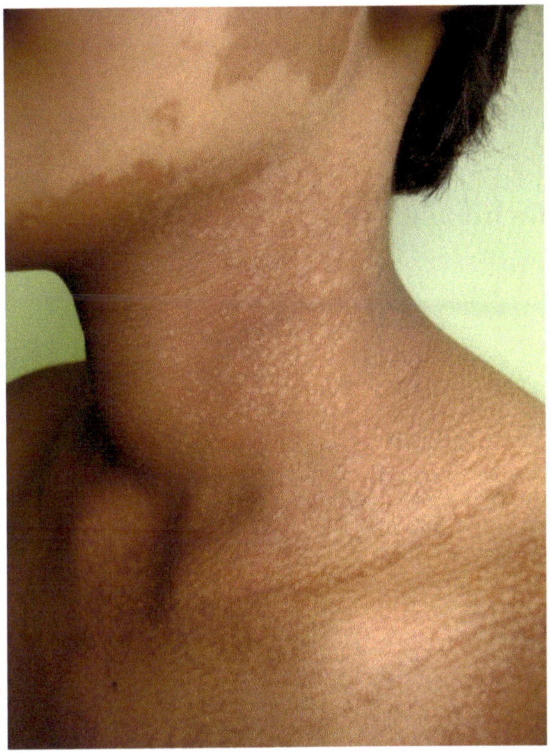

FIGURE 88.2 Hypopigmented pityriasis versicolor FST5.

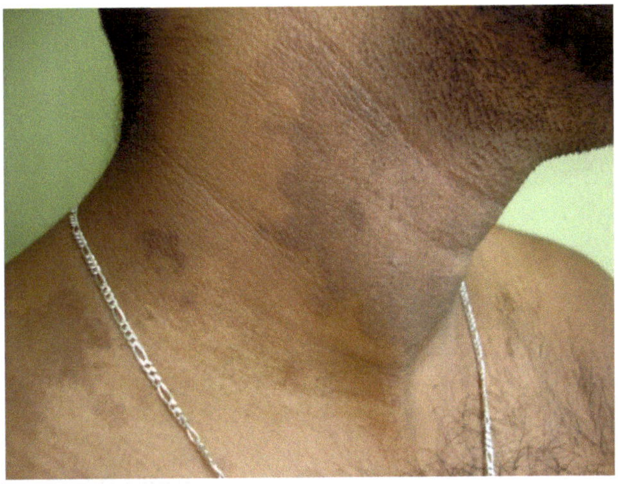

FIGURE 88.3 Hyperpigmented pityriasis versicolor FST5.

89
PITYROSPORUM FOLLICULITIS

Introduction

Malassezia (Pityrosporum) folliculitis is due to the proliferation of the *Malassezia* yeast within the hair follicles. It presents most frequently on the back and upper trunk as a monomorphic acne-like eruption with many papules or pustules which itch. The lesions are often diffusely scattered on the shoulders and back. The itching and distribution distinguish them from acne vulgaris.

Epidemiology

Most often seen in teenagers or young adults.

Associated diseases

None reported.

Clinical characteristics in light skin (Fitzpatrick skin types I–III)

Pityrosporum folliculitis is a chronic condition of young and middle-aged adults, probably more frequent in males than in females (Figures 89.1 and 89.2). Seborrheic areas are mainly involved. Crops of monomorphic follicle-bound reddish papules appear that typically itch, a symptom distinguishing it from truncal acne (no comedones!). However, it may be observed after acne vulgaris and then pose differential diagnostic challenges. The disease is more frequent after long-term antibiotic, steroid, or immunosuppressive therapy. Pityrosporum folliculitis can be diagnosed with direct microscopic examination, fungal culture, and histopathology. Treatment involves topical and systemic antifungals.

Clinical characteristics in dark skin (Fitzpatrick skin types IV–V)

Minute papules and pustules of 1–2 mm in diameter are diffusely scattered on the shoulders and back of the trunk (Figure 89.3). These start at puberty and appear as discrete lesions, which leave post-inflammatory hyperpigmentation. By the time they present to us, almost all the back is covered with post-inflammatory hyperpigmentation from previous lesions over the years. Rather than active papules and pustules, the patient's main concern is this hyperpigmentation, which takes years to resolve even after folliculitis is controlled effectively.

Investigations

This is a clinical diagnosis.

Treatments

- Topical antifungal shampoos and creams are generally helpful.
- Oral itraconazole short course is helpful in many cases.

Further reading

Chang CH, Stein SL (2021). *Malassezia*-Associated Skin Diseases in the Pediatric Population. *Pediatr Dermatol.* Sep–Oct;41(5):769–779.

Hay RJ (2024). Fungal Infections. In: Griffiths C, et al. (eds). *Rook's Textbook of Dermatology*, 10th ed. John Wiley & Sons Ltd., UK; 32.13.

Vlachos C, Henning MAS, Gaitanis G, et al. (2020). Critical Synthesis of Available Data in *Malassezia* Folliculitis and a Systematic Review of Treatments. *J Eur Acad Dermatol Venereol*;34(8):1672–1683.

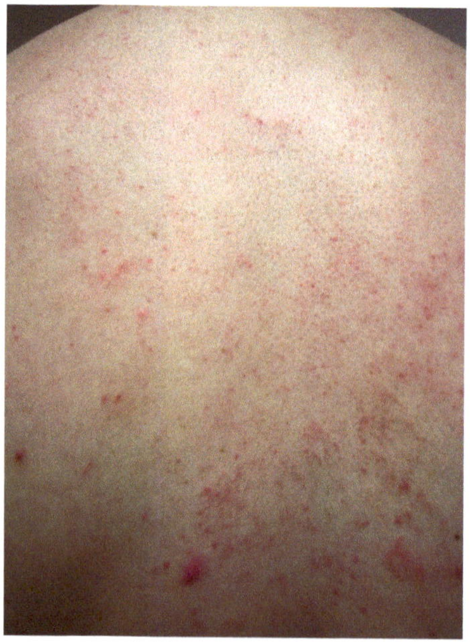

FIGURE 89.1 Pityrosporum folliculitis FST1. (Courtesy Prof. Ian Coulson, UK.)

DOI: 10.1201/9781003479512-89

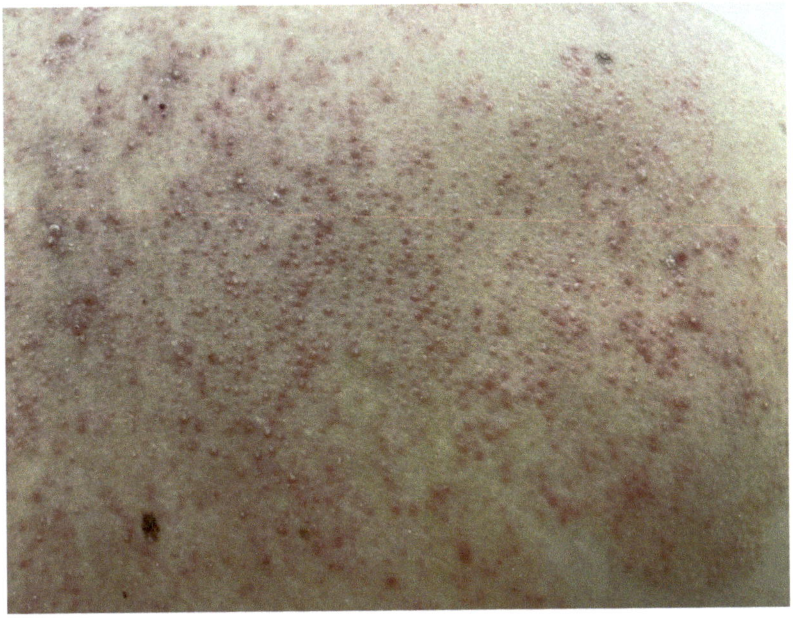

FIGURE 89.2 Pityrosporum folliculitis FST1: A closer view. (Courtesy Dr. Richard Ashton, UK.)

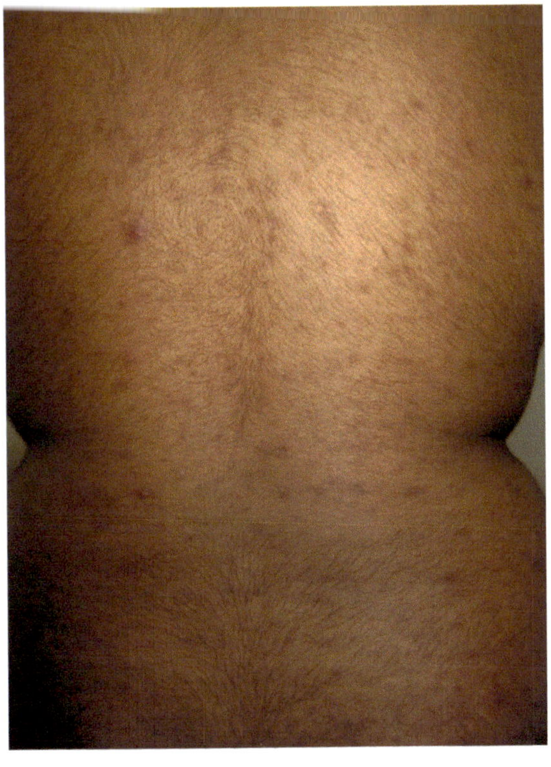

FIGURE 89.3 Pityrosporum folliculitis and post-inflammatory hyperpigmentation at the back of the trunk in a 17-year-old boy FST5.

90
POIKILODERMA

Introduction

Poikiloderma is a descriptive term, comprising atrophy, macular or reticulate pigmentation, and telangiectasia. There may be associated areas of scaling, hypopigmentation, petechiae, and signs of inflammation, such as lichenoid papules.

Poikiloderma can be congenital or acquired. Congenital poikiloderma is a feature of several inherited disorders, including Kindler syndrome, dyskeratosis congenita, Rothmund–Thomson and Weary syndromes, hereditary fibrosing poikiloderma, some types of xeroderma pigmentosum, and erythrokeratoderma variabile. Acquired poikiloderma may occur as a pattern of cutaneous response to injury by cold, heat, or ionizing radiation, as a particular form of cutaneous mastocytosis, and mycosis fungoides.

Associated diseases

Acquired poikiloderma is a feature of some systemic autoimmune diseases, such as dermatomyositis, lupus erythematosus, and rarely in systemic sclerosis. Poikiloderma atrophicans vasculare is an early presenting feature of cutaneous T-cell lymphoma (mycosis fungoides).

Clinical characteristics in light skin (Fitzpatrick skin types I–III)

The term poikiloderma literally means multicolored skin (Figures 90.1 and 90.2). This is due to macular and reticular pigmentation, irregular atrophy, and telangiectasias. In light skin, this may be very obvious and cosmetically embarrassing. Seeing a poikiloderma patient requires an exact diagnosis, as this may be part of a serious disease.

Congenital poikiloderma is a group of hereditary diseases that may or may not be associated with other symptoms like ophthalmologic signs such as premature cataract.

Poikiloderma is also a sign of dyskeratosis congenita, a severe inborn immunodeficiency disease with a characteristic Fanconi-like type of anemia.

Bloom syndrome is exceedingly rare and belongs to the group of DNA repair disorders.

We have seen a newborn girl with poikiloderma, who was later diagnosed with congenital rubella syndrome.

There is a macular variant of mastocytosis beginning with the clinical features of poikiloderma called telangiectasia macularis perstans.

Radio-dermatitis typically presents as circumscribed poikiloderma.

Chronic localized heat may cause reticular pigmentation and later transform to poikiloderma.

Poikiloderma is also a feature of late lupus erythematosus, dermatomyositis, and scleroderma.

Clinical characteristics in dark skin (Fitzpatrick skin types IV–V)

As in many other erythematous skin problems, poikiloderma is also not very well recognized in individuals with darker skin. Figure 90.3 shows a 57-year-old woman who presented with poikilodermatous mycosis fungoides.

Investigations

This is a clinical diagnosis.

Treatments

- Treat the underlying problem.
- Single-session pro-yellow laser treatment is a good treatment option for poikiloderma of Civatte (Sarac et al. 2022). The treatment of choice for poikiloderma of Civatte should address both pigmented and vascular lesions at the same time.

Further reading

Haneke E, Gutschmidt E (1979). Premature Multiple Bowen's Disease in Poikiloderma Congenitale with Warty Hyperkeratoses. *Dermatologica*;158:384–388.

Irvine AD, Mellerio JE (2024). Poikiloderma Syndromes. In: Griffiths C, et al. (eds). *Rook's Textbook of Dermatology*, 10th ed. John Wiley & Sons Ltd., UK; 75.1.

Rusciani A, Motta A, Fino P, et al. (2008). Treatment of Poikiloderma of Civatte Using Intense Pulsed Light Source: 7 Years of Experience. *Dermatol Surg*;34(3):314–319.

Sarac G, Kapicioglu Y, Cenk H (2022). A New Treatment Option for Poikiloderma of Civatte: 577 nm Pro-Yellow Laser. *J Cosmet Dermatol*;21(1):316–319.

DOI: 10.1201/9781003479512-90

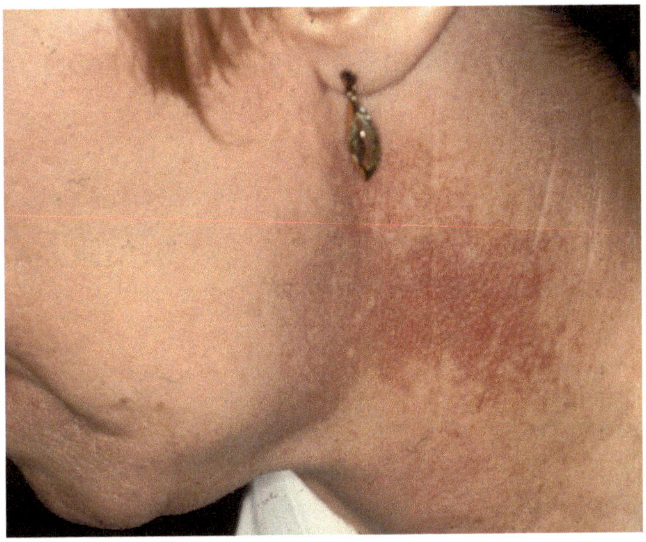

FIGURE 90.1 Poikiloderma of Civatte FST1. (Courtesy Dr. Richard Ashton, UK.)

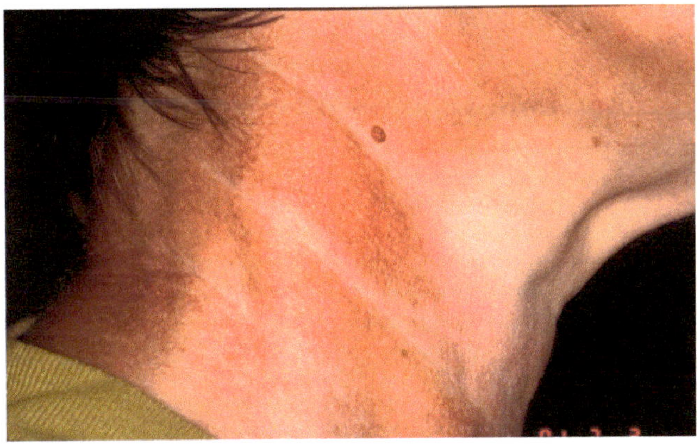

FIGURE 90.2 Poikiloderma of Civatte FST1. (Courtesy Dr. Richard Ashton, UK.)

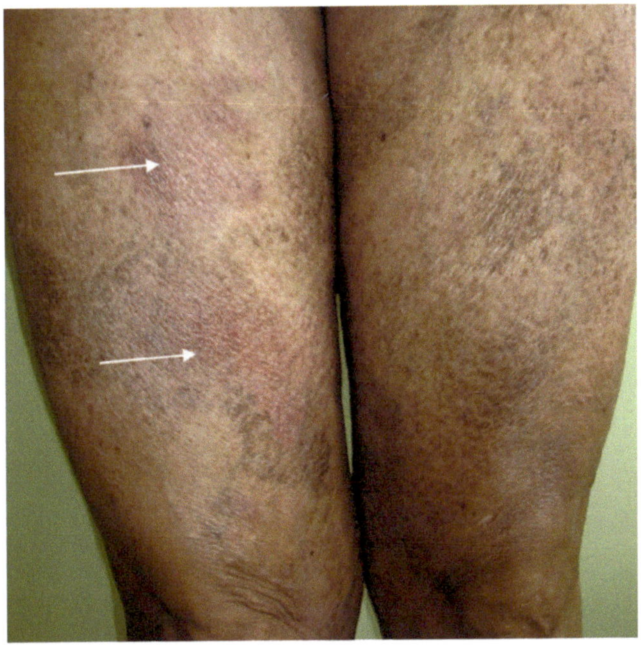

FIGURE 90.3 Poikilodermatous mycosis fungoides in a 57-year-old woman FST5.

91
POLYMORPHIC LIGHT ERUPTION

Introduction

Polymorphic light eruption (PLE) is a recurrent, delayed-onset, abnormal reaction to sunlight (or an artificial UVR source) that resolves without scarring. 'Polymorphic' means that it has several morphological variants. PLE affects sunlight-exposed sites exclusively: Face, upper trunk, dorsum of the hands, extensor surface of forearms, dorsum of feet, or scalp if bald-headed.

Epidemiology

Common all over the world, affecting all skin types, but worse in skin types I–III.

Associated diseases

Associated with lupus erythematosus (LE: Systemic, subacute cutaneous, and discoid), actinic prurigo, and photosensitive psoriasis.

Clinical characteristics in light skin (Fitzpatrick skin types I–III)

PLE is a polyetiological disease that is precipitated by (sun) light (Figures 91.1 and 91.2). It is mainly observed between March and June in the northern hemisphere. In Europe, both genders are equally affected. There is a lowered threshold to sunlight, although the minimal erythemal dose (MED) to ultraviolet B is not decreased. Erythematous and papular lesions, often with intense pruritus, appear after the first intense sun exposure. The lesions are monomorphic in the same patient but vary among different subjects.

Clinical characteristics in dark skin (Fitzpatrick skin types IV–V)

PLE is very common among older children who play outdoors in our settings (Figures 91.3 and 91.4). It is equally common among both boys and girls. The most common presentation is mildly scaly, well-demarcated, discrete hypopigmented macules on the face, dorsum of the hands, forearms and dorsum of the feet. Itchiness is not a constant finding. If untreated, some may develop into an eczematous rash. These heal without any sequelae. Other clinical variants, such as papulovesicular type, plaques, vesiculo-bullous, and erythema multiforme-like variants, are rare in dark skin.

Investigations

This is diagnosed clinically.

Treatments

- Photoprotection is advised; sunscreens if requested.
- Mild topical corticosteroid therapy if itching is a problem.
- Short course of systemic corticosteroid therapy if not responding to above.
- Patients with florid PLE often benefit from prophylactic desensitization treatment using narrow-band UVB phototherapy in early spring, an artificial method that induces a 'hardening' phenomenon.
- Janus kinase (JAK)1 and JAK3 inhibitors (tofacitinib) are effective in refractory cases of PLE (Sardana et al. 2024).

Further reading

Combalia A, Fernández-Sartorio C, Fustà X, et al. (2017). Successful Short Desensitization Treatment Protocol with Narrowband UVB Phototherapy (TL-01) in Polymorphic Light Eruption. *Actas Dermosifiliogr*;108(8):752–757.

Ibbotson S (2024). Cutaneous Photosensitivity Diseases. In: Griffiths C, et al. (eds). *Rook's Textbook of Dermatology*, 10th ed. John Wiley & Sons Ltd., UK; 126.2.

Kadurina M, Kazandjieva J, Bocheva G (2021). Immunopathogenesis and Management of Polymorphic Light Eruption. *Dermatol Ther*;34(6):e15167.

Sardana K, Mathachan SR, Khurana A (2024). Tofacitinib: A Treatment Option for Recalcitrant Polymorphic Light Eruption and Its Mechanistic Rationale. *Dermatitis*;35(3):246–249.

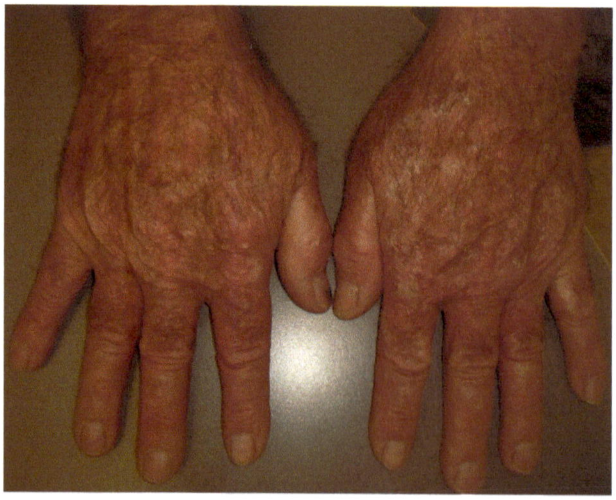

FIGURE 91.1 Actinic keratosis in FST1. (Courtesy Prof. Uwe Wollina, Germany)

DOI: 10.1201/9781003479512-91

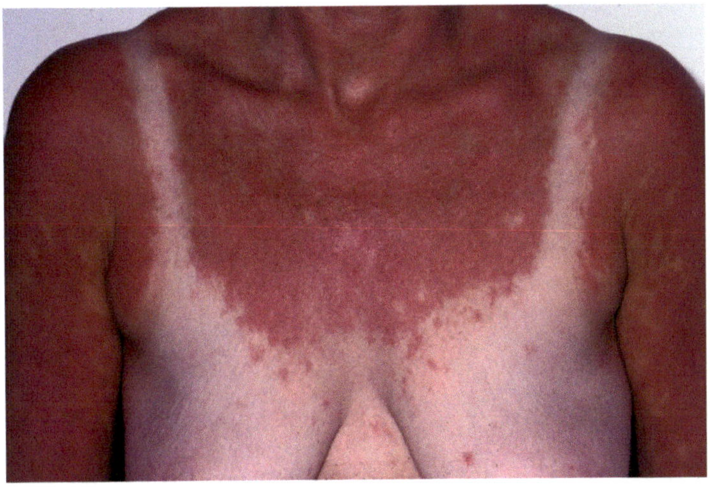

FIGURE 91.2 Erythema following acute UV radiation (intense natural sunlight) exposure ('sunburn') FST1. (Courtesy Dr. Richard Ashton, UK.)

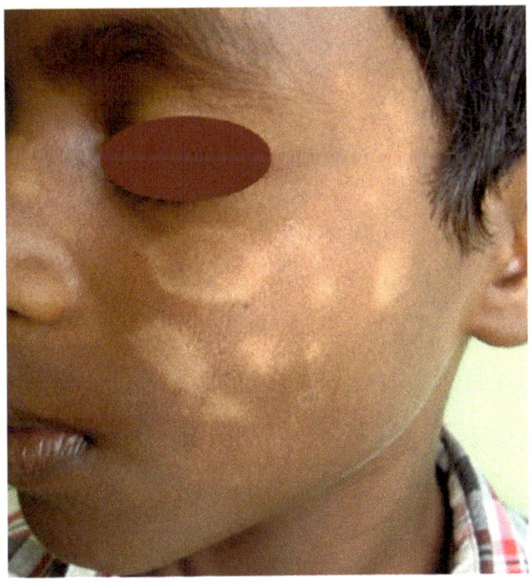

FIGURE 91.3 Polymorphic light eruption in a 9-year-old boy showing mildly scaly, well-demarcated, discrete hypopigmented macules, on the sun-exposed areas of the face FST5.

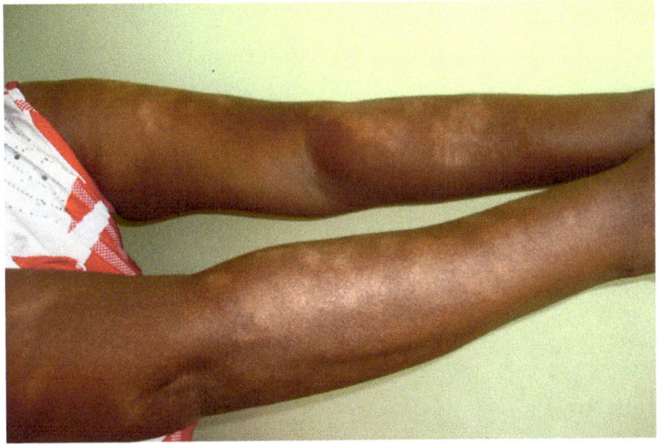

FIGURE 91.4 Polymorphic light eruption affecting the sun-exposed areas of the forearms and arms in a 32-year-old woman FST5.

92
PORT-WINE STAIN

Introduction

Port-wine stain (PWS) is a capillary malformation (CM). This is a homogenous, pink, red, or purple macule present at birth. These are usually located on the head and neck, but can also be seen on the trunk or limbs. A CM grows proportionately with the child and persists throughout life. The lesion darkens and often thickens with age, and the underlying tissues (skin, fat, muscle, and bone) can be hypertrophic. If untreated, PWSs thicken diffusely over time, with approximately two-thirds of patients developing hypertrophic or nodular lesions by age 50 years.

Epidemiology

It is the most common vascular malformation. It is present at birth in approximately 3 out of 1000 newborns.

Associated diseases

Sturge–Weber syndrome (SWS) is characterized by a CM located in the territory of the first or second branch of the trigeminal nerve, and may be associated with a leptomeningeal and/or retinal capillary–venous malformation on the same side. Patients with a periorbital PWS should also be tested for glaucoma.

Klippel–Trenaunay syndrome usually involves one leg with an extensive PWS unilateral varicosis, and bone hypertrophy.

Clinical characteristics in light skin (Fitzpatrick skin types I–III)

In fair skin, PWSs, also called nevi flammei, are quite obvious and may pose a serious cosmetic problem for the parents and the patient (Figures 92.1 and 92.2). It is due to a (functional) malformation of the capillaries and does not exhibit any tendency to grow; thus, X-ray and other radioactive treatment modalities such as thorium X lacquer are strictly contraindicated.

There is a clinical variant, the midline vascular nevus, also called nevus roseus or the stork bite, which is a pink spot in the midline forehead or nape of the neck. This usually fades with age but may be more visible in hot temperatures or during physical activity.

Clinical characteristics in dark skin (Fitzpatrick skin types IV–V)

Faint homogeneous pink macule detected at birth (Figures 92.3 and 92.4). In darker skin, this faint pink lesion may be obscure, but it may become apparent when hypertrophy or nodular lesions appear later in life. This becomes more erythematous and obvious when it is exposed to warm water, warm weather, spicy foods, or when crying.

Investigations

This is a clinical diagnosis.

Segmental lower extremity CMs need scaniometry at around 8 years of age to evaluate growth discrepancy.

If SWS is suspected, brain magnetic resonance imaging (MRI) and an ophthalmological evaluation of the fundus of the eye, as well as regular assessment of intraocular pressure, are required.

An abnormal MRI warrants a neurological evaluation.

Treatments

- Currently, the main treatments for PWS are pulsed dye laser (PDL) and photodynamic therapy (PDT). Pulsed-dye laser (PDL) is the first-line treatment, which reduces coloration in 75% of patients, with 6–8 treatments spaced at 4–6-week intervals.
- Poor prognostic factors include age over 1 year, central facial location, size >40 cm^2, nodular or hypertrophic lesions, vessels >400 μm below the dermal–epidermal junction, vessel diameter >20 μm, and more than five previous laser treatments.
- The nodular fibrous proliferations seen in patients over 40–50 years can be excised or treated with a carbon dioxide laser.

Further reading

Dompmartin A, Revencu N, Boon LM, et al. (2024). Disorders Affecting Cutaneous Vasculature. In: Griffiths C, et al. (eds). *Rook's Textbook of Dermatology*, 10th ed. John Wiley & Sons Ltd., UK; 71.3.

Messele F, Van Trigt W, Arkin L, et al. (2024). Port Wine Birthmark Therapy: A New Direction. *Lasers Surg Med*;56(6):529–531.

Nguyen L, Seeber N, Kautz G, et al. (2024). 532-nm Potassium Titanyl-Phosphate Laser versus 595-nm Pulsed Dye Laser for Port-Wine Birthmarks: A Prospective, Randomized, Split-Side Study. *J Eur Acad Dermatol Venereol*;38(6):1140–1146.

Tian R, Wang Q, Li S, et al. (2024). Non-Invasive Efficacy Assessment of Pulsed Dye Laser and Photodynamic Therapy for Port-Wine Stain. *Indian J Dermatol Venereol Leprol*;90(5):615.

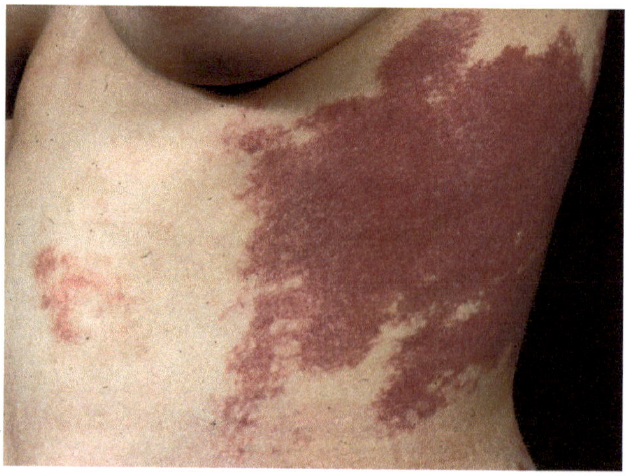

FIGURE 92.1 Port-wine stain FST1. (Courtesy Dr. Richard Ashton, UK.)

DOI: 10.1201/9781003479512-92

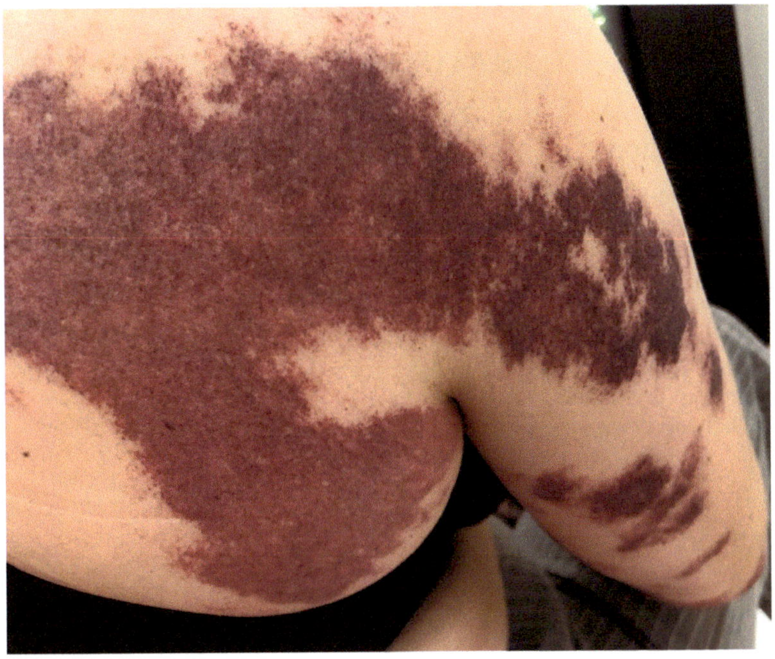

FIGURE 92.2 Extensive port-wine stain in a 43-year-old female FST2. (Courtesy Dr. Ivana Manola, Croatia.)

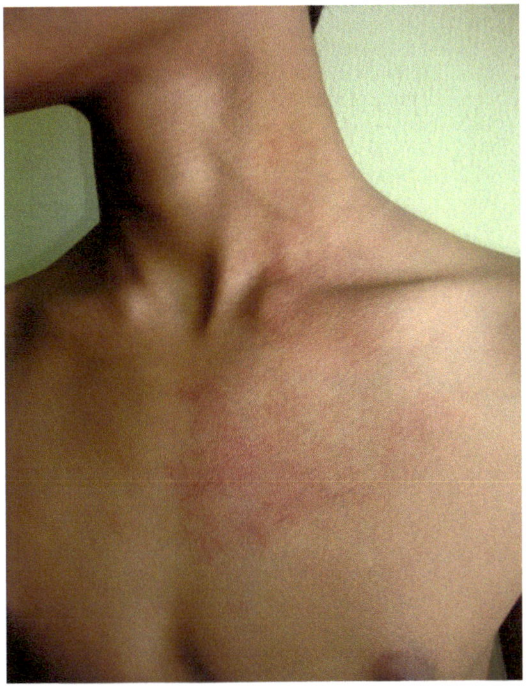

FIGURE 92.3 Port-wine stain in a 13-year-old boy FST5.

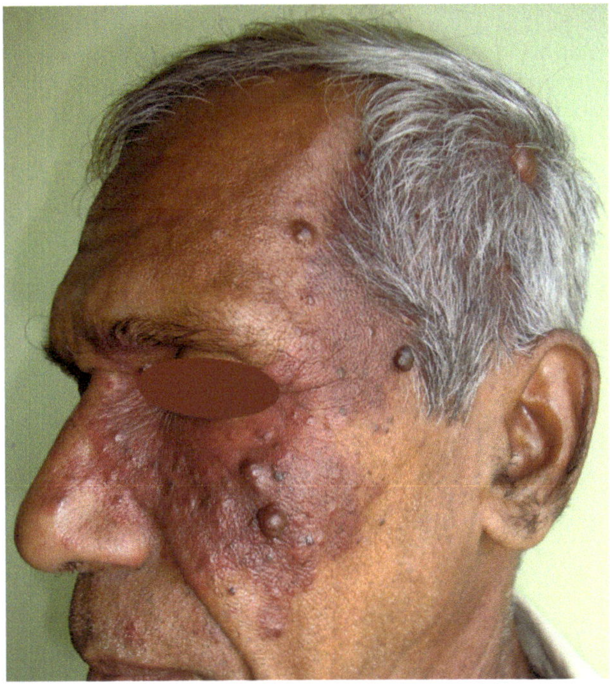

FIGURE 92.4 Untreated port-wine stain in a 65-year-old man FST5. PWSs thicken diffusely over time with hypertrophic or nodular lesions by age 50 years.

93
POST-INFLAMMATORY HYPERPIGMENTATION

Introduction

Post-inflammatory hypermelanosis is residual macular pigmentation resulting from prior skin inflammation. The pattern and distribution of the pigmentation depend on the respective skin disease, as in lichen planus, herpes zoster, tinea infection, drug rash, papular urticaria, acne, etc. Post-inflammatory hyperpigmentation may also occur following trauma to the skin, including procedures such as dermabrasion, laser therapy, skin peeling, and liquid nitrogen cryotherapy, particularly in darker skin types. The skin lightens slowly over time spontaneously or with therapy, usually over 6–12 months, but may take several years.

Epidemiology

Very common, can affect any age and both sexes. More common in darker skin types.

Clinical characteristics in light skin (Fitzpatrick skin types I–III)

Post-inflammatory hyperpigmentation is a characteristic sequela of any type of inflammation; however, compared to skin types IV–VI, it is less frequent in types I–III and rarely becomes as dark. It also has a better tendency to disappear spontaneously. Sun protection is necessary (Figures 93.1 and 93.2).

Clinical characteristics in dark skin (Fitzpatrick skin types IV–V)

This is a very common concern in dark skin following any inflammatory disease (Figures 93.3 and 93.4). However, in dark skin, post-inflammatory hyperpigmentation is cosmetically more acceptable than hypopigmentation.

Investigations

This is a clinical diagnosis.
Investigations depend on the primary disease.

Treatments

- Early treatment of underlying etiology to prevent inflammation and pigmentation.
- Sun protection.
- A variety of topical treatments may be effective, including hydroquinone 2–4%, retinoids, azelaic acid, α-hydroxy acid, glycolic acid, preferably in combination therapy.
- Laser therapy (Q-switched ruby, alexandrite, Nd:YAG) yields limited results.

Further reading

Alexis A, Del Rosso JQ, Forman S, et al. (2024). Importance of Treating Acne Sequelae in Skin of Color: 6-Month Phase IV Study of Trifarotene with an Appropriate Skincare Routine Including UV Protection in Acne-Induced Post-Inflammatory Hyperpigmentation. *Int J Dermatol*;63(6):806–815.

Fonseka S (2021). Acne. In: Ranawaka RR, et al. (eds). *Atlas of Dermatoses in Pigmented Skin*. Springer, Singapore; 503.

Garg S, Vashisht KR, Garg D, et al. (2024). Advancements in Laser Therapies for Dermal Hyperpigmentation in Skin of Color: A Comprehensive Literature Review and Experience of Sequential Laser Treatments in a Cohort of 122 Indian Patients. *J Clin Med*;13(7):2116.

Mar K, Khalid B, Maazi M, et al. (2024). Treatment of Post-Inflammatory Hyperpigmentation in Skin of Colour: A Systematic Review. *J Cutan Med Surg*;12034754241265716.

Paasch U, Zidane M, Baron JM, et al. (2022). S2k Guideline: Laser Therapy of the Skin. *J Dtsch Dermatol Ges*;20(9):1248–1267.

Rajendiran P (2021). Hyperpigmentary Disorders. In: Ranawaka RR, et al. (eds). *Atlas of Dermatoses in Pigmented Skin*. Springer, Singapore; 851.

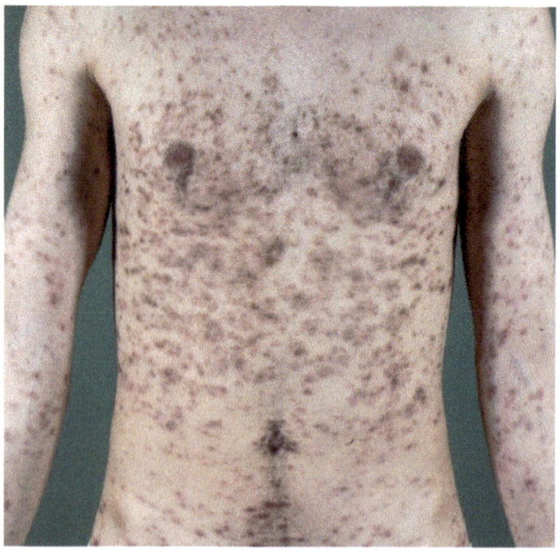

FIGURE 93.1 Post-inflammatory hyperpigmentation following lichen planus FST1. (Courtesy Dr. Richard Ashton, UK.)

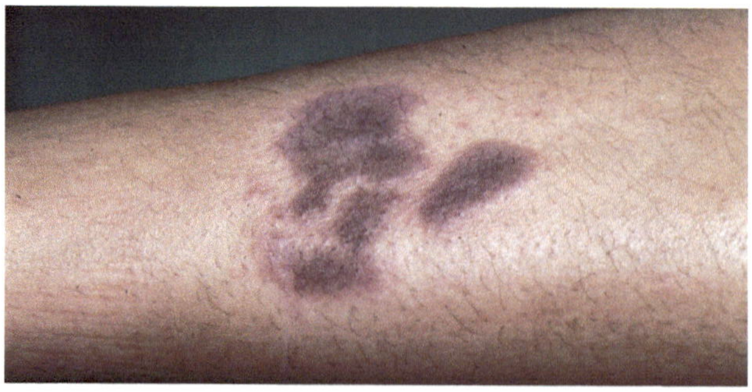

FIGURE 93.2 Post-inflammatory hyperpigmentation following lichen planus FST1. (Courtesy Dr. Richard Ashton, UK.)

DOI: 10.1201/9781003479512-93

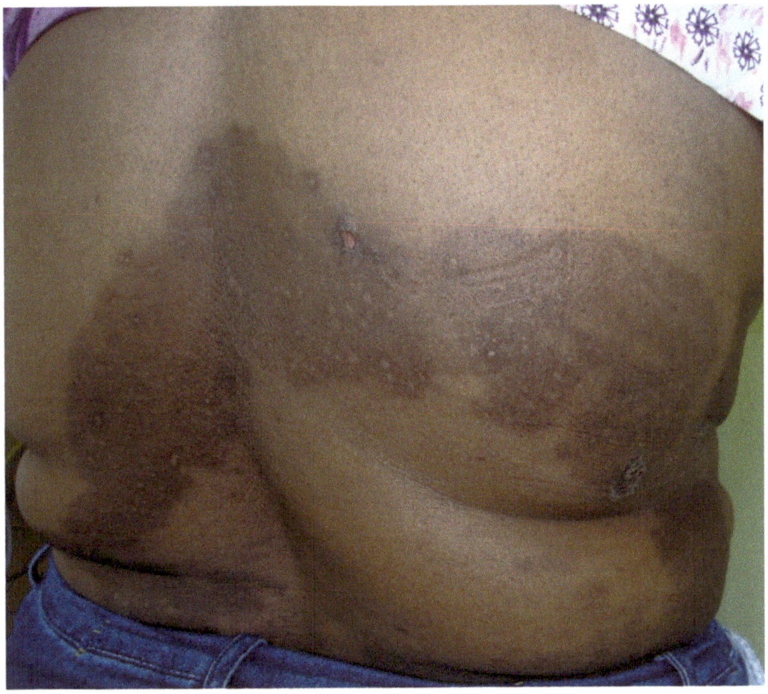

FIGURE 93.3 Post-inflammatory hyperpigmentation following extensive tinea infection FST5.

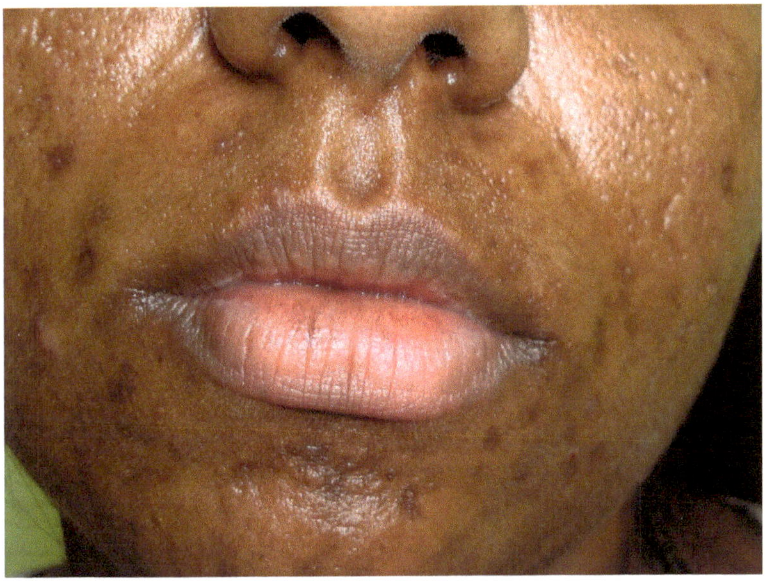

FIGURE 93.4 Post-inflammatory hyperpigmentation following acne FST5.

94
POST-INFLAMMATORY HYPOPIGMENTATION

Introduction

Hypomelanotic areas occur following the resolution of an inflammatory skin disease, such as eczema, psoriasis, pityriasis lichenoides chronica, polymorphic light eruption, lichen striatus, superficial fungal infection, pityriasis versicolor, and leprosy, etc. This is very common in dark-skinned infants with nappy rash, infantile seborrheic dermatitis, drooping saliva, dry skin, or atopic eczema.

Epidemiology

Males and females are equally predisposed

Clinical characteristics in light skin (Fitzpatrick skin types I–III)

This is rarely a problem in light skin, although it may occur (Figure 94.1). Spontaneous resolution is the rule except when it is associated with scarring. In pityriasis versicolor, the etiological fungus secretes substances that inhibit melanocyte function. It takes several months after successful therapy for the melanocytes to recover.

Clinical characteristics in dark skin (Fitzpatrick skin types IV–V)

Post-inflammatory hypopigmentation is very common in dark skin. This is very common in dark-skinned infants that causes major concern to parents (Figures 94.2 to 94.7).

Investigations

A skin biopsy can be helpful in investigating possible underlying causes, particularly if hypopigmented mycosis fungoides is suspected.

Treatments

- Identify the causative inflammatory disease and treat it.
- Post-inflammatory hypomelanosis is reversible, but in some, it may take years to regain normal skin color.

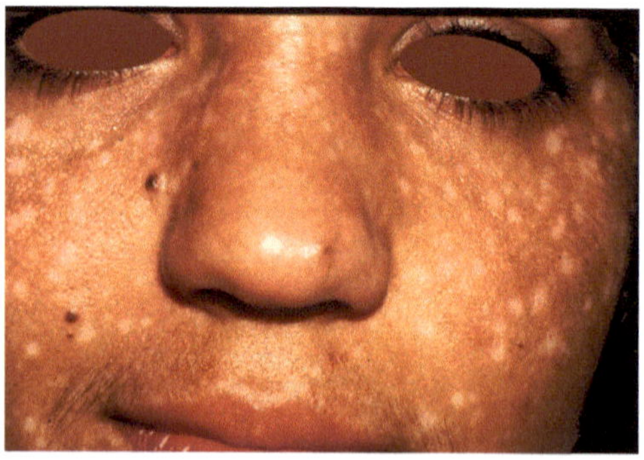

FIGURE 94.2 Post-inflammatory hypopigmentation following monobenzylether of hydroquinone FST4. (Courtesy Dr. Richard Ashton, UK.)

Further reading

Ceresnie MS, Gonzalez S, Hamzavi IH (2023). Diagnosing Disorders of Hypopigmentation and Depigmentation in Patients with Skin of Color. *Dermatol Clin*;41(3):407–416.

Chan LKW, Lee KWA, Hung LC, et al. (2024). Treating Hypertrophic Scar, Post-Inflammatory Hyperpigmentation, and Post-Inflammatory Hypopigmentation with Intense Pulsed Light. *Skin Res Technol*;30(6):e13823.

Gammanpila RR, Kannanagara AP (2023). Postinflammatory Hypopigmentation. In: *Paediatric Cases in Coloured Skin*. CRC Press; 80.

Jablon K, Theisen E, Hsu SH, et al. (2024). Fractional Non-Ablative Assisted Bimatoprost Delivery: A Synergistic Approach for Treating Post-Inflammatory Hypopigmentation Following Cosmetic Procedures in Skin of Color Patients. *Lasers Surg Med*;56(1): 11–13.

Rao M, Young K, Jackson-Cowan L, et al. (2023). Post-Inflammatory Hypopigmentation: Review of the Etiology, Clinical Manifestations, and Treatment Options. *J Clin Med*;12(3):1243.

van Geel N, Speeckaert R (2024). Acquired Pigmentary Disorders. In: Griffiths C, et al. (eds). *Rook's Textbook of Dermatology*, 10th ed. John Wiley & Sons Ltd., UK; 86.43.

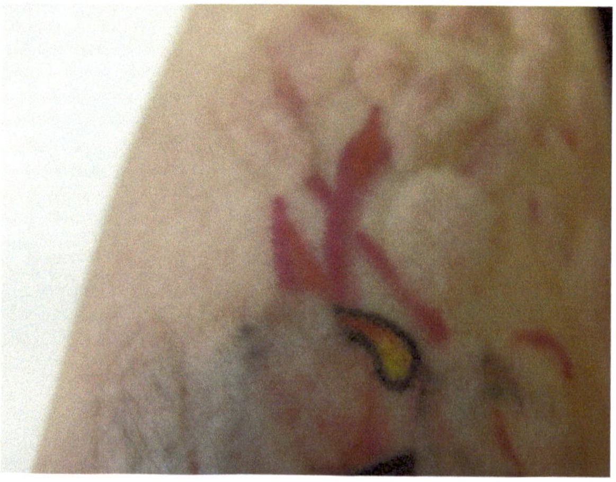

FIGURE 94.1 Post-inflammatory hypopigmentation.

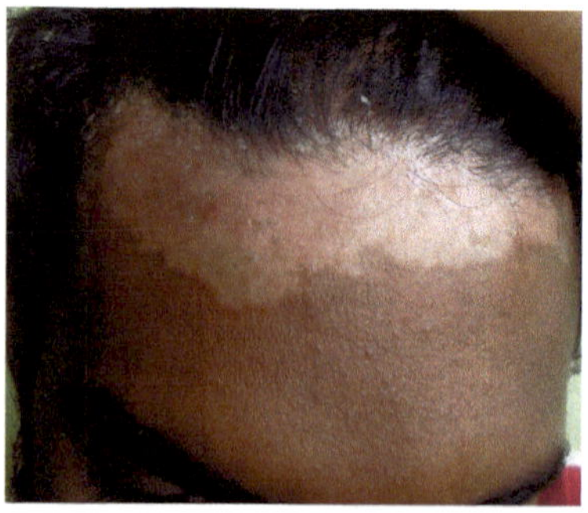

FIGURE 94.3 Post-inflammatory hypopigmentation in psoriasis FST5.

DOI: 10.1201/9781003479512-94

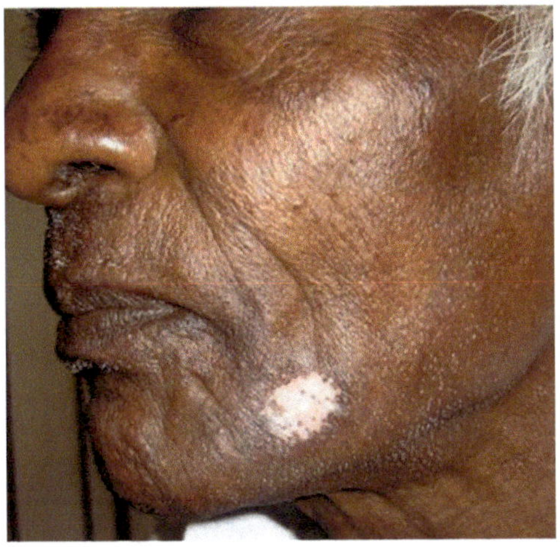

FIGURE 94.4 Post-inflammatory depigmentation following liquid nitrogen cryotherapy applied on cutaneous leishmaniasis FST5.

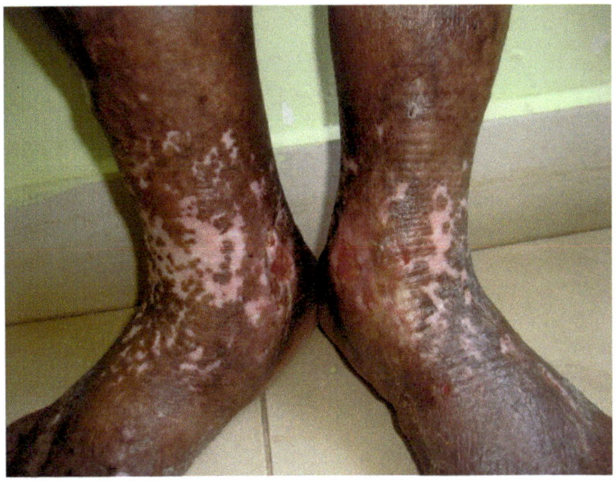

FIGURE 94.5 Post-inflammatory hypo- or depigmentation in chronic venous eczema FST5.

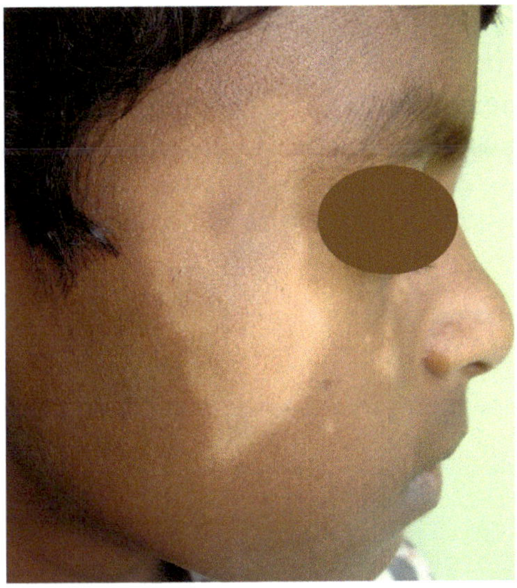

FIGURE 94.6 Post-inflammatory hypopigmentation in polymorphic light eruption FST5.

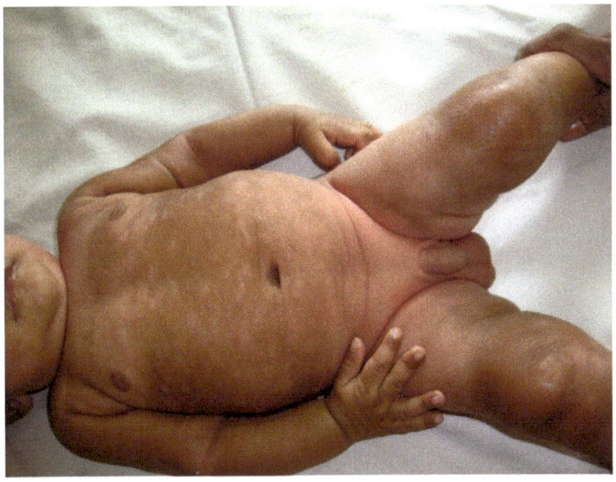

FIGURE 94.7 Post-inflammatory hypopigmentation in infantile seborrheic dermatitis FST5.

95
PROGRESSIVE MACULAR HYPOMELANOSIS

Introduction

Progressive macular hypomelanosis (PMH) is a common acquired dermatosis characterized by ill-defined nummular hypopigmented macules, mainly affecting the trunk. It has been postulated that different subtypes of *Cutibacterium* (formerly *Propionibacterium*) species might be responsible for PMH.

Epidemiology

A very common skin disorder in adolescents and young adults with darker skin. It has an equal incidence in both sexes.

Associated diseases

Benign condition and not associated with other diseases.

Clinical characteristics in light skin (Fitzpatrick skin types I–III)

PMH mostly presents as acquired, non-scaly, confluent, hypopigmented macules on the trunk, with no history of inflammation or infection. The patches are inconspicuous in light skin (Figure 95.1).

Clinical characteristics in dark skin (Fitzpatrick skin types IV–V)

PMH is very common in our settings in adolescents and young adults and is equal incidence in both sexes (Figures 95.2 and 95.3). Patients seek treatment early in fear of extensive pityriasis versicolor or vitiligo. They present with ill-defined nummular hypopigmented non-scaly macules on the back and front of the trunk. This condition typically starts in areas rich in sebaceous glands, in and around the midline, and then coalesces to form large hypopigmented patches. This mimics hypopigmented mycosis fungoides (HMF) in dark-skinned individuals.

Investigations

This is diagnosed clinically.

Wood's lamp examination: Orange-red fluorescence in some, but absence does not exclude PMH.

Skin biopsy if HMF is clinically suspected.

Treatments

- This condition generally resolves spontaneously within a few years.
- Topical application of 5–10% benzoyl peroxide hydrogel and 1% clindamycin lotion or gel alternatively for 2–3 months gives very good results, removing the lesions and regaining normal skin pigmentation.
- Phototherapy (both UVA and narrow-band UVB) has been shown to be effective.

Further reading

Leonard N, Krueger S, Rashighi M (2020). Successful Treatment of Progressive Macular Hypomelanosis. *Dermatol Reports*;12(2):8509.

Mitchell KN, Tay YK, Heath CR, et al. (2021a). Review Article: Emerging Issues in Pediatric Skin of Color, Part 1. *Pediatr Dermatol*;38 Suppl 2:20–29.

Mitchell KN, Tay YK, Heath CR, et al. (2021b). Review Article: Emerging Issues in Pediatric Skin of Color, Part 2. *Pediatr Dermatol*;38 Suppl 2:30–36.

Paquette GM, Sherman S, Akabane A, et al. (2023). Adolescent Extra-Truncal Progressive Macular Hypomelanosis. *Pediatr Dermatol*;40(4):702–705.

Petersen RL, Scholz CF, Jensen A, et al. (2017). *Propionibacterium Acnes* Phylogenetic Type III is Associated with Progressive Macular Hypomelanosis. *Eur J Microbiol Immunol*;7(1):37–45.

Ranawaka RR (2021). Hypopigmentary Disorders. In: Ranawaka RR, Kannagara AP, Karawita A (eds). *Atlas of Dermatoses in Pigmented Skin*. Springer, Singapore.

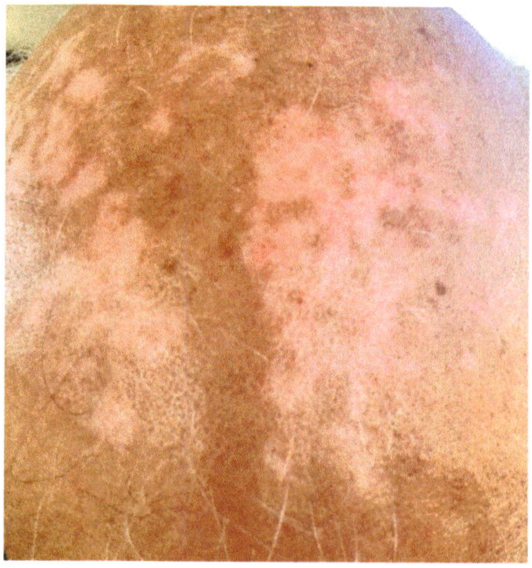

FIGURE 95.1 Progressive macular hypomelanosis in a suntanned FST3. (Courtesy Prof. Eckart Haneke, Germany.)

DOI: 10.1201/9781003479512-95

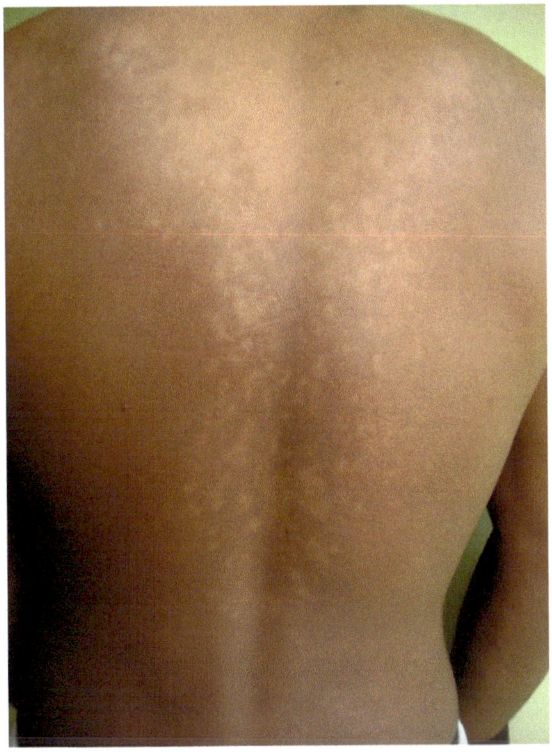

FIGURE 95.2 Progressive macular hypomelanosis in a 25-year-old man showing the back of the trunk FST5.

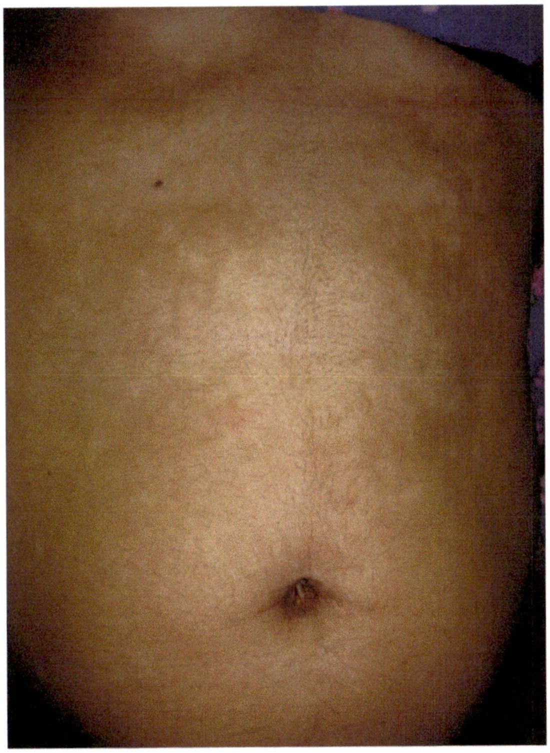

FIGURE 95.3 Progressive macular hypomelanosis affecting chest and abdomen in a 21-year-old woman FST5.

96
PRURIGO NODULARIS

Introduction

Prurigo nodularis (PN) is characterized by the presence of numerous symmetrically distributed hyperkeratotic or eroded nodules. Nodules in PN are intensely itchy, and thus a vicious itch–scratch cycle may evolve. It may occur in a broad variety of diseases that induce pruritus; dermatological, systemic, neurological, and psychiatric diseases. Most patients have either an atopic predisposition or atopic eczema as an important cause of PN.

Epidemiology

PN affects patients of all ages, including children, but is more common in older patients and in women.

Associated diseases

May occur in a broad variety of diseases that induce pruritus.

- *Dermatological*: Atopic eczema, atopic predisposition, nummular eczema, psoriasis, Grover disease, lichen planus, epidermolysis bullosa acquisita, dermatitis herpetiformis, bullous pemphigoid, lymphoma, untreated scabies.
- *Systemic diseases*: Uremia, diabetes mellitus, hyperbilirubinemia, biliary disease.
- *Neurological*: Brachioradial pruritus, chronic pain syndrome, restless legs syndrome, etc.
- *Psychiatric diseases*: Delusional parasitosis, emotional stress and psychological disorders, depression, anxiety.

Clinical characteristics in light skin (Fitzpatrick skin types I–III)

PN is a characteristic disease in light skin (Figures 96.1 and 96.2). It may occur spontaneously or in the context of the above-mentioned diseases. Atopy is most frequent.

Single hard nodules and papules with a hyperkeratotic to verrucous surface or scratched-out surface are seen particularly in areas where the patient can easily reach the skin; thus, the central back is virtually always spared. However, some patients also have genital lesions, which is a particularly severe burden as the urge to scratch is usually insurmountable. There is a close relation to lichen simplex chronicus (plaque-type PN?).

Clinical characteristics in dark skin (Fitzpatrick skin types IV–V)

The typical lesion of PN is a blackish nodule with a hyperpigmented border (Figures 96.3 and 96.4). The lesion may have a hyperkeratotic or eroded surface. In most patients, the PN lesion starts as a small erythematous papule and then develops into a blackish nodule.

Investigations

The aim of examination and investigations is to identify any underlying dermatoses that may be masked by the presence of PN.

Treatments

- Therapy must be multimodal, including treatment of the underlying disease and the use of topical emollients (especially for dry skin, atopic predisposition).
- Topical substances for short-term relief of itch (e.g., menthol).
- Specific systemic antipruritic therapy.
- Cryosurgery, intralesional steroids, or excimer laser have been used on individual lesions.
- If necessary, psychosomatic counseling.
- Gabapentin, pregabalin, naltrexone, aprepitant, ciclosporin, thalidomide, and PUVA have been used with variable success.
- Recently, dupilumab was approved for the treatment of PN. Janus kinase inhibitors are now being tested with promising results.

Further reading

Andersen TP, Fogh K (2011). Thalidomide in 42 Patients with Prurigo Nodularis Hyde. *Dermatology*;223(2):107–112.

Hanly A, Watsky KL (2023). Prurigo Nodularis: Moving Forward. *Cutis*;112(6):262–263.

Mazza M, Guerriero G, Marano G, et al. (2013). Treatment of Prurigo Nodularis with Pregabalin. *J Clin Pharm Ther*;38(1):16–8.

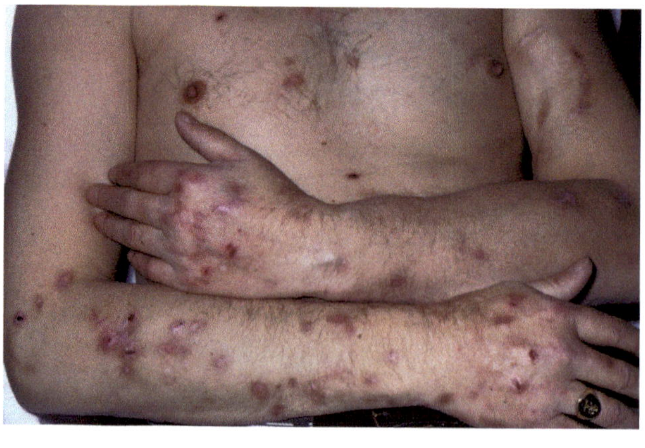

FIGURE 96.1 Excoriations following nodular prurigo FST1. (Courtesy Dr. Richard Ashton, UK.)

DOI: 10.1201/9781003479512-96

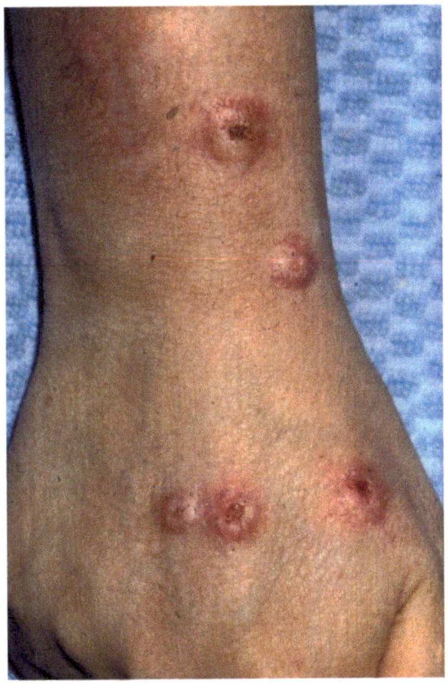

FIGURE 96.2 Nodular prurigo FST2. (Courtesy Dr. Richard Ashton, UK.)

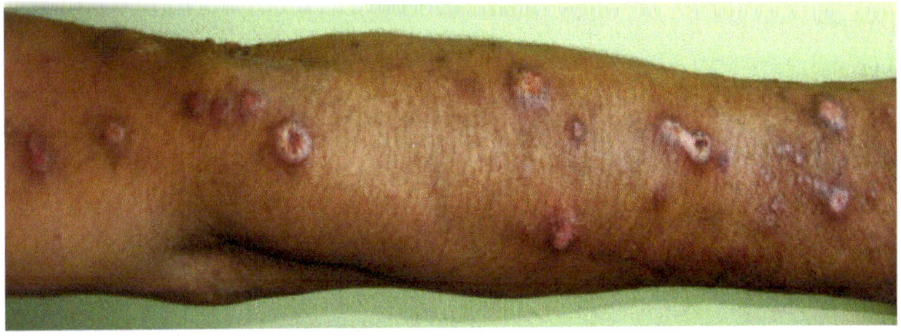

FIGURE 96.3 Nodular prurigo, acute stage, in a 56-year-old woman FST5.

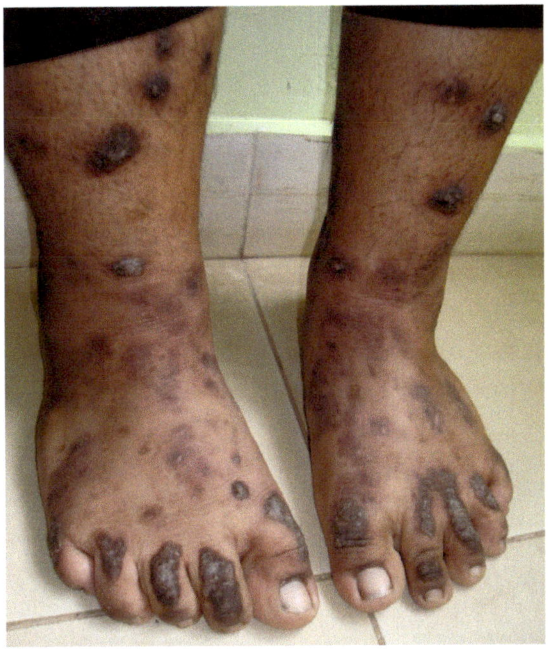

FIGURE 96.4 Nodular prurigo, chronic stage, in a 17-year-old girl FST5.

97
ERYTHRODERMIC PSORIASIS

Introduction

In erythrodermic psoriasis, most or all of the body surface is affected by psoriasis. It can be acute or chronic. In the chronic form, the individual may be systemically well, the clinical characteristics of psoriasis are retained, and there are usually some areas of uninvolved skin. Mild topical treatments are well tolerated, and the overall prognosis is good.

In the acute form, the patient may be febrile and systemically ill. The entire skin may be affected, and the clinical characteristics of psoriasis are often lost. Complications are those of skin failure, including sepsis, hypothermia or hyperthermia, hypoalbuminemia, anemia, dehydration, and high output cardiac failure.

Epidemiology

Erythrodermic psoriasis is uncommon, occurring in 1–2% of patients.

Associated diseases

The acute form is often precipitated by environmental or therapeutic triggers, including systemic illness, alcoholism, antimalarials, irritating topical treatments, ultraviolet radiation, withdrawal of systemic corticosteroids, or break-through under systemic steroids, ciclosporin, or methotrexate.

Clinical characteristics in light skin (Fitzpatrick skin types I–III)

Erythrodermic psoriasis is a life-threatening disease (Figure 97.1). It can develop *de novo* on previously unaffected skin, or classical psoriasis can aggravate to cover the entire integument. This is important as the *de novo* psoriatic erythroderma is a very serious, potentially lethal disease and carries the risk of developing pustules. However, the clinical aspect of the skin is not different. The entire skin is red and scaly, including the face, scalp, palms, and soles. There is usually an ectropion. The fingertips tend to fissure and are painful. All long-standing erythrodermas develop dermopathic lymph node swelling.

Chronic psoriatic erythroderma has to be differentiated from malignant lymphoma and drug-induced erythroderma. In children, Netherton syndrome is an important, though rare differential diagnosis.

Clinical characteristics in dark skin (Fitzpatrick skin types IV–V)

Erythroderma may not be apparent in individuals with darker skin (Figures 97.2 and 97.3). This may lead to morbidity and mortality in inexperienced hands. They present with generalized illness and tender, swollen skin. Erythema may be more conspicuous upon applying pressure on the skin.

Investigations

Skin biopsy is performed if the underlying cause of erythroderma is not identified. Other investigations are based on anticipated systemic complications.

Treatments

- The treatment of erythrodermic psoriasis often requires inpatient dermatological management with topical and usually systemic drug therapy, general supportive measures, and removal of possible provocative factors.
- Excessive heat loss must be prevented by maintaining an adequate ambient temperature.
- Fluid intake should be increased so that the daily urine volume remains adequate.
- Appropriate antibiotics.
- PUVA is highly effective for generalized pustular or erythrodermic psoriasis. Narrow-band (TL-01) UVB (NB-UVB) can be used to treat all variants except generalized pustular and erythrodermic psoriasis.
- Ciclosporin may have a place when urgent, rapid control of potentially lethal generalized pustular or erythrodermic psoriasis is needed.
- TNF-α inhibitors (adalimumab, etanercept, and infliximab) are limited to moderate/severe disease when other treatments (methotrexate, ciclosporin, and phototherapy) have been ineffective or are contraindicated. Their use is often further restricted because of their greater cost than traditional systemic treatments.

Further reading

Burden AD, Kirby B, Burden AD (2024). Psoriasis and Related Disorders. In: Griffiths C, et al. (eds). *Rook's Textbook of Dermatology*, 10th ed. John Wiley & Sons Ltd., UK; 35.14.

Heinrich M, Cook E, Roach J, et al. (2019). Erythrodermic Psoriasis Secondary to Systemic Corticosteroids. *Proc Bayl Univ Med Cent*;33(1):113–114.

Licata G, Rizzo D, Frazzitta M, et al. (2024). Successful Treatment of Sub-Erythrodermic Psoriasis with Bimekizumab: A Case Report and Literature Review. *Int J Dermatol*;63(8):1105–1107.

Shi H, Chen D, Si J, et al. (2024). Efficacy and Safety of Oxymatrine in the Treatment of Patients with Erythrodermic Psoriasis. *Dermatol Ther*; 14(6):1659–1670.

DOI: 10.1201/9781003479512-97

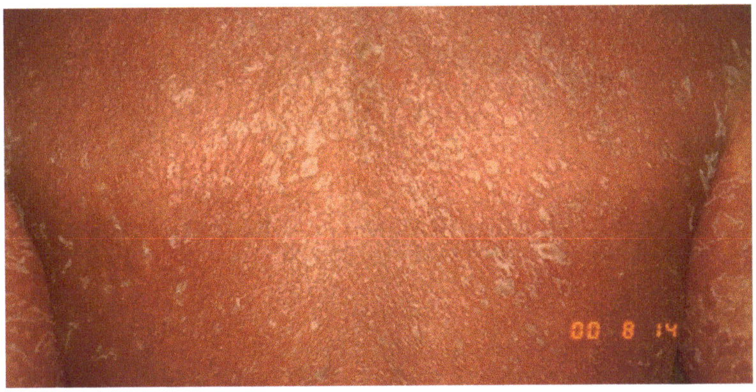

FIGURE 97.1 Erythrodermic psoriasis FST1. (Courtesy Dr. Richard Ashton, UK.)

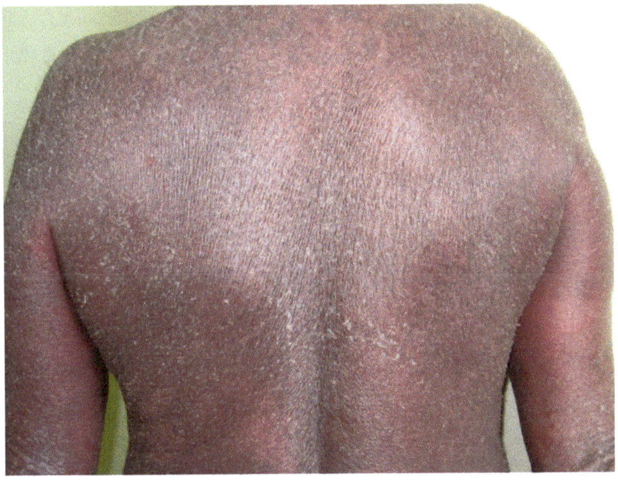

FIGURE 97.2 This 48-year-old man, who is a known psoriatic, presented with erythroderma following a viral fever. His plaque psoriasis has disappeared. Note erythema is hidden in darker skin FST5.

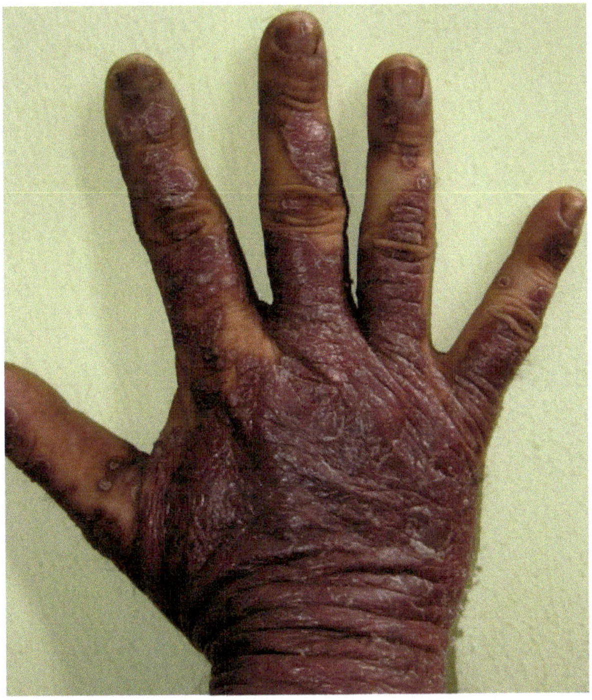

FIGURE 97.3 The same man's hands show features of plaque psoriasis FST5. Note islands of unaffected skin on fingers.

98
PSORIASIS GUTTATA

Introduction

The sudden onset of a shower of small psoriatic lesions appears diffusely over the body. It frequently follows several weeks after a pharyngitis caused by group A Streptococci. The lesions usually resolve in about 3 months. A minority of patients with acute guttate psoriasis subsequently develop plaque psoriasis.

Epidemiology

It is more common in children and young adults.

Clinical characteristics in light skin (Fitzpatrick skin types I–III)

Psoriasis guttata, mainly occurring in children and young adults, is an acute-onset type of psoriasis characterized by small red papules that rapidly enlarge from drop-shaped (*gutta* [Latin] drop) to lesion of 1–2 cm diameter with silvery-white scales (Figure 98.1). They have a tendency to heal spontaneously or may transform into common plaque-type psoriasis vulgaris. Many patients have a history of an acute streptococcal infection some 4–6 weeks prior to the onset of guttate psoriasis; however, intense sun exposure may also precipitate this psoriatic manifestation.

Treatment should be as bland as possible and avoid all harsh treatment regimens. Some drugs are known to aggravate psoriasis, particularly chloroquine and hydroxychloroquine. Other drugs may precipitate psoriasis, such as some biologics, and both COVID-19 and COVID mRNA vaccine were observed to induce psoriasis.

Clinical characteristics in dark skin (Fitzpatrick skin types IV–V)

The lesions are from 2–3 mm to 1 cm in diameter, round or slightly oval (Figure 98.2). They are scattered more or less evenly over the trunk and proximal part of the limbs. They have the normal characteristics of plaque psoriasis: Well-demarcated plaques with silvery scales; erythema may be unnoticeable in darker skin.

Investigations

This is a clinical diagnosis. Histopathology may confirm psoriasis in doubtful cases.

Treatments

- Good prognosis in many cases, usually resolves in about 3 months.
- Antihistamines if itchy. Otherwise, emollients will suffice.

Further reading

Barisić-Drusko V, Rucević I (2004). Trigger Factors in Childhood Psoriasis and Vitiligo. *Coll Antropol*;28(1):277–285.

Kirby B, Burden AD (2024). Psoriasis and Related Disorders. In: Griffiths C, et al. (eds). *Rook's Textbook of Dermatology*, 10th ed. John Wiley & Sons Ltd., UK; 35.12.

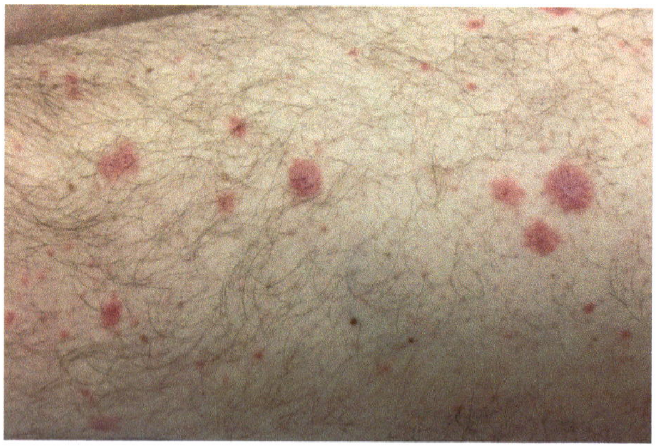

FIGURE 98.1 Guttate psoriasis in FST1. (Courtesy Prof. Eckart Haneke, Germany.)

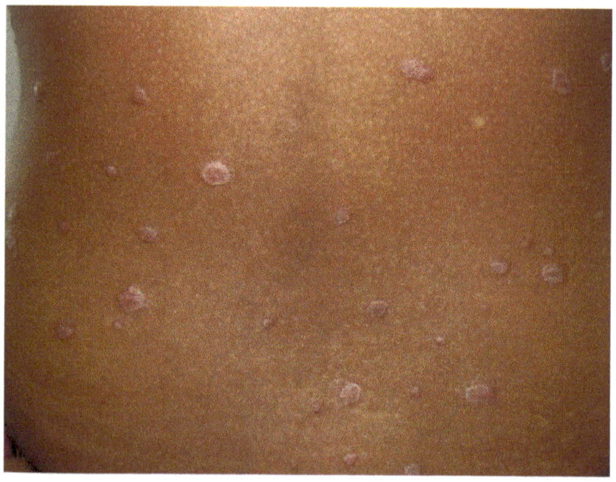

FIGURE 98.2 Guttate psoriasis in a 14-year-old girl FST5.

DOI: 10.1201/9781003479512-98

99
PSORIASIS PUSTULOSA

Introduction

Pustular psoriasis is reserved for those forms of the disease in which macroscopic pustules appear in a patient with extensive psoriasis. This is separated into localized and generalized pustular psoriasis, but there is clinical overlap. In the localized forms, the disease is usually confined largely to the hands and feet and tends to be chronic. In the generalized forms, the whole body may be involved and the course is subacute, acute or even fulminating and life-threatening. Factors that may trigger or exacerbate generalized pustular psoriasis include infection, topical or systemic corticosteroids, psychological stress, pregnancy, and hypocalcemia.

Generalized pustular psoriasis has four clinical variants:

1. Acute generalized pustular psoriasis (von Zumbusch).
2. Subacute annular and circinate pustular psoriasis.
3. Acute generalized pustular psoriasis of pregnancy.
4. Infantile and juvenile generalized pustular psoriasis.

Localized pustular psoriasis has two clinical variants:

1. Palmoplantar pustular psoriasis.
2. Acrodermatitis continua suppurativa of Hallopeau.

Epidemiology

Generalized pustular psoriasis is rare. The incidence peaks between 40 and 59 years of age, but infantile and juvenile cases are also reported.

Associated diseases

The reported co-morbidities included obesity (43%), hypertension (26%), dyslipidemia (26%), and diabetes (24%). Inflammatory polyarthritis is common in this condition.

Clinical characteristics in light skin (Fitzpatrick skin types I–III)

Generalized pustular psoriasis is a potentially life-threatening disease (Figures 99.1 and 99.2). The skin is diffusely red, scaling, and studded with innumerable small, very superficial yellow pustules. The patients are severely ill and require skilled in-patient treatment. Often, the primary care physician misdiagnoses the pustules as an infection and institutes antibiotic treatment, which, of course, fails to improve the condition. The clinical features of generalized pustular psoriasis in infants and children are not fundamentally different from those in adults.

Subacute annular and circinate psoriasis usually has pustules on the outer margin of the figurate lesions. This type may develop during topical treatment with high-potency corticosteroids.

Pustular psoriasis of pregnancy is also called herpes gestationis. It usually begins in the middle of pregnancy or the last trimester and tends to resolve after delivery, sometimes only after the lactation period.

Palmar plantar pustular psoriasis is a chronic psoriasis of the palms and soles with pustulation. It may be associated with nail lesions.

Acrodermatitis continua suppurativa of Hallopeau is a chronic type of pustular psoriasis localized on the tips of the fingers and toes, particularly under and around the nails. Its clinical expression can be extremely variable, with some cases demonstrating fiercely red digital tips insidiously destroying the entire nail apparatus until it then subsides, and other cases just exhibiting a chronic erythema with occasional pustules on a single digit. All grades between these two extremes may be observed.

The pustular psoriasis forms are also grouped into the class of deficiency of interleukin-36 receptor antagonist (DITRA).

Palmoplantar pustulosis is distinct from palmar plantar psoriasis by its genetic profile, clinical course and appearance, HLA types, immune reactions, and histopathology.

Clinical characteristics in dark skin (Fitzpatrick skin types IV–V)

Pre-existing lesions become fiery and develop pinpoint pustules. Sheets of erythema and pustulation spread to involve previously unaffected skin, the flexures and genital regions being particularly affected. Waves of pustulation may succeed each other, subsiding into exfoliation of the dried pustules.

Investigations

Histopathology is performed if the diagnosis is in doubt.

Treatments

The treatment of acute generalized pustular psoriasis often requires inpatient dermatological management with topical and usually systemic drug therapy, general supportive measures, and removal of possible provocative factors.

- Excessive heat loss must be prevented by maintaining an adequate ambient temperature.
- Fluid intake should be increased so that the daily urine volume remains adequate.
- Appropriate antibiotics.
- Weak corticosteroid creams may be helpful in subacute forms.
- Tar and dithranol are contraindicated.
- Oral retinoids (acitretin, not in pregnancy) are the treatment of choice, as are ciclosporin and methotrexate.
- Second-line therapies are infliximab, adalimumab, etanercept, and prednisolone (prednisolone is prescribed in special circumstances only).
- Third-line therapy is Anakinra (an IL-1 blocker).
- New and emerging biologic therapeutics target the IL-36 pathway, as most cases of pustular psoriasis have an inborn deficiency of the IL-36 receptor antagonist.

DOI: 10.1201/9781003479512-99

Further reading

Abbas O, Itani S, Ghosn S, et al. (2013). Acrodermatitis Continua of Hallopeau Is a Clinical Phenotype of DITRA: Evidence That It Is a Variant of Pustular Psoriasis. *Dermatology*;226(1):28–31.

Djawari D, Deinlein E, Hornstein OP (1980). Zur Immunologie des Bakterid Andrews. I. Immunreaktionen [Immunology of the pustular bacterid of Andrews. I Immune responses (author's transl.)]. *Dermatol Monatsschr*;166(5):297–304.

Gooderham MJ, Van Voorhees AS, Lebwohl MG (2019). An Update on Generalized Pustular Psoriasis. *Expert Rev Clin Immunol*;15(9):907–919.

Seishima M, Fujii K, Mizutani Y (2022). Generalized Pustular Psoriasis in Pregnancy: Current and Future Treatments. *Am J Clin Dermatol*;23(5):661–671.

Vilaça J, Yilmaz O, Torres T (2024). New and Emerging Treatments for Generalized Pustular Psoriasis: Focus on IL-36 Receptor Inhibitors. *Pharmaceutics*;16(7):908.

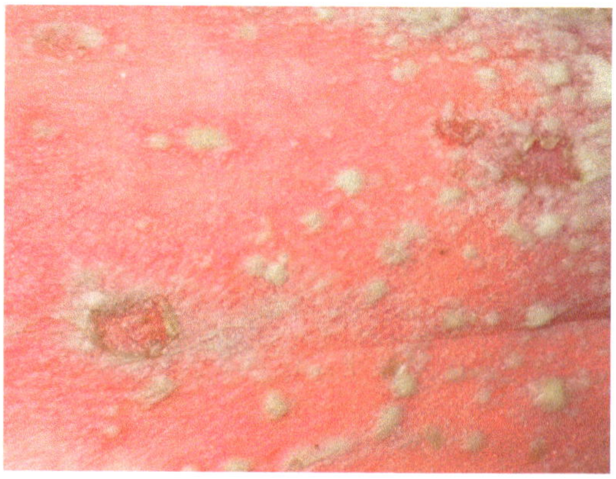

FIGURE 99.1 Pustular psoriasis FST1. (Courtesy Prof. Ian Coulson, UK.)

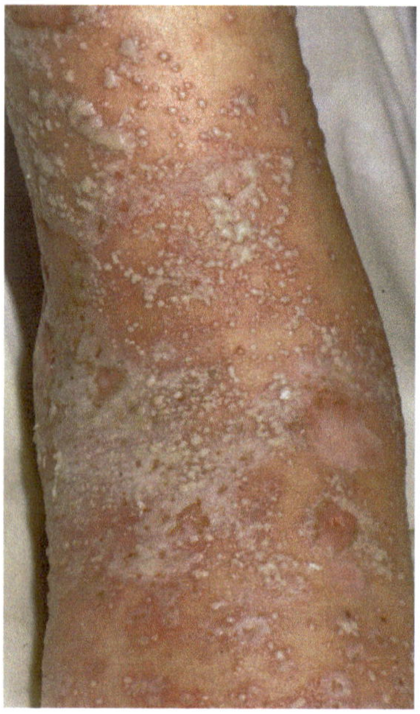

FIGURE 99.2 Generalized pustular psoriasis FST1. (Courtesy Dr. Richard Ashton, UK.)

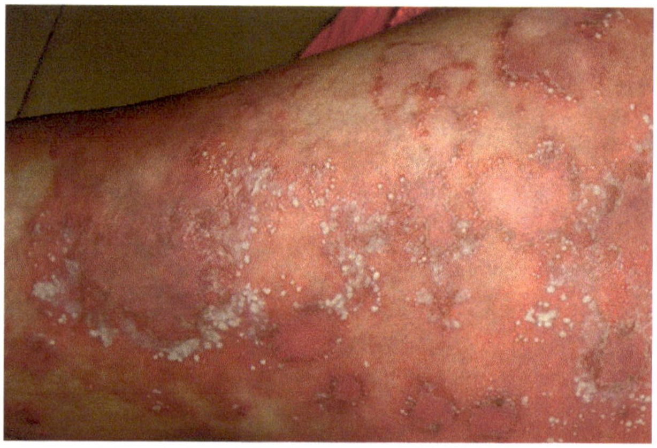

FIGURE 99.3 Pustular psoriasis in a 39-year-old woman FST5.

100
PSORIASIS VULGARIS

Introduction

Plaque psoriasis is the most common type of psoriasis, accounting for about 80–90% of all cases. Typical lesions are scaly plaques, which are remarkably well demarcated from unaffected skin, with sharply delineated edges. Psoriasis lesions are surmounted by silvery-white scales, which vary considerably in thickness. The amount of scaling may be minimal in partially treated disease and in the flexures. The scalp is one of the most common areas to be affected by plaque psoriasis and is often the site first affected, extending a short distance beyond the hairline and around the ears.

Epidemiology

This is common and affects approximately 2–3% of the world population. There are two peak ages of incidence, the first occurring between 16 and 22 years and the second between 57 and 62 years of age. There is equal sex distribution in adults.

Associated diseases

The prevalence of metabolic syndrome (truncal obesity, hyperlipidemia, hypertension, and insulin resistance) was, at 34%, found to be significantly elevated in patients with psoriasis compared with 26% of the unaffected population. Psoriatic arthritis occurs in up to 40% of patients with moderate to severe psoriasis.

Clinical characteristics in light skin (Fitzpatrick skin types I–III)

Psoriasis is a very frequent disease with the prevalence being higher in Nordic countries. Globally, approximately 2–3% of the population is affected. Psoriasis is a genetic disease of immune and cell regulation with a strong influence from environmental factors.

Classical psoriasis vulgaris starts with a red papule that enlarges and develops a silvery-white scale (Figure 100.1). This may be just a few layers thick but sometimes mimics an oyster shell. Scales on seborrheic skin, particularly the scalp and in the midline of the trunk, tend to be yellow and greasy. The papules grow to form large plaques that are sharply delimited. Characteristically, psoriasis plaques are located on the elbows, knees, at the nape of the neck – border to the occipital hair, in the rima ani, and extensor surfaces of the extremities. Involvement of flexor surfaces is called psoriasis inversa. Here, the axillae, umbilicus, groin, and genitals may be involved with a serious negative impact on quality of life.

Psoriasis on the face is stigmatizing and extremely embarrassing. Psoriasis of the hands may interfere with many types of manual work. Many national psoriasis guidelines mention these as particular localizations that deserve therapy with biologics.

Although often not mentioned, itching may be intense and disturbing (actually, the term psoriasis is derived from the Greek word for *itch*).

Psoriasis, once called the skin disease of the healthy, is now often linked to metabolic syndromes such as obesity and type 2 diabetes. In fact, there is a significant difference in alcohol and tobacco abuse and hyperalimentation between psoriatics and atopics, with the latter tending to be more abstinent than the former.

Clinical characteristics in dark skin (Fitzpatrick skin types IV–V)

Erythema is less marked in dark skin (Figures 100.2 and 100.3). Therefore, the psoriasis area severity index (PASI) score is lower and misleading compared to an equally affected white-skinned patient. Post-inflammatory hypo- and hyperpigmentation are common.

Investigations

Diagnosed clinically.

Treatments

Treatment depends upon many variables, including age, gender, occupation, personality, general health, intelligence, and resources, as well as the type, extent, site, duration, and natural history of the disease. Therefore, treatment should be tailored to the individual. It should not be more unpleasant, intolerable, or dangerous than the disease itself. Reassurance and emotional support are invaluable.

- Topical therapies are the mainstay of treatment for psoriasis of limited extent: Emollients, corticosteroids, vitamin D and its analogues, coal tar, dithranol, and retinoids.

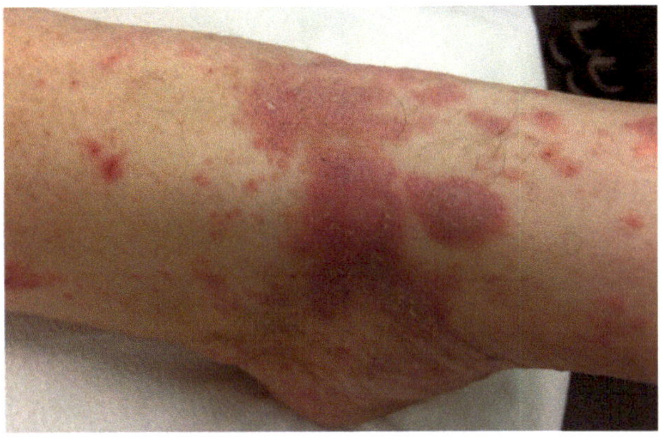

FIGURE 100.1 Plaque psoriasis in FST1. (Courtesy Prof. Eckart Haneke, Germany.)

DOI: 10.1201/9781003479512-100

- Phototherapy with narrow-band UVB or PUVA (psoralens and long-wave ultraviolet radiation) is the recommended first-line therapy for most patients with moderate to severe psoriasis.
- Systemic treatment is used for more extensive disease that is not responsive to topical therapy or phototherapy, including acitretin, apremilast, ciclosporin, fumaric acid esters, and methotrexate.
- Biological treatments are now well established for moderate to severe psoriasis: Adalimumab, etanercept, infliximab, secukinumab, ustekinumab, and ixekizumab.

Further reading

Alajroush WA, Alrshid AI, Alajlan AH, et al. (2024). Psoriasis and Metabolic Disorders: A Comprehensive Meta-Analysis of Million Adults Worldwide. *Cureus*;16(1):e52099.

Mallawaarachchi K (2021). Psoriasis. In: Ranawaka RR, Kannangara AP, Karawita A (eds). *Atlas of Dermatoses in Pigmented Skin*. Springer, Singapore; 91.

Poizeau F, Leducq S, Fardet L, et al. (2024). Psoriasis Research Group (GRPso) and the Centre of Evidence of the French Society of Dermatology. Treatment of Moderate-to-Severe Psoriasis in Adults: An Expert Consensus Statement Using a Delphi Method to Produce a Decision-Making Algorithm. *Ann Dermatol Venereol*;151(3):103287.

Ruggiero A, Potestio L, Camela E, et al. (2022). Bimekizumab for the Treatment of Psoriasis: A Review of the Current Knowledge. *Psoriasis*;12:127–137.

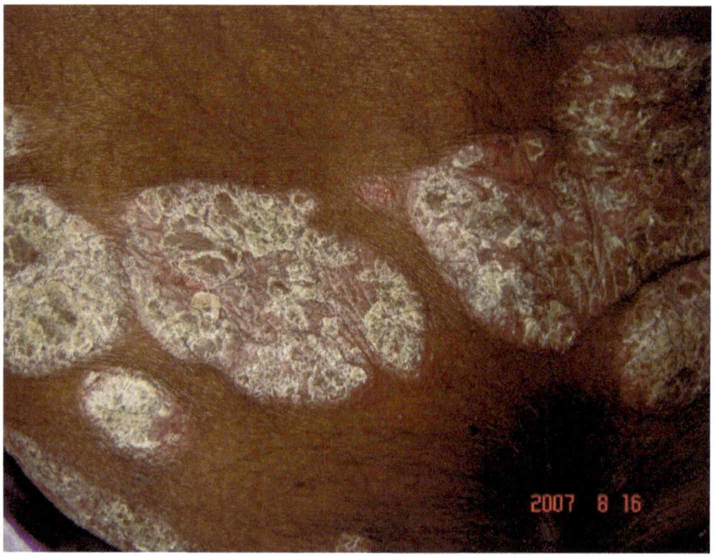

FIGURE 100.2 Plaque psoriasis in a 60-year-old man FST5. Note erythema is hidden in dark skin.

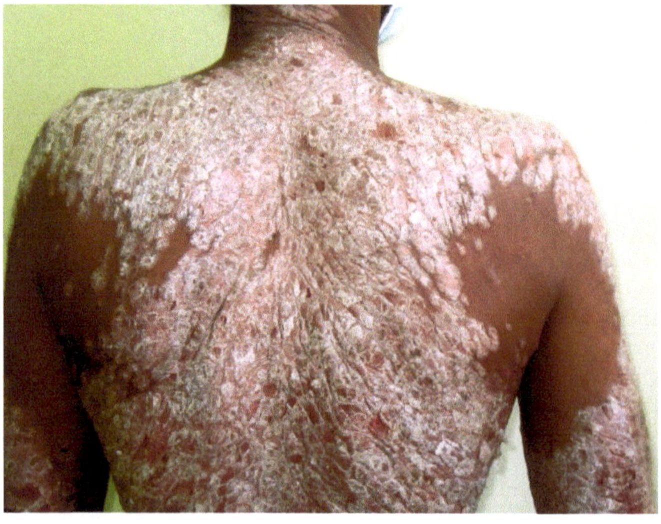

FIGURE 100.3 Extensive plaque psoriasis in a 47-year-old man FST5. Note erythema is inconspicuous in dark skin implying false assessment in severity and a false PASI score.

101
PURPURA FULMINANS

Introduction

Purpura fulminans is a true dermatological emergency and requires immediate diagnosis and management. It is rapidly progressive and is often accompanied by disseminated intravascular coagulation (DIC) and circulatory collapse. It occurs in neonates, children, and adults.

There are three different types of purpura fulminans – neonatal, acute infectious, and idiopathic.

Neonatal purpura fulminans is usually due to a genetically transmitted thrombophilic disorder: Most commonly homozygous deficiency of protein C or, less frequently, protein S. However, it may be caused by acute infections, particularly with endotoxin-associated, Gram-negative bacteria such as *Neisseria meningitidis*.

Acute infectious purpura fulminans is the most common type. In older children and adults, purpura fulminans is a highly characteristic feature of meningococcal septicemia, where it results from an acquired deficiency of protein C or S. It can rarely occur due to infections such as group B *Streptococcus, Streptococcus pneumoniae, Streptococcus pyogenes, Haemophilus influenzae*, methicillin-resistant *Staphylococcus aureus*, Gram-negatives (*Klebsiella pneumoniae, Escherichia coli, Pseudomonas aeruginosa, Proteus mirabilis*), viral infections (varicella, measles, Rubeola virus, West Nile virus), *Plasmodium falciparum*, fungal infections (*Cryptococcus neoformans, Aspergillus* spp., *Fusarium* spp.). This condition starts as rapidly progressive purpura a few days to weeks after a febrile illness. This type is found in splenectomy (physical or functional) patients.

Idiopathic purpura fulminans is thought to be a post-infectious autoimmune disorder, often occurring 7–10 days after an initiating febrile illness (usually varicella or scarlet fever), which later leads to rapidly progressive purpura. In this form, a relative deficiency of protein S is believed to be causative. This type is very rare.

Presentation is with more or less symmetrical and well-defined 'lakes' of confluent ecchymosis, without petechiae. Retiform (stellate) purpura and necrosis are the most typical cutaneous findings that results from thrombosis within the cutaneous microvasculature. There is surrounding erythema, and the lesions are tender. The lesions occur most often on the limbs, particularly at sites of pressure, but may also appear on the trunk, face, and scalp. The onset is sudden, and the lesions enlarge rapidly, with coalescence and the development of hemorrhagic bullae and central necrosis leading to necrotizing fasciitis. There is a substantial danger of internal hemorrhage, thrombosis in the central nervous system and in the retinal vessels, shock, and death.

Diagnosis is often evident, based on the observation of characteristic skin changes within a consistent clinical context (septic shock) and a consistent laboratory pattern. However, in situations where the diagnosis is not clear, the following differential diagnoses should be considered:

1. Catastrophic antiphospholipid syndrome (CAPS).
2. Heparin-induced thrombocytopenia.
3. Necrotizing fasciitis.
4. Warfarin-induced skin necrosis: Severe acquired protein C dysfunction.
5. Vasculitis (e.g., Henoch–Schonlein purpura, cryoglobulinemic vasculitis).
6. Thrombotic thrombocytopenic purpura (TTP).
7. Cocaine/levamisole toxicity.

Epidemiology

The frequency of homozygous protein C deficiency is estimated at 1 in 250,000–500,000 births.

The peak incidence of warfarin-induced skin necrosis is between the ages of 60–70 years, and is four times higher in women.

Associated diseases

Homozygous deficiency of either protein C or protein S is associated with cerebral and ophthalmic vessel thrombosis. Purpura fulminans has been associated with lupus anticoagulant activity and with autoantibodies to protein S.

Clinical characteristics in light skin (Fitzpatrick skin types I–III)

Purpura fulminans is an acute life-threatening disease that requires immediate intensive treatment. As the term implies, this condition progresses extremely fast. The patients are

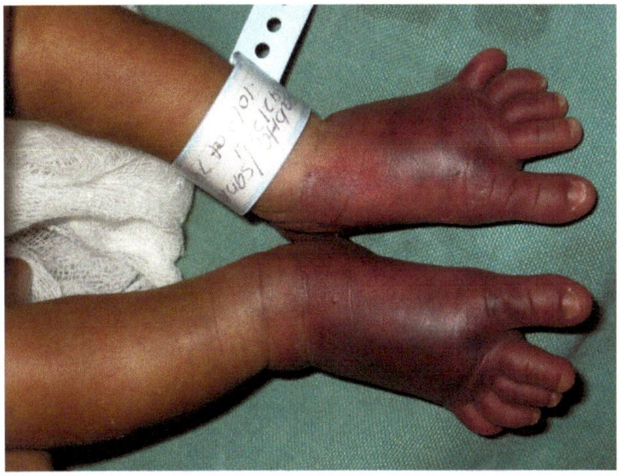

FIGURE 101.1 Purpura fulminans in a 5-day-old baby with meningococcal septicemia FST5. (Courtesy Prof. Archana Singal, India.)

DOI: 10.1201/9781003479512-101

severely ill with fever, they develop erythema, and soon multiple bleeding from several sites occurs. Hypotension develops rapidly. Large skin bleedings are visible; the toes, fingers, and skin often become necrotic. Sometimes, amputations are inevitable to save the patient's life. Pain out of proportion should make one consider necrotizing fasciitis. Septic shock is often fatal. Surviving patients frequently remain mutilated.

The pathogenesis is widespread intravascular coagulation due to toxins, mostly of meningococci and *Streptococcus pneumoniae*.

Clinical characteristics in dark skin (Fitzpatrick skin types IV–V)

In the early stage, erythema may go unnoticed in dark skin, leading to delayed diagnosis and, therefore, increased morbidity and mortality in inexperienced settings (Figures 101.1 to 101.3).

Investigations

1. *Partial thromboplastin time (PTT)*: Elevated 1–3 times.
2. *INR*: Normal or elevated.
3. *D-dimer*: Elevated in the range of 5000–30,000/mL (this is perhaps the most *sensitive* lab abnormality in purpura fulminans).
4. *Fibrinogen level*: Low, normal, or high (normal fibrinogen level excludes neither DIC nor purpura fulminans).
5. *Thrombocytopenia*: 25,000–150,000 ng/mL.
6. *Protein C levels*: Reduced below <40% of normal.
7. *Skin biopsy*: Early biopsy of retiform purpuric lesions shows microvascular occlusion with fibrin and perivascular hemorrhage with minimal to no inflammation.

Skin biopsy may be used to differentiate purpura fulminans from other conditions (e.g., vasculitis). In purpura fulminans, the biopsy will show dermal vessel thrombosis without vasculitis. Skin biopsy is usually unnecessary. In situations where the diagnosis of purpura fulminans is extremely likely based on clinical context, avoid delaying therapy while waiting for a skin biopsy.

Treatments

- In patients with sepsis, DIC, and retiform (occlusion) purpura, it seems reasonable to assume severe protein C deficiency in the acute setting and to treat it appropriately.
- The treatment of all types of purpura fulminans starts with supportive care and adequate hydration. This is important because the widespread thrombosis associated with this disease can lead to damage of multiple end organs.
- Early surgical debridement for areas that have become necrotic has been shown to decrease mortality.
- Fresh frozen plasma (FFP) should be given urgently in a dose of 10–15 mL/kg/12 h to replace deficient protein C or S.
- If protein C deficiency is confirmed, ongoing therapy with protein C concentrate or activated protein C should continue until the skin lesions have healed.
- If these are not available, heparin therapy is recommended.
- Plasma exchange has also been successfully used to replace protein C in purpura fulminans.
- Longer-term treatment is with oral anticoagulants.
- Liver transplantation can be curative in neonatal type.
- Any concomitant infection needs to be treated as well.
- In cases of post-infectious purpura fulminans, replacement of protein S activity is difficult, presumably because this condition is not due to the simple clearing of protein S but rather to the inhibition of protein S function by an antibody. Such antibody-mediated dysfunction is difficult to overcome by the replacement of the factor, and concentrated sources of protein S are unavailable.

Further reading

Edlich RF, Cross CL, Dahlstrom JJ, et al. (2008). Modern Concepts of the Diagnosis and Treatment of Purpura Fulminans. *J Environ Pathol Toxicol Oncol*;27(3):191–196.

Perera TB, Murphy-Lavoie HM (2023). Purpura Fulminans. July 17. In: *StatPearls* [Internet]. StatPearls Publishing, Treasure Island, FL.

Shah VH, Kharkar VD (2021). Pediatric Dermatological Emergencies in Tertiary Health Care. *Int J Res Dermatol*;7:58–63.

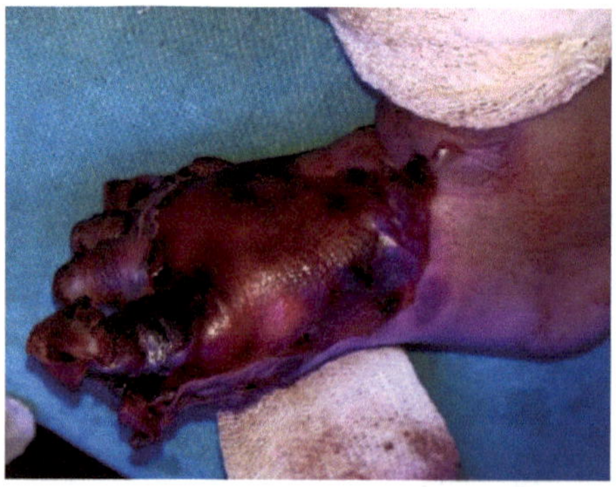

FIGURE 101.2 Purpura fulminans in a newborn FST5. (Courtesy Prof. Archana Singal, India.)

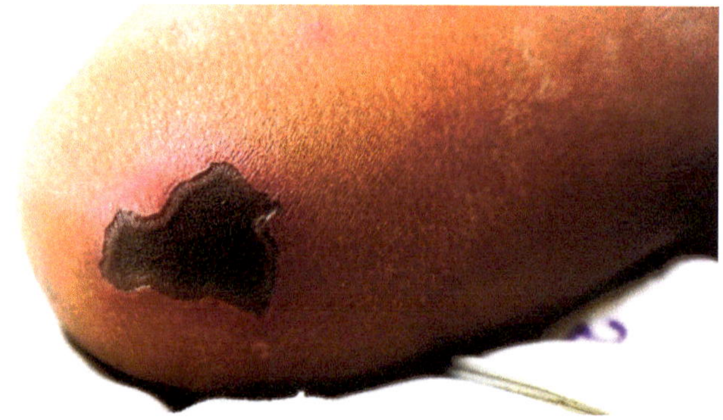

FIGURE 101.3 Retiform purpuric lesions in blood culture positive meningococcal septicemia in a 7-month-old baby FST5. Retiform (stellate) purpura and central necrosis is the most typical cutaneous finding. There is surrounding erythema and the lesions are tender.

102
SENILE PURPURA

Introduction

Bateman purpura (also known as senile purpura) is ecchymotic patches on photodamaged extensor surfaces of the arms and dorsal hands that appear with or without antecedent trauma. These lesions are not seen on the flexor surfaces of the arms nor on any sun-protected sites.

In addition to intrinsic and extrinsic aging, Bateman purpura is likely attributable to antecedent trauma and anticoagulant medications such as aspirin, heparin, warfarin, and other new antiplatelet agents, as well as oral and topical corticosteroids. Resolution is often slow, and the condition is recurrent.

Epidemiology

As its name implies, this is a condition of the elderly. Both men and women are equally affected.

Associated diseases

May be associated with diseases necessitating anticoagulant medications and antiplatelet agents.

Clinical characteristics in light skin (Fitzpatrick skin types I–III)

Light skin tends to develop actinic damage on any skin areas exposed to long-term sunlight. Thus, it is seen on the extensor surfaces of the forearms, dorsa of the hands, lower half of the upper arms, lower legs, and dorsa of the feet (Figure 102.1). The skin may develop further signs of actinic damage such as actinic keratoses, squamous and basal cell carcinoma, and severe actinic elastosis of the dermal connective tissue. When this – in susceptible persons – also involves the perivascular connective tissue, large ecchymoses develop and are seen as very obvious violaceous spots. Slight shearing forces lead to rupture in the reticular dermis level and finally major skin abrasions that take a long time to heal with white superficial scars that may look stellate (*pseudo-cicatrices stellaires*). If this process is exaggerated, the condition is called dermatoporosis.

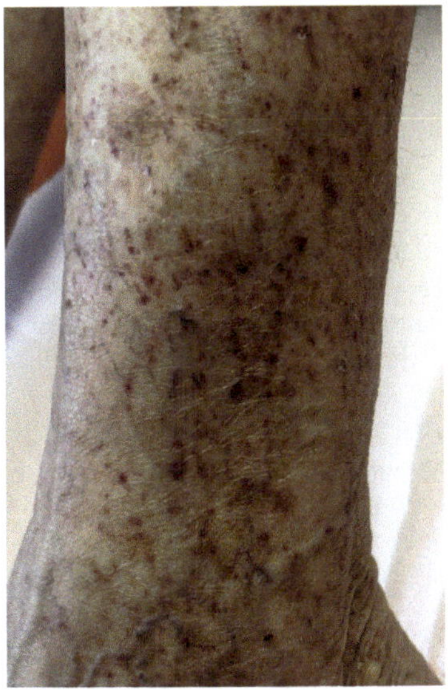

FIGURE 102.1 Stasis pupura on the leg in a 92-year-old man FST1. (Courtesy Prof. Eckart Haneke, Germany.)

Clinical characteristics in dark skin (Fitzpatrick skin types IV–V)

Senile purpura described in photodamaged skin is almost unseen in our setting (Figure 102.2).

Spontaneous purpura appearing in the elderly is not uncommon in those over 90 years. Additionally, it appears commonly in the middle-aged and elderly who are on anticoagulant therapy. Asymptomatic erythematous patches may appear anywhere on the body. These tend to change their appearance to purplish blue and then resolve with post-inflammatory hyperpigmentation that resolves spontaneously over weeks. Patients notice these when multiple bluish patches appear on the skin. Erythematous stage often goes unnoticed in darker skin.

Investigations

This is a clinical diagnosis. Further investigations are performed if any bleeding disorder is suspected.

Treatments

- No therapy is available; reassurance.
- Microneedle radiofrequency therapy and intense pulsed light (IPL) have been tried with a favorable response.

Further reading

Baek G, Kim MH, Jue MS (2022). Efficacy of Microneedle Radiofrequency Therapy in the Treatment of Senile Purpura: A Prospective Study. *Skin Res Technol*;28(6):856–864.

McKnight B, Seidel R, Moy R (2015). Topical Human Epidermal Growth Factor in the Treatment of Senile Purpura and the Prevention of Dermatoporosis. *J Drugs Dermatol*;14(10):1147–1150.

Pedersen EA, Fisher GJ, Voorhees JJ, et al. (2024). Skin Ageing. In: Griffiths C, et al. (eds). *Rook's Textbook of Dermatology*, 10th ed. John Wiley & Sons Ltd., UK; 156.5.

Siperstein R, Wikramanayake TC (2021). Intense Pulsed Light as a Treatment for Senile Purpura: A Pilot Study. *Lasers Surg Med*;53(7):926–934.

Whiting C, Azim SA, Friedman A (2024). What's Old Is New: An Emerging Focus on Dermatoporosis. *J Drugs Dermatol*;23(2): 113–114.

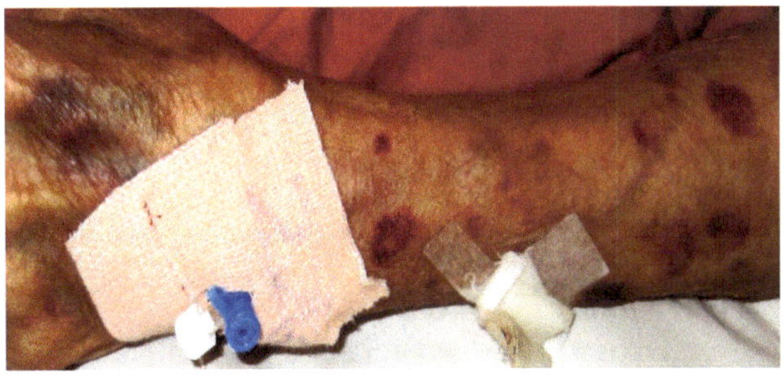

FIGURE 102.2 Senile pupura on the forearm in a 94-year-old man FST5. Note he has ecchymoses on the dorsum of the hand due to cannulation.

DOI: 10.1201/9781003479512-102

103
PYODERMA GANGRENOSUM

Introduction

Pyoderma gangrenosum (PG) is a rare non-infectious neutrophilic dermatosis. For classical PG, the following major criteria must be met: Rapid progression of a painful necrolytic cutaneous ulcer with an irregular, violaceous, and undermined border; and the exclusion of other causes of cutaneous ulceration. Rapid response to systemic corticosteroids is a minor criterion for diagnosis. A history suggestive of pathergy and the clinical finding of cribriform scarring favor the clinical diagnosis.

Clinical presentation depends on the clinical variant of PG.

1. **Classical ulcerative PG** is the most common and occurs most often on the legs (in 70%) but may affect any body site including the genitals and mucosae. It presents with small, tender, red-blue papules, plaques or pustules that evolve into painful ulcers with characteristic violaceous undermined edges. Healing is protracted and usually occurs with an atrophic cribriform scar.
2. **Parastomal or peristomal PG** may arise as a pathergy response to the trauma of appliances and fecal irritation.
3. **Pustular PG** is a variant that often occurs during acute exacerbations of inflammatory bowel disease. Discrete painful pustules, with a surrounding halo of erythema, develop on normal skin.
4. **Bullous PG** is an atypical presentation that presents with rapidly arising, superficial, hemorrhagic bullae, often located on the arms. It shares clinical and histopathological findings with Sweet syndrome, but typically ulcerates and heals with scarring. Bullous PG is especially associated with myeloproliferative disorders.
5. **Granulomatous superficial PG** is a superficial lesion with a granulomatous histology. Most cases begin as a single superficial ulcer with granulations and an elevated edge.

Epidemiology

PG is more common in females and in old age, with a median age of 59 years.

Associated diseases

Pustular form of PG may be associated mainly with inflammatory bowel disease (IBD) with a similar incidence of Crohn's disease and ulcerative colitis, 20–30%.

The bullous form may be associated with hematological malignancies.

Rheumatoid arthritis and other seronegative arthritides occur in about 10% of cases; hematological malignancy or monoclonal gammopathy in approximately 5%; and other visceral malignancies in 5%.

Clinical characteristics in light skin (Fitzpatrick skin types I–III)

PG is the prototype of a deep dermal neutrophilic dermatosis. It is a rare and often misdiagnosed condition. Typically, it is a secondary disease associated with inflammatory bowel diseases such as Crohn's disease and ulcerative colitis. These patients are therefore usually slender and malnourished. The lesions predominantly located on the lower extremities start as a dark red-brown tender infiltrate with a characteristic violaceous hue until it soon ulcerates and develops a malodorous putrid-hemorrhagic ulcer with overhanging margins (Figures 103.1 to 103.3). Next to bowel diseases and rheumatological disorders, various malignancies have to be looked for, particularly hematological ones that are associated with immunosuppression. It also has a strong association with hidradenitis suppurativa (OR 26.56). The diagnosis is made by exclusion of other well-defined diseases, both clinically as well as histopathologically.

Post-operative PG is a well-known condition in dermatology but unfortunately less known among surgeons. The author has seen a female patient who had been serially amputated on both legs up to the mid-thighs for 'non-healing ulcers.'

Clinical characteristics in dark skin (Fitzpatrick skin types IV–V)

Classic ulcerative PG presents with small, tender, red-blue papules, plaques, or pustules that evolve into painful ulcers with characteristic violaceous undermined edges (Figures 103.4 and 103.5). Lesions may be solitary or multiple and occur most commonly on the legs (in 70%). Healing usually occurs with an atrophic cribriform scar.

Investigations

Mostly clinical diagnoses.

Histopathological findings (sterile dermal neutrophilia, with or without mixed inflammation or lymphocytic vasculitis) are a minor criterion for diagnosis.

Treatments

- For smaller lesions, potent topical corticosteroids, intralesional corticosteroids, and topical tacrolimus.
- For more severe disease, corticosteroids are the most frequently used and the mainstay of therapy.
- Cyclosporine, combined prednisolone and cyclosporine, methotrexate, thalidomide, azathioprine, mycophenolate mofetil are second-line treatments.
- Anti-TNF therapies infliximab, adalimumab, etanercept, ustekinumab, and topical platelet-derived growth factor are third-line therapies. Anti-TNF biologic therapy should be considered more often as a first-line therapy, particularly for those with associated IBD.
- Intravenous immunoglobulin is useful as an adjunct therapy for refractory pyoderma gangrenosum.

Further reading

El-Kehdy J, Haneke E, Karam PG (2013). Pyoderma Gangrenosum: A Misdiagnosis. *J Drugs Dermatol*;12(2):228–230.

Maronese CA, Pimentel MA, Li MM, et al. (2022). Pyoderma Gangrenosum: An Updated Literature Review on Established and Emerging Pharmacological Treatments. *Am J Clin Dermatol*;23(5):615–634.

DOI: 10.1201/9781003479512-103

Schnetter D, Haneke E (1994). Pyoderma gangraenosum vegetans. Neue Aspekte in der Differentialdiagnose des Pemphigus vegetans Hallopeau (Pyodermite végétante Hallopeau) und Vorschlag einer neuen Klassifizierung [Pyoderma gangraenosum vegetans. New aspects in the differential diagnosis of pemphigus vegetans Hallopeau (Pyodermite végétante Hallopeau) and proposal for a new classification]. *Z Hautkr*;69:605–612.

Schnetter D, Haneke E (1995). Pyoderma gangraenosum vegetans. Eine zusammenfassende Betrachtung chronisch vegetierender Pyodermien und des Pyoderma gangraenosum [Pyoderma gangrenosum vegetans. An overview of chronic pyoderma vegetans and pyoderma gangrenosum]. *Hautarzt*;45:635–638.

Wijenayake BKS (2021). Neutrophilic Dermatoses. In: Ranawaka RR, et al. (eds). *Atlas of Dermatoses in Pigmented Skin*. Springer, Singapore; 219.

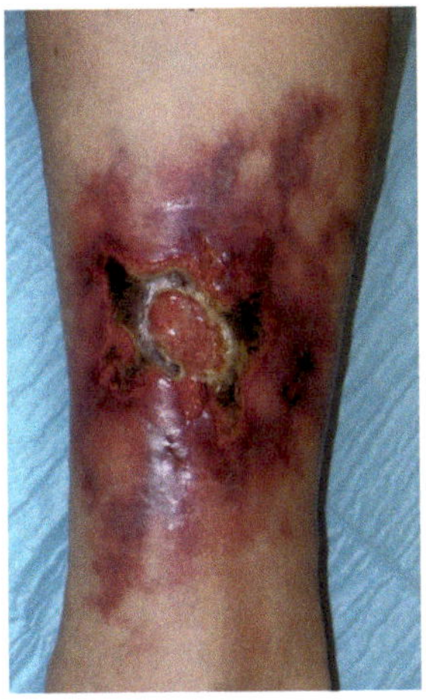

FIGURE 103.1 Ulcerative pyoderma gangrenosum FST1. (Courtesy Prof. Uwe Wollina, Germany.)

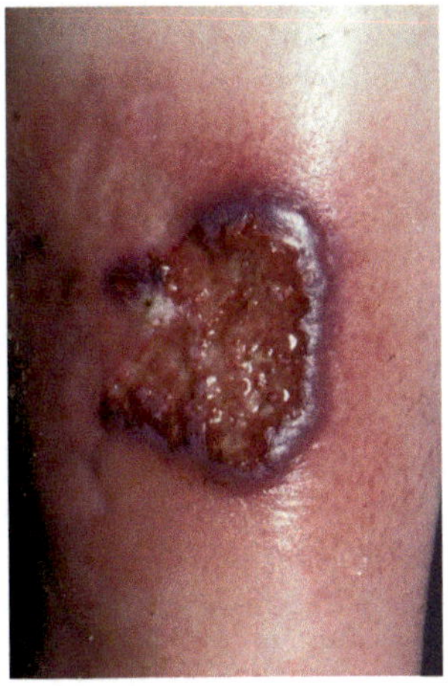

FIGURE 103.2 Classical ulcerative pyoderma gangrenosum FST1. (Courtesy Dr. Richard Ashton, UK.)

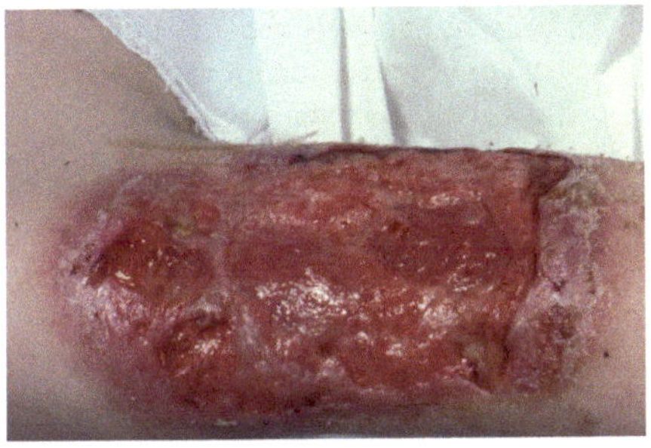

FIGURE 103.3 Bullous pyoderma gangrenosum FST1. (Courtesy Dr. Richard Ashton, UK.)

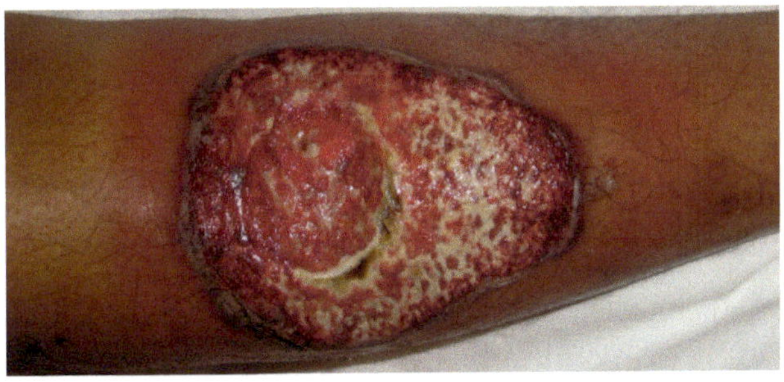

FIGURE 103.4 Classical ulcerative pyoderma gangrenosum in a 35-year-old woman FST5. Note characteristic violaceous undermined edges.

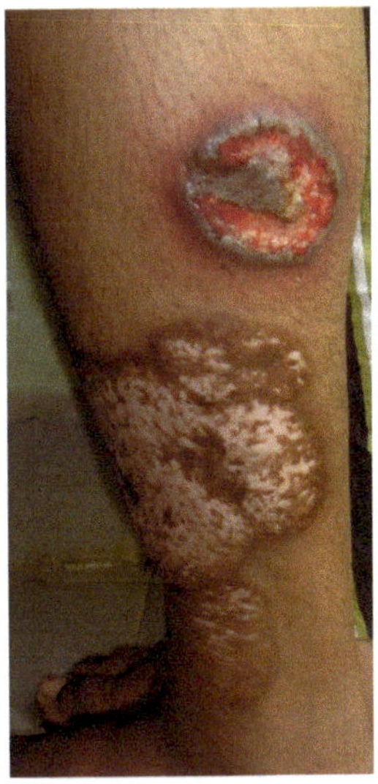

FIGURE 103.5 Recurrent pyoderma gangrenosum in a 29-year-old woman FST5. Note the previous lesion which had healed leaving a scar.

104
PYOGENIC GRANULOMA

Introduction

Pyogenic granuloma is a common acquired benign vascular tumor. It is bright red to brownish-red or blue-black in color. It is partially compressible but cannot be completely blanched, does not show pulsation, and may bleed very easily. Spontaneous disappearance is rare.

This vascular nodule develops rapidly, often at the site of a recent injury. Lesions are not painful; patients mainly complain about the appearance or recurrent bleeding. The common sites are the hands, especially the fingers, the feet, lips, head and upper trunk, and the mucosal surfaces of the mouth and perianal area.

This can clinically mimic keratoacanthoma and other epithelial neoplasms such as inflamed seborrheic keratoses, melanocytic nevi, melanoma, Spitz nevi, viral warts, molluscum contagiosum, angioma, glomus tumor, eccrine poroma, Kaposi sarcoma, and metastatic carcinoma.

Pyogenic granulomatous-like lesions may occur in severe acne, acne fulminans, result from treatment with isotretinoin, or in association with hidradenitis suppurativa. These lesions may respond to clobetasol propionate cream applied topically twice daily and carefully to the lesions over a 2–3-week period.

Epidemiology

This is very common. There is a peak in the second decade of life and is common in males.

Associated diseases

Pyogenic granulomas may occur within a port-wine stain.

Multiple lesions closely resembling pyogenic granulomas have been reported after systemic and topical treatments with retinoids.

When it is multiple, bacillary angiomatosis can be clinically and histologically difficult to distinguish.

Clinical characteristics in light skin (Fitzpatrick skin types I–III)

The term pyogenic granuloma is a misnomer as it is not a granuloma but an eruptive lobular angioma, and it is not pyogenic as it is not infectious although, when eroded the surface is seldom sterile. It must not be mistaken for granulation tissue, as is often the case.

After a minor trauma, a rapidly developing reddish nodule is seen that grows to the size of a pea or even bigger and usually becomes eroded, then oozing and bleeding. It may be pedunculated with a narrow base and a collarette of macerated epidermis (Figure 104.1).

Histopathology shows a lobulated angioma with a feeder artery in the depth. This has to be ligated or coagulated to avoid recurrence.

Clinical characteristics in dark skin (Fitzpatrick skin types IV–V)

This is a very common vascular lesion, bright red to brownish-red or blue-black in color (Figure 104.2). It is partially compressible but cannot be completely blanched and does not show pulsation. The size is commonly between 5 and 10 mm. The base is often pedunculated, but it may have a wide base.

Investigations

Excised lesion is sent for histopathology to exclude amelanotic melanoma and secondary deposits, which can clinically mimic pyogenic granuloma.

Treatments

- Simple excision is the treatment of choice. Local recurrence may be seen after incomplete excision.
- The pedunculated lesions are easy to treat by curettage with cauterization or diathermy coagulation of the base.
- Nd:YAG laser, cryosurgery, intralesional steroids, flash lamp pulsed dye laser, sclerotherapy with sodium tetradecyl sulfate, and even injection of absolute ethanol are effective treatments.

Further reading

Calonje E, Zlatko Maruko M (2024). Soft-tissue Tumours and Tumour-like Conditions. In: Griffiths C, et al. (eds). *Rook's Textbook of Dermatology*, 10th ed. John Wiley & Sons Ltd., UK; 136.25.

Eily N, Shah RR, Tariq Z, et al. (2024). Sclerotherapy as a Treatment Option for Pyogenic Granuloma. *Dermatol Surg*;Dec 1;50(12): 1219–1220.

Gaghan LJ, Sluder IT, Sampath A, et al. (2024). Spontaneous Multifocal Pyogenic Granulomas. *Pediatr Dermatol*;Nov–Dec; 41(6):1134–1140.

Ranawaka RR (2021). Vascular Tumours and Malformations. In: Ranawaka RR, et al. (eds). *Atlas of Dermatoses in Pigmented Skin*. Springer, Singapore; 73.

DOI: 10.1201/9781003479512-104

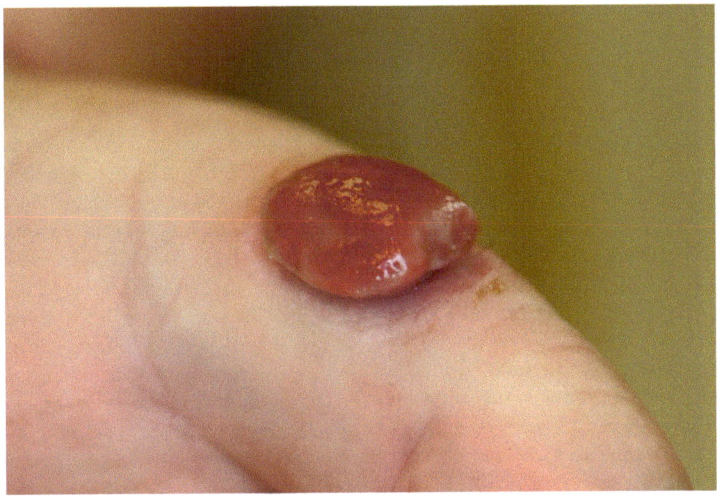

FIGURE 104.1 Pyogenic granuloma on the finger FST1. (Courtesy Dr. Richard Ashton, UK.)

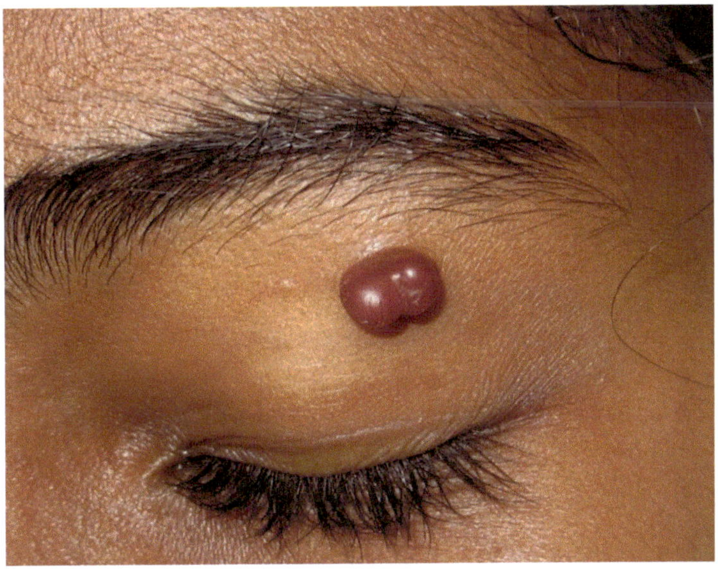

FIGURE 104.2 Pyogenic granuloma in a 10-year-old girl FST5.

105
RAYNAUD PHENOMENON

Introduction

The Raynaud phenomenon is defined as episodic digital ischemia occurring in response to cold or emotional stimuli. This is characterized by sequential color changes: White (pallor), blue (cyanosis), and red (rubor). Pallor is essential for the diagnosis. The Raynaud phenomenon affects the hands and, less often, the feet.

Primary Raynaud phenomenon (or Raynaud disease) is idiopathic and occurs as an isolated harmless disorder. This is usually symmetrical and involves several digits, is more common in women (5:1), occurs in those under 25 years of age, has a history of cold intolerance since childhood, and the nail fold capillaries are normal.

Causes of secondary Raynaud phenomenon are many; trauma or vibration, connective tissue diseases and vasculitis, obstructive arterial disease, neurological disease, hematological disease, drugs, and toxins. In secondary Raynaud phenomenon, only one or a few digits are affected, and asymmetry is not unusual. Severe cases, which are usually of the secondary type, may be complicated by telangiectases of the nail fold, thinning and ridging of the nail, and atrophy or sclerosis of the fingers (sclerodactyly). Skin necrosis is extremely rare in primary Raynaud phenomenon but not uncommon in secondary Raynaud phenomenon and may result in the destruction of the digits.

Epidemiology

The age of onset is usually under 40 years.

Primary Raynaud phenomenon is more common in women.

Associated diseases

Secondary Raynaud phenomenon has associations with many connective tissue diseases and vasculitis, such as systemic sclerosis, systemic lupus erythematosus, rheumatoid arthritis, Sjögren syndrome, mixed connective tissue disease, dermatomyositis, temporal arteritis, and hepatitis B antigen vasculitis. It also may appear in neurological diseases: Thoracic outlet syndrome (cervical rib), carpal tunnel syndrome, hypothenar hammer syndrome, reflex sympathetic dystrophy, and several hematological diseases: Cryoglobulinemia, cold agglutinins, paroxysmal hemoglobinuria, and Waldenstrom macroglobulinemia.

Clinical characteristics in light skin (Fitzpatrick skin types I–III)

The distinction between Raynaud phenomenon and Raynaud disease is somewhat artificial. By definition, Raynaud phenomenon is functional and defined by the recurrent appearance of painful vascular spasms elicited by cold or sometimes by stress, with white fingers and toes (Figure 105.1). From the digital tips, the whitening progresses to the base of the digit. It may become blue and then red; this last phase is often accompanied by pain. These attacks occur at variable intervals. Most patients are women over 20 years of age. They often have a personal history of cold and sweaty hands and feet since childhood or adolescence. Long-term Raynaud may lead to gradual stiffening and hard edema of the digits. Radiologically, distal acro-osteolysis may be seen.

Raynaud is also observed in association with a variety of other diseases. In recent times, COVID toes were described that look like chronic Raynaud's or chilblain lupus.

Many patients are advised to use hot-cold baths for treatment: This is wrong as the vasospasm will be even more aggravated by this maneuver; instead, twice daily hot hand-forearm-foot baths for 10 minutes until the patient feels the whole body is warmed up are recommended. Performing this regimen for a whole year will reduce or completely prevent cold extremities in the following cold season.

Clinical characteristics in dark skin (Fitzpatrick skin types IV–V)

Primary Raynaud phenomenon is rare in our setting, possibly due to the hot climate. In our skin clinics, this is mostly seen in patients with systemic sclerosis and is the presenting feature in some (Figure 105.2). They complain of a burning and tingling sensation of distal digits following exposure to cold water or cold weather. Some may notice pallor or mild cyanosis, which is also rare; but redness or rubor is never a feature in dark skin.

Investigations

This is a clinical diagnosis. Investigations are directed toward detecting an underlying cause.

Treatments

- Conservative management includes taking measures to keep the hands and feet warm, reducing cold exposure, and also emotional stress.
- Calcium-channel antagonists, such as nifedipine, can be useful in decreasing the frequency, duration, and severity of attacks, specifically in primary Raynaud.
    - Nifedipine ranges from 30 to 180 mg daily, and for amlodipine between 5 and 20 mg daily.
- Intravenous infusion of vasodilatory prostaglandins can reverse ischemic complications in Raynaud phenomenon.
- For severe cases, botulinum toxin injections or sympathectomy surgery can be used to control symptoms.

Further reading

Bashir SJ, Chew AL (2024). Cutaneous Reactions to Cold and Heat. In: Griffiths C, et al. (eds). *Rook's Textbook of Dermatology*, 10th ed. John Wiley & Sons Ltd., UK; 124.10.

Pauling JD, Hughes M, Pope JE (2019). Raynaud's Phenomenon: An Update on Diagnosis, Classification and Management. *Clin Rheumatol*;38(12):3317–3330.

Ture HY, Lee NY, Kim NR, et al. (2024). Raynaud's Phenomenon: A Current Update on Pathogenesis, Diagnostic Workup, and Treatment. *Vasc Specialist Int*;Jul 23;40:26.

Wiąk-Walerowicz K, Wielosz E, Majdan M (2024). The Usefulness of Nailfold Capillaroscopy in Scleroderma-Spectrum Disorders: A Single-Centre Observational Study. *Postepy Dermatol Alergol*;41(3):296–300.

DOI: 10.1201/9781003479512-105

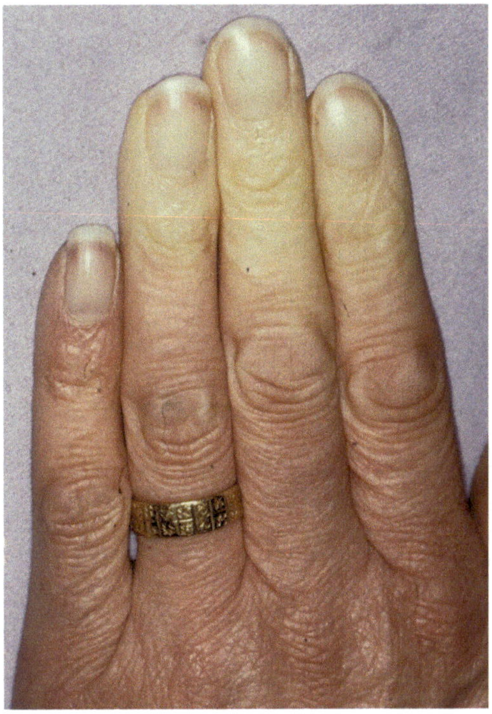

FIGURE 105.1 Raynaud phenomenon FST1 (digiti mortui). (Courtesy Dr. Richard Ashton, UK.)

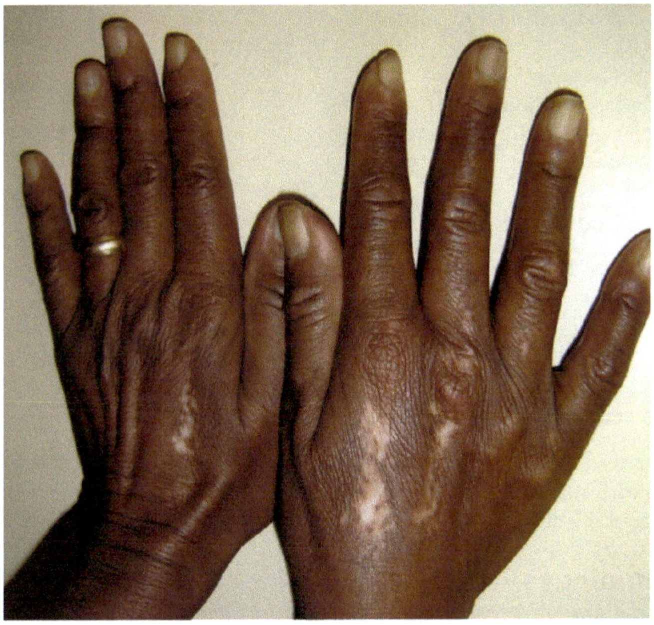

FIGURE 105.2 This 66-year-old woman FST5, who has systemic sclerosis complains of a burning sensation on her distal fingers when exposed to cold water or cold weather (Raynaud phenomena), but skin changes are not visualized except for mild fingertip pallor. Note sclerodactyly and speckled vitiligo on the fingers and dorsum of hands.

106
ROSACEA

Introduction

The term rosacea is used to include a broad spectrum of clinical features, many of which are not exclusive or specific to rosacea. The cause of rosacea is not exactly known. It is a chronic disorder that primarily affects the face with a tendency to facial erythema and involvement of the eye.

Patients present a spectrum of clinical features that differ according to each subtype (Fonseka 2021). A common feature in the majority of patients is the presence of facial erythema.

Erythematotelangiectatic rosacea

Patients with erythematotelangiectatic rosacea (ETTR) usually complain of a gradual increase in facial redness. This affects the central face but is not confined to this region, with the lateral cheeks, the ears, and sometimes the sides of the neck also being affected.

Papulopustular rosacea

Patients with papulopustular rosacea (PPR) give a history of developing groups of 'spots, red bumps, or pimples' that are located principally on the proximal cheeks, central chin, nose, and central forehead. The presence of oily skin, open and closed comedones, cystic lesions, and scarring are features supporting the diagnosis of acne vulgaris.

You can still sometimes find the term 'acne rosacea.' This is wrong. Acne vulgaris is a disease of the sebaceous follicle, while rosacea is rather a vascular abnormality. Although they do not exclude each other, comedones do not belong to rosacea.

Phymatous rosacea

Rhinophyma is the most common form of phymatous rosacea (PR) and is typically seen in male patients. It may appear *de novo* (without preceding inflammatory changes) or occur in a patient with pre-existing PPR.

Ocular rosacea

Patients who develop ocular rosacea (OR) frequently complain of a sensation of dryness with slight itch or a 'gritty' feeling of the eyes in the early stage of the disease.

Epidemiology

Rosacea is a disorder that usually presents in middle age, with peak onset between 35 and 50 years. Up to 25% of patients have a family history of the condition, indicating a significant genetic predisposition in some individuals. Male patients are said to develop more severe rosacea than women and are much more likely to develop rhinophyma than females.

Associated diseases

These patients sometimes have associated facial seborrheic dermatitis. A possible link between rosacea and gastrointestinal abnormalities has been suggested.

Clinical characteristics in light skin (Fitzpatrick skin types I–III)

Rosacea is a very common condition in fair-skinned people, particularly in the so-called Celtic type with red hair and blue to green eyes (Figures 106.1 and 106.2). The peak of the disease is between 30 and 50 years. There may be pronounced seborrhea. The condition often starts with flushes that have an increasing duration (rosacea erythematosa). With time, the erythema becomes stable and develops visible 'burst vessels' (rosacea telangiectatica). Then red papules develop that may also turn pustular. These may develop into indurated red infiltrates. The skin changes are mainly located in the central face with sparing of the upper lip and eyelid region (in contrast to lupus miliaris disseminatus faciei, which has to be differentiated from lupoid rosacea). Extra-facial rosacea is possible but very rare. Particularly, men may develop a fibro-sebaceous hypertrophy of the nose (rhinophyma), rarely the chin (mentophyma), central forehead (prosopophyma), or ear (otophyma), which can take on a disfiguring aspect.

Eye involvement may cause blepharitis, conjunctivitis, iridocyclitis, and hypopyon iritis, with the risk of becoming blind.

Rosacea is often erroneously treated with topical steroids, which first leads to diminished redness due to the vasoconstrictive effect of the corticosteroid; however, soon the rosacea worsens again, transforming into so-called steroid rosacea.

Rosacea conglobata is a rare complication with huge inflammatory abscesses and hemorrhagic infiltrates. When this occurs peracutely, it is called rosacea fulminans, a condition requiring intensive treatment with systemic steroids and synthetic retinoids.

Rosacea was often said to be associated with gastrointestinal disease; this could not be convincingly proven. However, precipitating factors such as sunlight, heat, stress, coffee, etc. should be avoided. Although ivermectin has been demonstrated to be effective for rosacea treatment, rosacea is different from demodicosis.

Clinical characteristics in dark skin (Fitzpatrick skin types IV–V)

ETTR patients present with persistent erythema on the lateral cheeks, the ears, and sometimes the sides of the neck that flush with environmental temperature changes (Figures 106.3 to 106.5). This type may go unnoticed in dark skin except for frequent flushing they notice, provoked by hot liquids, spicy foods, or alcohol.

PPR gives a history of 'acne or pimples' that are located principally on the proximal cheeks, central chin, nose, and central forehead and do not respond to conventional anti-acne treatments.

Rhinophyma patients are not uncommon and complain of a thickening of the skin on their distal nose with increased prominence of the 'pores' (follicular openings). They remark that their nose is increasing in size and that the distal end is becoming bulbous.

DOI: 10.1201/9781003479512-106

Even though the erythema is not as marked in darker skin as in white skin, the persistent erythema on these patients' faces is significantly visible.

Investigations

This is a clinical diagnosis.

Treatments

Management differs according to the clinical type. The following are general measures for all the clinical types:

- Avoid unnecessary sun exposure.
- Use sun-protective measures (apply daily sunblock cream all year round and wear a hat) as chronic UV damage will contribute to facial erythema, especially in patients with ETTR. Physical sunscreens based on zinc or titanium are best tolerated.
- Many patients with rosacea have dry, easily irritated skin. The daily application of a moisturizing cream is important for such patients.
- Avoidance of potential irritants (abrasive soaps, adstringents, perfumes, aftershave lotions, and skin-peeling preparations) is important as they tend to aggravate the facial erythema.
- Patients with a tendency to flushing (mainly those with ETTR) should avoid agents that provoke flushing, such as hot drinks, spicy foods, alcohol, some drugs, and precipitating or exacerbating factors (e.g., stress, temperature).
- For active inflammatory lesions, select a topical agent such as metronidazole 0.75% gel or cream, azelaic acid 15% gel, ivermectin 1% cream, or sodium sulfacetamide 10% and sulfur 5% preparations.
- The JAK1 inhibitors upadacitinib and abrocitinib may be promising medical options for patients with refractory rosacea.

Further reading

Fonseka, S. (2021). Rosacea. In: Ranawaka RR, et al. (eds). *Atlas of Dermatoses in Pigmented Skin*. Springer, Singapore; 511.

Li L, Hajam I, McGee JS, et al. (2024). Comparative Transcriptome Analysis of Acne Vulgaris, Rosacea, and Hidradenitis Suppurativa Supports High-Dose Dietary Zinc as a Therapeutic Agent. *Exp Dermatol*;33(7):e15145.

van Zuuren EJ, Tan J, van der Linden MMD, et al. (2024). Rosacea. In: Griffiths C, et al. (eds). *Rook's Textbook of Dermatology*, 10th ed. John Wiley & Sons Ltd., UK; 89.1.

Wu Y, Yan Y, Zhang L, et al. (2024). Positive Results of Intense Pulsed Light-Photodynamic Therapy for Moderate-to-Severe Rosacea: A Prospective, Single-Arm Study. *J Am Acad Dermatol*; Nov;91(5):943–945.

Zhang T, Liu X, Zhang L, et al. (2024). Treatment of Rosacea with Upadacitinib and Abrocitinib: Case Report and Review of Evidence for Janus Kinase Inhibition in Rosacea. *Front Immunol*;Jul 9;15:1416004.

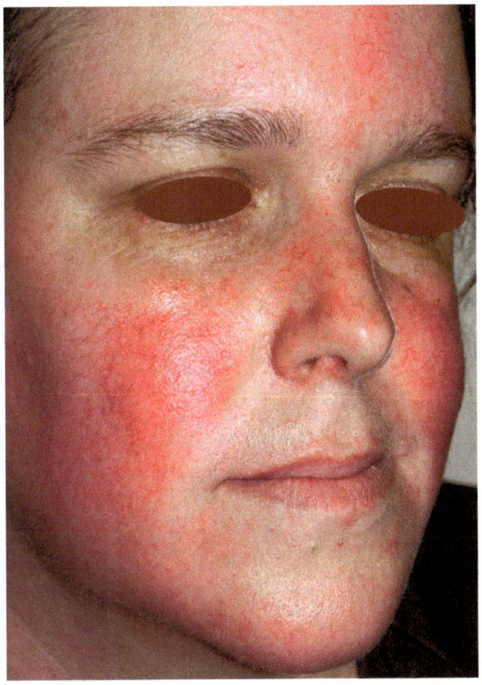

FIGURE 106.1 Erythematotelangiectatic rosacea FST2. (Courtesy Prof. Ian Coulson, UK.)

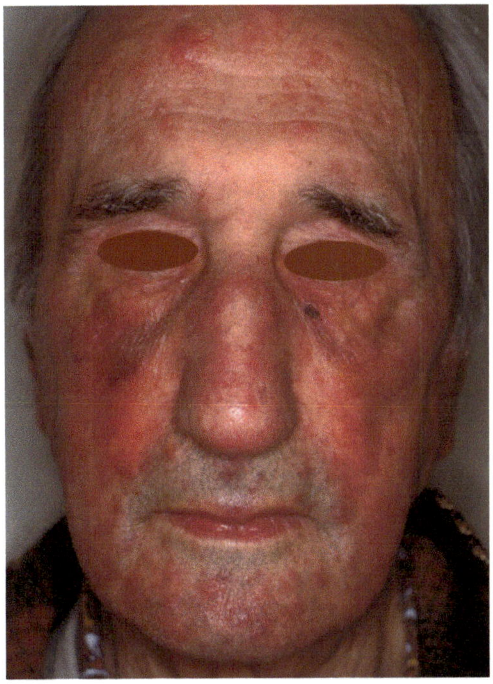

FIGURE 106.2 Steroid rosacea FST1. (Courtesy Prof. Ian Coulson, UK.)

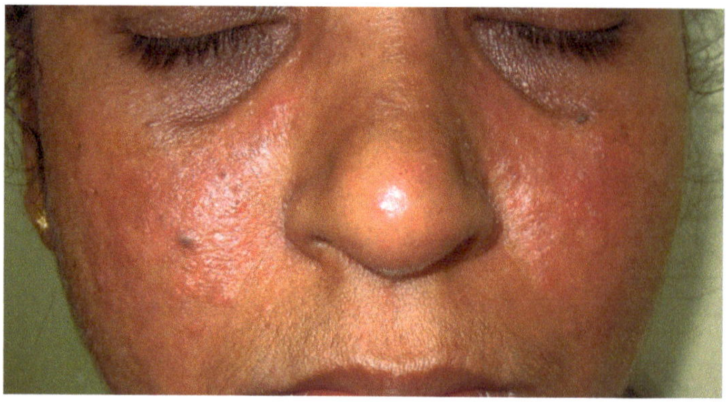

FIGURE 106.3 Erythematotelangiectatic rosacea in a 39-year-old woman FST5. In dark skin, erythema is not obvious at rest, but it becomes more obvious in hot climates, after hot water baths, and after eating hot spicy foods.

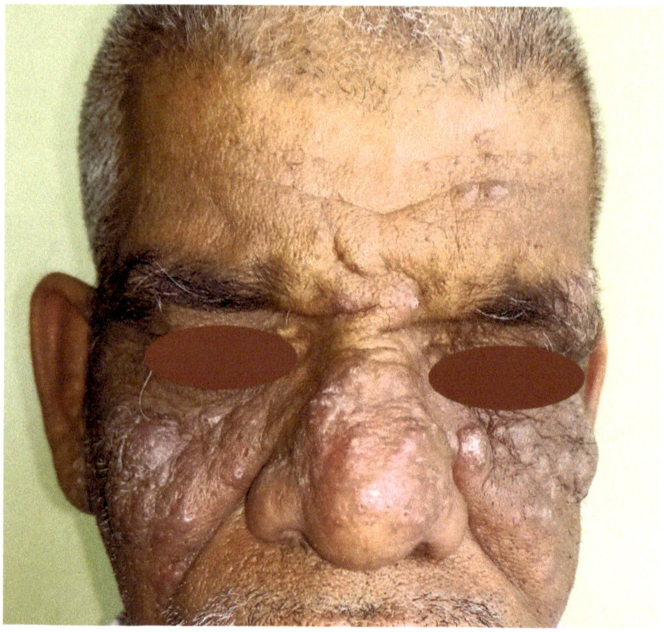

FIGURE 106.4 Papulopustular rosacea in a 57-year-old man FST5.

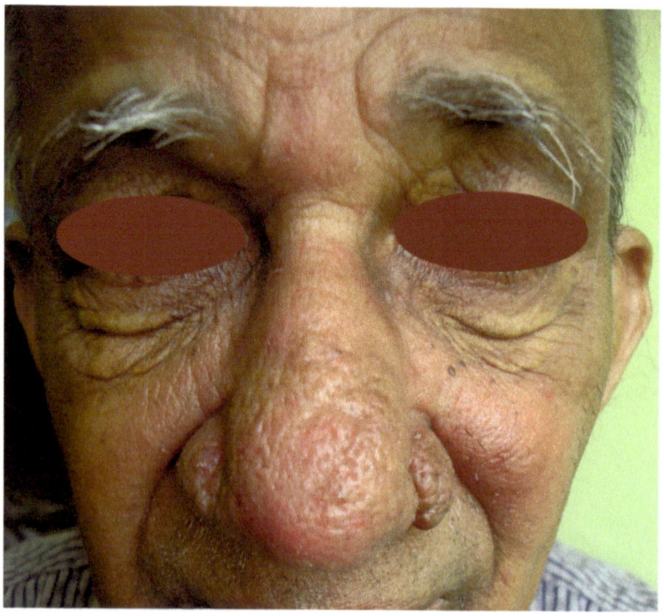

FIGURE 106.5 Rhinophyma in a 74-year-old man FST5.

107
SEBORRHEIC DERMATITIS IN ADULTS

Introduction

Seborrheic dermatitis (SD) is a common, relapsing dermatitis that is characterized by itchy, superficial scaling.

It occurs in two age groups: Babies in their first 3 months of life and adults 40 years and older. It is localized in sebaceous gland-rich areas like the scalp, face, midline of the trunk, and anogenital region.

In babies, it is also called *crusta lactea*. It starts on the scalp with a yellowish greasy scab of scales and serous crusts and is usually not itchy. This is in contrast to similar, but more oozing lesions in early infant atopic dermatitis. SD in babies differs in clinical manifestation and response to therapy from adult SD; therefore, is not discussed in this chapter.

SD in adults affects areas with a high density of sebaceous glands: The scalp, face, central chest, and anogenital areas. Facial SD typically affects the cutaneous folds, nasolabial folds, ear creases, eyelids, glabellar area, and medial eyebrows. Dandruff or pityriasis capitis is usually considered the mildest form of SD.

The cause remains unknown, but commensal lipophilic yeasts of the genus *Malassezia* (previously known as *Pityrosporum*) have long been associated with SD and dandruff.

Epidemiology

SD is a common dermatosis affecting 1–3% of the adult population and is common in males above the age of 20.

Associated diseases

The prevalence of SD is higher in patients with human immunodeficiency virus (HIV), human T-cell leukemia virus (HTLV) infection, Parkinson's disease, and in iatrogenic immunosuppression.

Clinical characteristics in light skin (Fitzpatrick skin types I–III)

In adults, it is frequently localized in the face, with the borders of hairy skin particularly involved, such as the fronto-temporal and occipital hairline, eyebrows, and mustache or beard, but also in skin creases like the nasolabial fold (Figures 107.1 and 107.2). The skin is red and covered with fine yellow greasy scales. Often, the patients link the onset with periods of particular stress; however, it is probably more associated with the increased sweating during these phases of life and sweating is accompanied by higher sebaceous gland activity.

Many patients use topical steroids, which indeed attenuate the erythema and inflammation but also favor the growth of the probably etiologically involved yeasts of *Malassezia* spp.

Clinical characteristics in dark skin (Fitzpatrick skin types IV–V)

Fine flaking of the skin with localized mild erythema is present around the alar creases and nasal side walls (Figures 107.3 and 107.4). Involvement of the scalp ranges from mild flaking without underlying erythema to a more inflammatory eruption with thicker, yellow, greasy scales and crusts resembling psoriasis. Similar changes can occur in the beard. Inflammation of the anterior eyelid margin (anterior blepharitis) may occur in SD and presents with flaky debris on the eyelashes. In men, involvement of the presternal area is typical with petaloid (petal-shaped) lesions that may be localized. More widespread involvement may extend to the upper back, umbilicus, axillae, groin, and submammary area. Erythema is inconspicuous in dark skin, and itchy inflammation is the prominent feature.

Investigations

This is diagnosed clinically.

Treatments

There is no definitive cure for SD. Long-term maintenance treatment may be required. Some patients only use treatment intermittently for acute symptomatic flares.

- Keratolytic agents – urea, propylene glycol, and lactic acid can reduce scaling and inhibit the growth of fungi.
- Topical antifungals are the mainstay of therapy – azoles, ciclopirox olamine, zinc pyrithione, coal tar, and selenium sulfide.
- Topical corticosteroids may be used in combination with antifungals for their additional anti-inflammatory effects. Short-term use of a mild topical corticosteroid is recommended.
- Maintenance treatment with twice-weekly 0.1% tacrolimus has also been reported to be effective.
- Oral antifungal therapy is occasionally advocated for recalcitrant or widespread SD, e.g., itraconazole

Further reading

Dessinioti C, Katsambas A (2013). Seborrheic Dermatitis: Etiology, Risk Factors, and Treatments: Facts and Controversies. *Clin Dermatol*;31(4):343–351.

Massiot P, Reygagne P, Chagnoleau C, et al. (2023). Maintenance Effect of a Once-Weekly Regimen of a Selenium Disulfide-Based Shampoo in Moderate-to-Severe Scalp Seborrheic Dermatitis after Initial Treatment with Topical Corticosteroid/Salicylic Acid. *Eur J Dermatol*;33(S1):13–18.

Paulino LC (2017). New Perspectives on Dandruff and Seborrheic Dermatitis: Lessons We Learned from Bacterial and Fungal Skin Microbiota. *Eur J Dermatol*;27(S1):4–7.

Vano-Galvan S, Reygagne P, Melo DF, et al. (2024). A Comprehensive Literature Review and an International Expert Consensus on the Management of Scalp Seborrheic Dermatitis in Adults. *Eur J Dermatol*;34(S1):4–16.

DOI: 10.1201/9781003479512-107

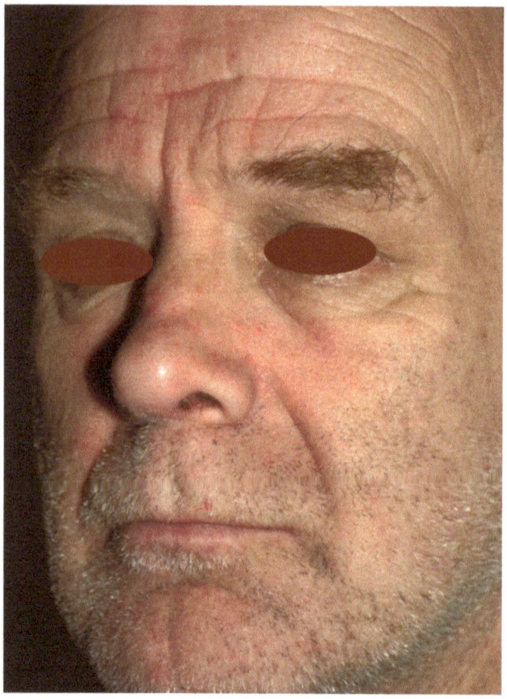

FIGURE 107.1 Seborrheic dermatitis on nasolabial folds and face FST1. (Courtesy Prof. Ian Coulson, UK.)

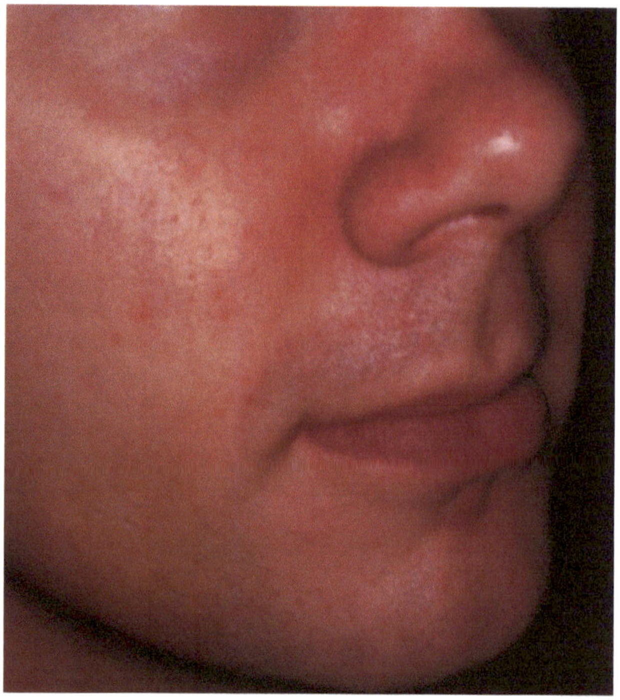

FIGURE 107.2 Seborrheic dermatitis on nasolabial folds FST1. (Courtesy Prof. Ian Coulson, UK.)

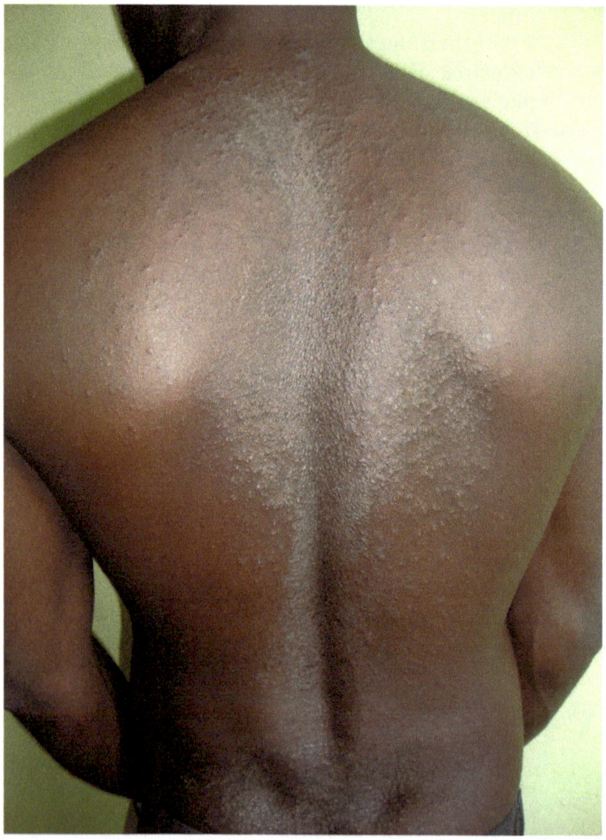

FIGURE 107.3 Extensive seborrheic dermatitis in a 32-year-old man; back of the trunk FST5.

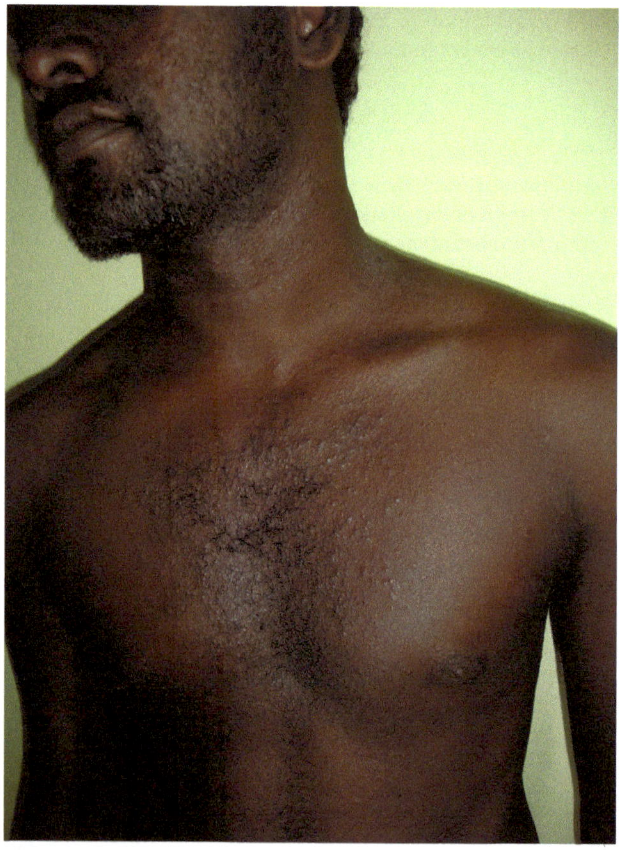

FIGURE 107.4 Extensive seborrheic dermatitis in a 32-year-old man; anterior chest and the face FST5.

108
SEBORRHEIC KERATOSIS AND DERMATOSIS PAPULOSA NIGRA

Introduction

Seborrheic keratosis (SK) is a benign tumor of epidermal keratinocytes that is usually asymptomatic. It can present with varying morphological features, from pale superficial patches (flat SK) to darkly pigmented verrucous plaques. SKs can be pedunculated or acanthotic. It has a typical 'stuck-on' appearance with loosely adherent greasy keratin on the surface.

Dermatosis papulosa nigra (DPN) is a variant of SK and is most common among individuals with darker skin complexion.

Epidemiology

SK is common in the elderly, approximately 75% of subjects over the age of 70 years, and both males and females are equally affected. DPN is more common in females and appears after 10 years of age, after which it increases steadily in frequency, number, and size.

Associated diseases

Eruptive SKs (Leser–Trélat sign) is a cutaneous paraneoplastic syndrome that warrants evaluation for a possible underlying malignancy, primarily gastrointestinal adenocarcinomas but also squamous cell carcinomas (SCC), leukemias, and lymphomas. The Leser–Trélat sign is characterized by the sudden onset of multiple SKs or an unusually rapid increase in the size and number of preexisting SK.

Clinical characteristics in light skin (Fitzpatrick skin types I–III)

SKs were once called 'senile warts.' This term implies that they increase with age both in number as well as in size and often also in color (Figures 108.1 to 108.3). In light-skinned people, they are often extremely frequent, with some having hundreds of SKs on the trunk, in the face, and on the proximal parts of the extremities, but indeed no body part is spared except for skin without hair follicles. This hints at their origin from the follicle (some believe them to be the benign counterpart of basal cell carcinoma [BCC]). An SK commonly begins as a small light brown papule that grows to a flat plaque and then further to its individual morphology, either as a brown keratotic plaque, a dark brown papillomatous growth, or sometimes a pedunculated large tumor. When present in the hundreds, the patient looks like they are splattered with brown mud. In contrast, DPN is a variant with innumerable but very small dark brown papules mainly on the face; this is a rarity in light skin.

Treatment is usually for cosmetic concerns and consists of superficial removal, as the lesions are always **on** the skin, not **in** the skin. Methods leading to scarring have to be avoided.

Clinical characteristics in dark skin (Fitzpatrick skin types IV–V)

SKs are usually asymptomatic but can be pruritic. In dark skin, it can have pleomorphic features varying from brown superficial patches to blackish pigmented verrucous plaques. This is a very common cosmetic issue in the elderly (Figures 108.4 to 108.6).

DPN is considered a variant of SK where the lesions are small, ranging in size from 1 to 3 mm. DPN is a very common cosmetic issue in dark skin where both men and women are affected equally, and the lesions may appear at any age after puberty. Unless removed, the number of lesions increases with time and spontaneous resolution is unlikely.

Investigations

Mostly a clinical diagnosis.

In doubtful cases, a skin biopsy can be performed to exclude mimics such as lentigo maligna, actinic keratosis, and pigmented BCC. An inflamed SK may be confused with a malignant melanoma, and an irritated SK can mimic early invasive SCC in histopathology.

Treatments

- Primarily for cosmetic reasons: Curettage, cryotherapy, ablative or non-ablative lasers, medium depth chemical peel.
- Electrocautery, curettage, and ablative or non-ablative lasers are effective on DPN.

Further reading

Ranawaka RR (2021). Benign Skin Proliferations. In: Ranawaka RR, et al. (eds). *Atlas of Dermatoses in Pigmented Skin*. Springer, Singapore; 955.

DOI: 10.1201/9781003479512-108

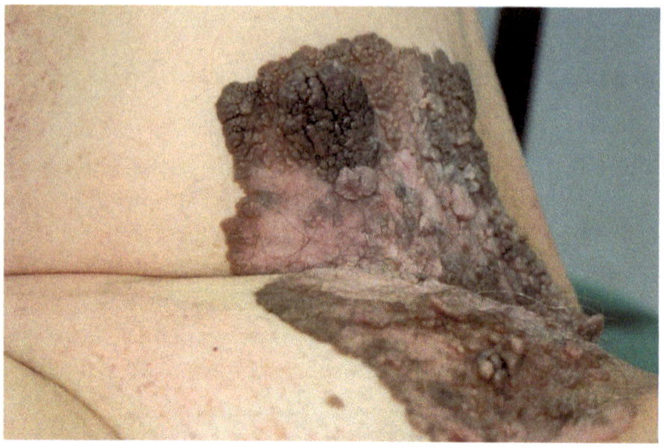

FIGURE 108.1 Seborrheic keratosis FST1. Since this was a large single lesion, skin biopsy was performed to exclude Buschke Lowenstein tumor. (Courtesy Prof. Uwe Wollina, Germany.)

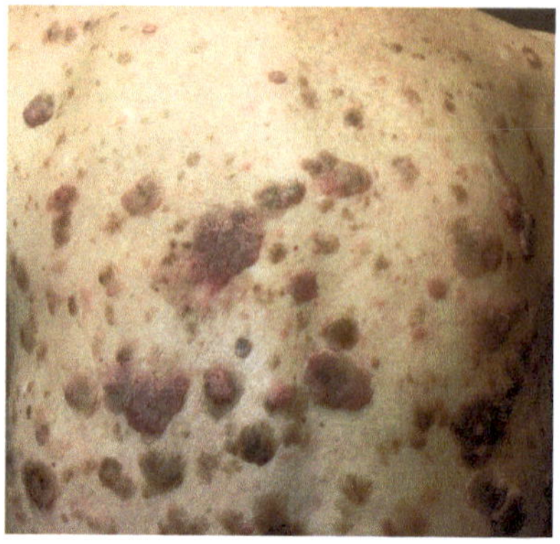

FIGURE 108.2 Multiple seborrheic keratosis on the back of the trunk FST1. (Courtesy Dr. Richard Ashton, UK.)

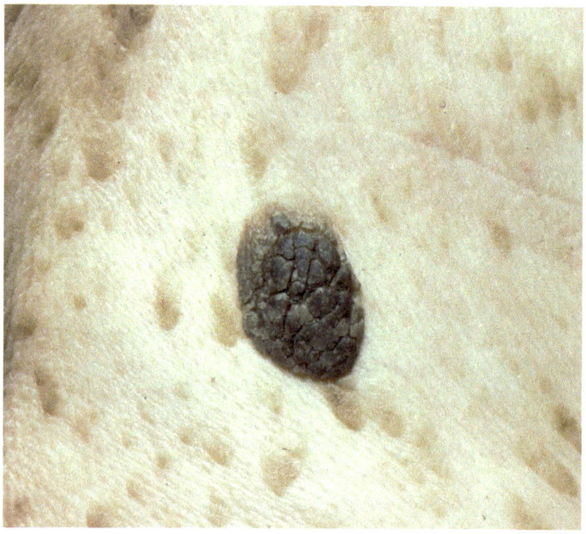

FIGURE 108.3 Seborrheic keratosis: A closer view FST1. (Courtesy Dr. Richard Ashton, UK.)

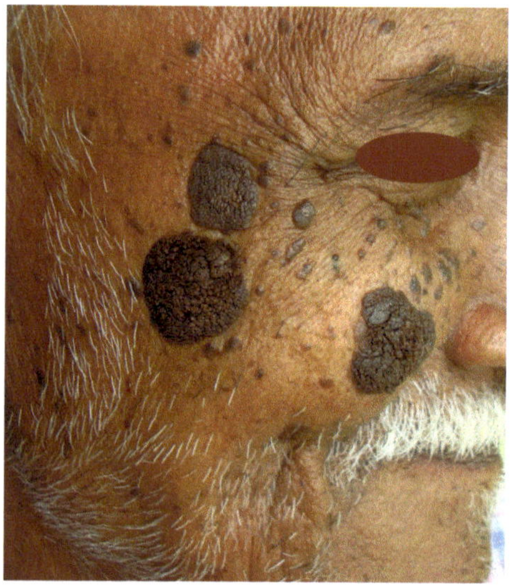

FIGURE 108.4 Multiple seborrheic keratoses and dermatosis papulose nigra in an 86-year-old farmer FST5. This is a very common cosmetic issue in advancing age in our setting.

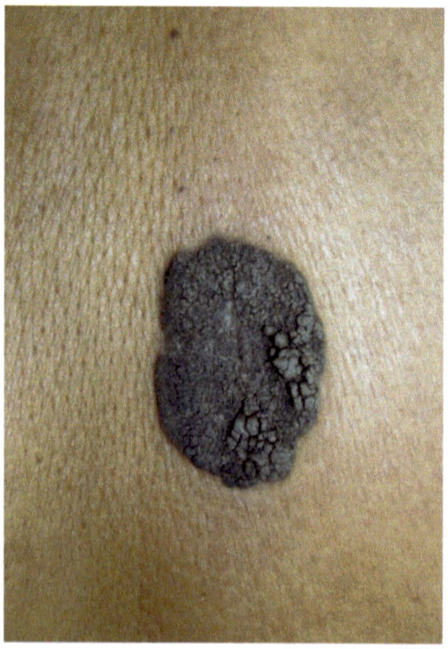

FIGURE 108.5 Seborrheic keratosis (closer-view) showing typical 'stuck-on' appearance with a loosely adherent greasy keratin on the surface FST5.

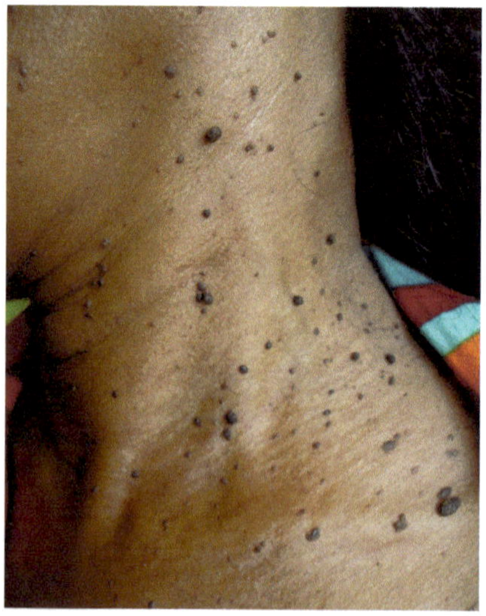

FIGURE 108.6 Numerous dermatosis papulosa nigra lesions in a 35-year-old woman FST5. This is considered a variant of seborrheic keratosis.

109
SKIN TESTING, PATCH TEST

Introduction

The diagnosis of allergic contact dermatitis may be made by patch testing.

Indications for patch testing are:

- Eczematous disorders where contact allergy is suspected or is to be excluded (including occupational).
- Eczematous disorders failing to respond to treatment as expected (including occupational).
- Chronic hand and foot eczema.
- Persistent or intermittent eczema of the face, eyelids, ears, and perineum.
- Varicose eczema.

The patch test is applied to normal skin, usually on the upper back where the tests are least likely to be disturbed. Other sites (e.g., the lateral aspect of the upper arm) may be considered when this is not practicable, for example, when there is pre-existing inflammation or other skin changes on the back. The test site has to be clear of eczema for at least a fortnight. Patch testing should be delayed for 4 weeks following sunbathing, and the patches should not be exposed to the sun or other sources of UV light. Corticosteroids and other immunosuppressive drugs should be stopped (if this is feasible) before patch testing.

The patient should be instructed not to bathe or shower for the duration of the tests and to avoid exercise or other activities likely to dislodge the patches. They should avoid excessive sweating during the test period.

After 48 hours, the first readings are taken 1 hour after removal of the patches, and again 48 hours later (that is, on day 2 and day 4). A single day 2 reading is not advised as it may lead to the labeling of some marginal irritants as allergens, and positive reactions to more poorly absorbed allergens may be missed.

Once they have developed, positive allergic reactions often persist for several days. The strength of the reaction depends on the degree of allergy to the tested substance(s), skin barrier function, the presence or absence of sweating, atmospheric humidity, test material, technique, and the reactivity of the individual.

Clinical characteristics in light skin (Fitzpatrick skin types I–III)

The epicutaneous patch test procedure is independent of the degree of skin pigmentation (Figure 109.1). Readings are made after 48 hours and (72 hours) 96 hours. The reactivity is commonly classified as 0 for non-reactivity, + for slight erythema, ++ palpable erythema, +++ raised erythema with small vesicles, and ++++ for vesiculo-bullous reactions. These allergic reactions tend to increase in intensity and spread beyond the immediate test patch contact area after 48–96 hours. Toxic reactions decrease after 48 hours and are thus weaker than at the first reading; they remain sharply delimited. Sometimes, the entire test area may become erythematous and render an exact reading virtually impossible; this is called the angry back syndrome. However, the 96-hour reading often allows for the evaluation of single test reactions as the surrounding redness usually diminishes after the removal of all test patches.

Weak test reactions with just mild erythema may be difficult to evaluate in dark skin in contrast to light skin.

Clinical characteristics in dark skin (Fitzpatrick skin types IV–V)

According to the author's experiences there are some drawbacks with this test on dark skin (Figure 109.2). Firstly, staying 2–4 days without a shower is almost impossible in hot humid climates, such as in Sri Lanka. However, there are water-resistant patch test kits available, which are more expensive. Secondly, sweating is inevitable in a hot, humid climate. Thirdly, allergens in different socio-cultural areas differ, and patch test kits should be tailored to the local environment and customs. Fourthly, erythema, which is an important marker of the patch-test reaction scoring system, is obscured in darker skin, giving false negative results. Therefore, the scoring system should be tailored to different skin colors, especially brown (FST 5) and black (FST 6) skin types. Furthermore, the penetration of the allergen depends on the barrier function of the skin. The measurement of transepidermal water loss (TEWL) as a marker of skin barrier function showed greater TEWL in black skin compared to white skin, while Asian skin was equal to black skin. Therefore, patch test kits should be tailored to different skin colors, cultures, and local environments.

Further reading

Orton D, Stone N (2024). Allergic Contact Dermatitis. In: Griffiths C, et al. (eds). *Rook's Textbook of Dermatology*, 10th ed. John Wiley & Sons Ltd., UK; 127.1.

Wesley NO, Maibach HI (2003). Racial (Ethnic) Differences in Skin Properties: The Objective Data. *Am J Clin Dermatol*;4(12):843–860.

DOI: 10.1201/9781003479512-109

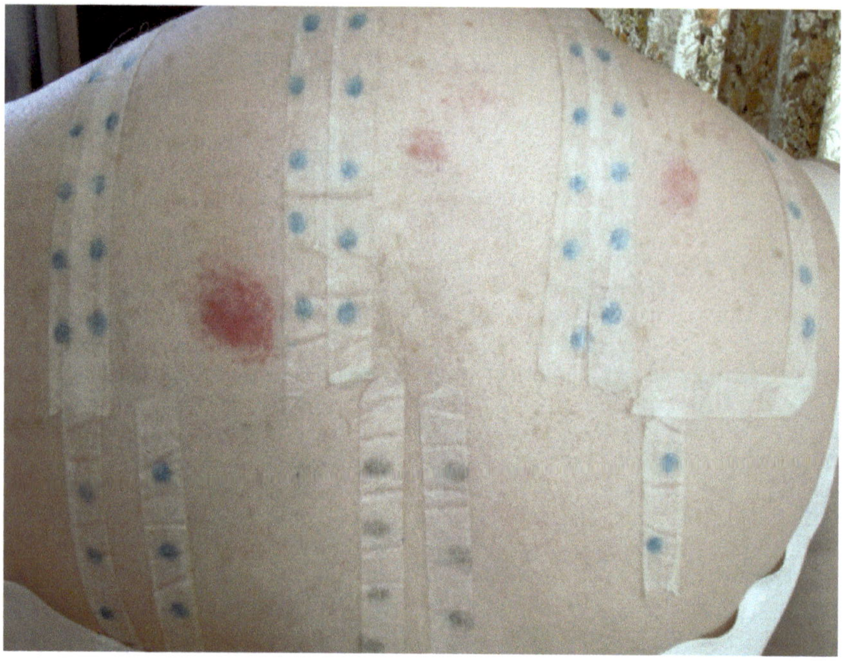

FIGURE 109.1 Skin patch test showing positive results FST1. (Courtesy Prof. Ian Coulson, UK.)

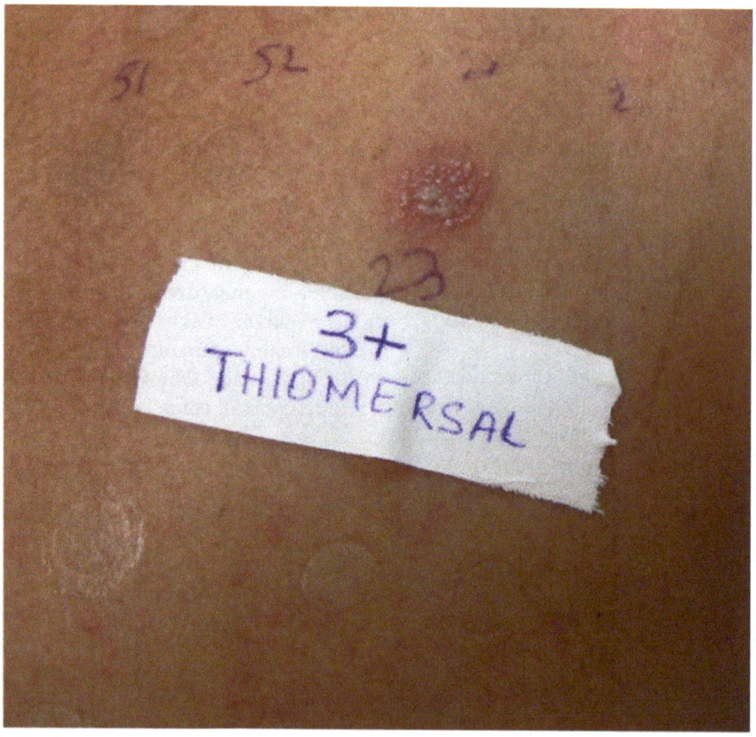

FIGURE 109.2 Weak test reactions with just a mild erythema may be difficult to evaluate in dark skin. (Courtesy Prof. Archana Singal, India.)

110
SQUAMOUS CELL CARCINOMA

Introduction

Squamous cell carcinoma (SCC) is a malignant tumor arising from epidermal keratinocytes or its appendages. SCC is the second most common skin cancer after basal cell carcinoma (BCC) in the white population. This is predominantly a disease of white populations and is especially prevalent in this group in areas of high ambient sun exposure. Fitzpatrick skin types I and II, particularly those with freckling, are most at risk.

Although the incidence is low in non-white populations, SCC is the most common skin cancer among them. In non-white populations, SCC is mostly secondary to trauma, albinism, burn scars, ionizing radiation, chronic inflammation, and chronic discoid lupus erythematosus. There is a high incidence of SCC in albinos in Nigeria but no evidence of an increased incidence in the vitiliginous skin of black people.

Epidemiology

The incidence of SCC increases with age. Males are more at risk of developing SCC, possibly due to outdoor employment, differences in sun avoidance behavior, and more frequent traumas, particularly to the lower legs.

Associated diseases

Precursor lesions are actinic keratosis and Bowen disease in white skin. HIV infection, immunosuppressive therapies, immune suppressive diseases, and PUVA therapy are highly susceptible to SCC development.

Clinical characteristics in light skin (Fitzpatrick skin types I–III)

SCC is very common in skin types I–III. (Figures 110.1 and 110.2) Its etiopathogenesis is different from that in dark-skinned people in that most cases are localized in areas of chronic sun exposure. Therefore, white people living in tropical and subtropical climates are at an extremely high risk. Most of these SCCs develop from a precursor lesion, an actinic keratosis. Taking actinic keratoses and SCCs together, they are even more frequent than BCC. However, there is another rarer variant developing *de novo*, which is known for its much more malignant behavior.

In the face, on the bald scalp, ear lobes, dorsa of the hands, and upper torso, hard keratoses grow on a red base, enlarge, and slowly become nodular and hyperkeratotic. With time, they may ulcerate. Metastases develop late except for the lower lips, ears, and genital which have a different growth kinetic.

Treatment is surgical with three-dimensional margin control (Mohs surgery). 'Blind methods' are not recommended.

Clinical characteristics in dark skin (Fitzpatrick skin types IV–V)

The author has not seen actinic keratosis in dark skin. Sunlight exposure is not a risk factor for SCC in dark skin. Recent growth on existing discoid lupus erythematosis (DLE), burn scar, radiation scar, or at site of previous ionizing radiation should arouse suspicion of SCC. Non-healing plaque-like, verrucous, tumid lesions, or ulcers should be excluded for SCC (Figures 110.3 to 110.7). In an albino, any persistent growth should be excluded for skin cancer. Oral submucous fibrosis is a precancerous lesion common in India and Sri Lanka, where betel chewing is a popular habit among villagers. Cancers developing on untreated oral submucous fibrosis are the most common cause of oral cancer in Sri Lanka.

Investigations

Skin biopsy is performed on suspected lesions.

Oncologist referral for further investigations and management; however, SCC is treated by dermatologists in most Western countries.

Treatments

- Surgical excision, especially Mohs micrographic surgery, produces excellent cure rates and spares the maximal amount of tissue.
- Other modalities include electrodesiccation and curettage, cryosurgery, radiotherapy, topical medications, photodynamic therapy, and systemic therapy.

Further reading

Ranawaka RR (2021). Precursors of Skin Carcinoma. In: Ranawaka RR, et al. (eds). *Atlas of Dermatoses in Pigmented Skin*. Springer, Singapore; 971.

Ranawaka RR, de Silva K, Abeygunasekara PH (2021). Skin Carcinomas. In: Ranawaka RR, et al. (eds). *Atlas of Dermatoses in Pigmented Skin*. Springer, Singapore; 989.

Tilakaratne WM, Jayasinghe RD (2021). Oral Potentially Malignant Disorders (OPMDs). In: Ranawaka RR, et al. (eds). *Atlas of Dermatoses in Pigmented Skin*. Springer, Singapore; 879.

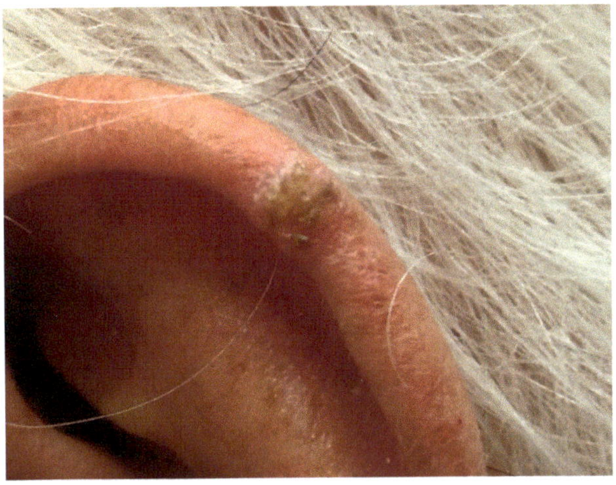

FIGURE 110.1 Squamous cell carcinoma in FST1. (Courtesy Prof. Eckart Haneke, Germany.)

DOI: 10.1201/9781003479512-110

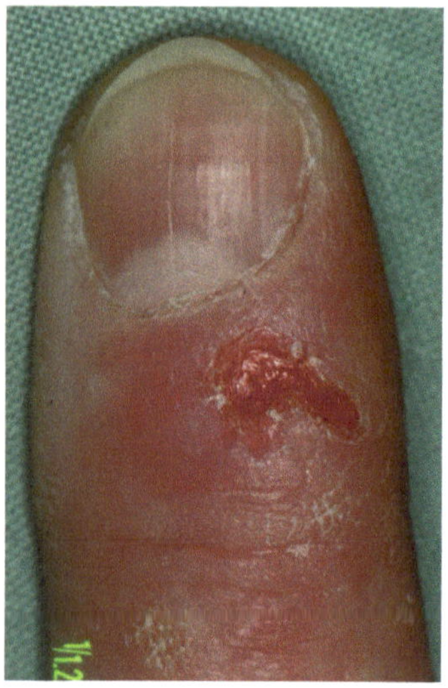

FIGURE 110.2 Ulcerated squamous cell carcinoma on the proximal nail fold of the index finger of a 58-year-old man FST1. (Courtesy Prof. Eckart Haneke, Germany.)

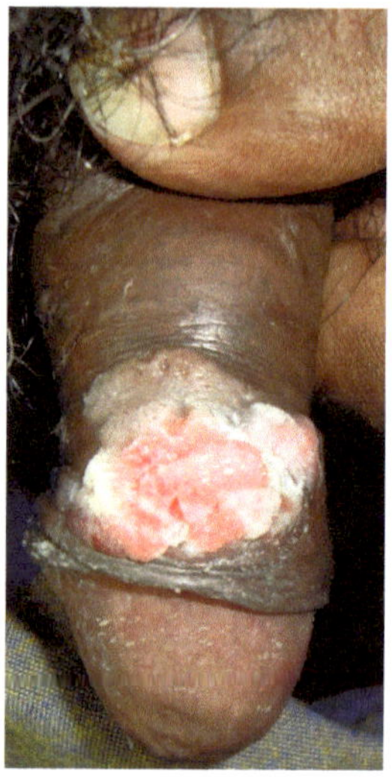

FIGURE 110.3 Non-healing ulcer on the penile skin in a 68-year-old man (FST5) was a squamous cell carcinoma.

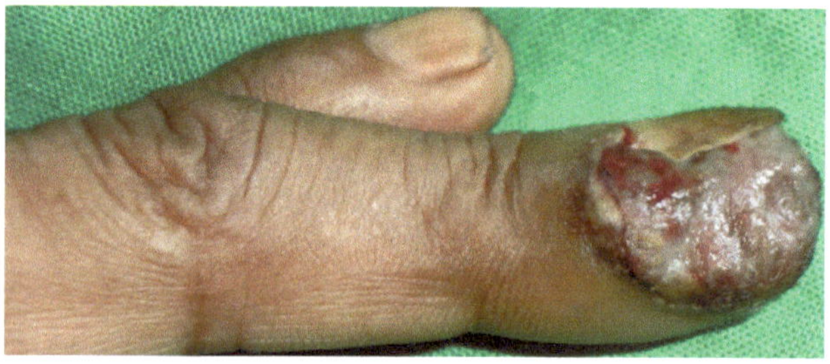

FIGURE 110.4 Non-healing ulcer on the fingertip in a 45-year-old woman (FST5) was a squamous cell carcinoma.

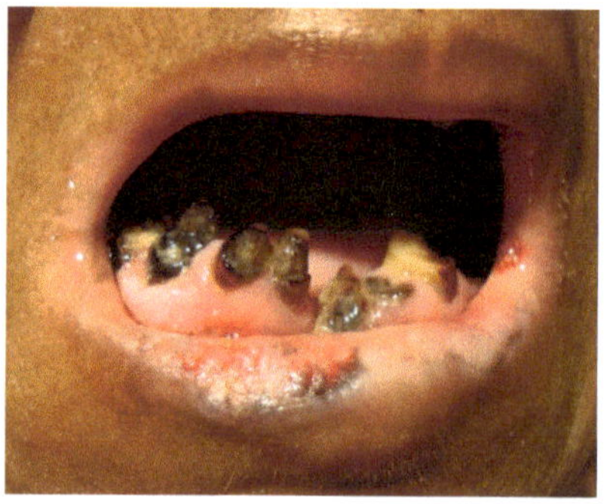

FIGURE 110.5 This 67-year-old woman had untreated oral submucous fibrosis for more than 10 years FST5. Note limited opening of the mouth and stained and decayed teeth due to betel chewing and poor oral hygiene. This ulcer that appeared on the lower lip was a squamous cell carcinoma.

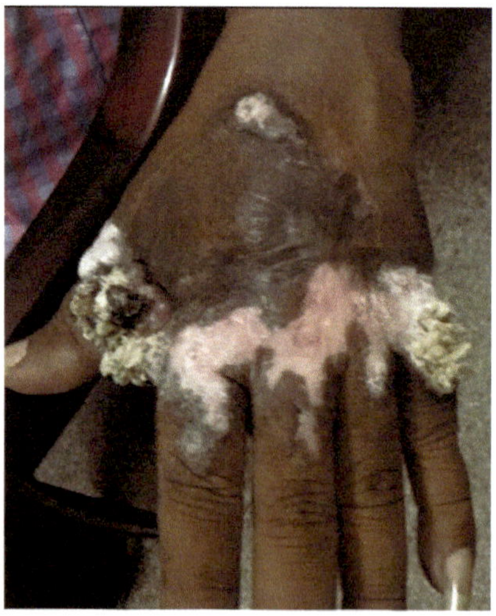

FIGURE 110.6 Squamous cell carcinoma arising on a burn scar (Marjolin's ulcer) in a 37-year-old man FST5. (Courtesy Dr. Kanishka de Silva, Sri Lanka.).

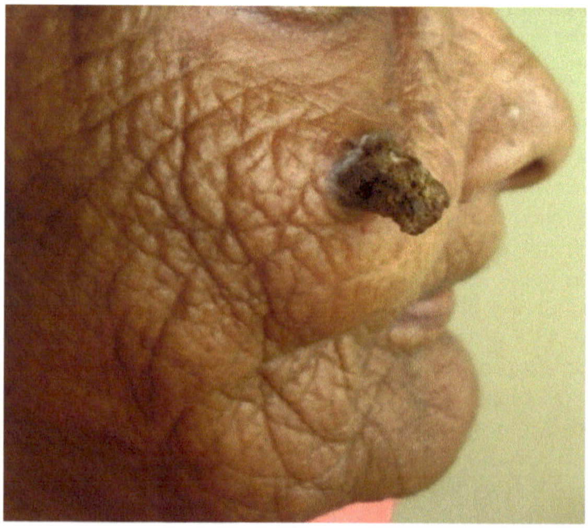

FIGURE 110.7 An 80-year-old woman presented with this recently enlarged warty growth on her right cheek FST5. Histopathology confirmed squamous cell carcinoma.

111
STAPHYLOCOCCAL SCALDED SKIN SYNDROME

Introduction

Staphylococcal scalded skin syndrome (SSSS) is an exfoliative dermatosis in which, classically, most of the body surface becomes tender and erythematous and the superficial epidermis strips off. SSSS is caused by epidermolytic toxin A and/or B of certain strains of *Staphylococcus aureus*, most commonly of phage group II, particularly strains 71 and 55. These toxins reach the skin via the circulation from a distant focus of infection, usually in the umbilicus, breast, conjunctiva, or the site of circumcision. Neonates are more prone, which is believed to reflect less efficient metabolism and excretion of the toxin. The rapid onset with marked cutaneous tenderness distinguishes it from most of the other causes of erythroderma in infancy. The main differential diagnosis is toxic epidermal necrolysis (TEN), but TEN shows mucosal involvement. Mortality is 2–10% in children with late diagnosis.

Epidemiology

Children (under the age of 6 years) and neonates are most commonly affected by the generalized form of SSSS. The localized form of the disease may be more frequent in older children and adults.

Associated diseases

Renal failure, malignancy, immunosuppression, and alcohol abuse have all been reported to predispose adults to the disease. Epidermolytic toxins are usually eliminated through the kidneys.

Clinical characteristics in light skin (Fitzpatrick skin types I–III)

SSSS is a life-threatening disease in newborns (*dermatitis exfoliativa neonatorum* of Ritter von Rittershain) (Figures 111.1 and 111.2). Variants occur in older children and adults that are much less widespread. Toxic shock syndrome is also caused by epidermolytic exotoxins, and some forms of impetigo may be seen as very limited forms.

In the classical form, the rash starts on the face and large flexures. The skin is very tender, intensely red, and exfoliates in large sheets. The infant is severely ill, developing fever, hypotension, and multiorgan failure. The mucosa is unaffected. The outcome in infants is generally good, with a mortality rate of about 5%, in contrast to adults, where it may be up to 60%.

Differential diagnoses comprise bullous impetigo, drug eruption, erythema multiforme, hemorrhagic shock, Kawasaki disease, meningococcemia, necrotizing fasciitis, scarlet fever, thermal burn, and toxic epidermal necrolysis.

Clinical characteristics in dark skin (Fitzpatrick skin types IV–V)

Extreme tenderness of the skin is an early feature in all skin types and may occur at a stage where cutaneous signs are not yet striking (Figures 111.3 and 111.4). The patient is pyrexial and distressed. Within the following 24–48 hours, the surface becomes wrinkled before starting to separate, leaving raw, red erosions (positive Nikolsky sign). Sites of predilection are the central part of the face, the axillae, and the groin.

The first sign of erythema or macular, orange-red, scarlatiniform eruption can be inconspicuous and can be easily missed in darker skin, leading to delayed diagnosis, more complications, and high mortality in an inexperienced setting.

Investigations

Mostly clinical diagnoses.

But basic investigations are performed to assess liver, renal, and hematological parameters, and blood cultures with antibiotic sensitivity (ABST).

Skin biopsy for histology; a frozen section provides rapid differentiation from TEN, where the level of the split in TEN is lower at the subepidermal level but is intraepidermal in SSSS.

Treatments

- Treatment is with either a penicillinase-resistant penicillin analogue, such as co-amoxiclav, or with a cephalosporin; adjustments have to be made according to ABST.
- Heat, fluid losses, and hyponatremia should be dealt with.
- Pain will also require treatment, and affected infants will generally be much more comfortable if the lesions are dressed rather than left open.

Further reading

Wootton C, Elliott I (2024). Bacterial Infections. In: Griffiths C, et al. (eds). *Rook's Textbook of Dermatology*, 10th ed. John Wiley & Sons Ltd., UK; 26.27.

DOI: 10.1201/9781003479512-111

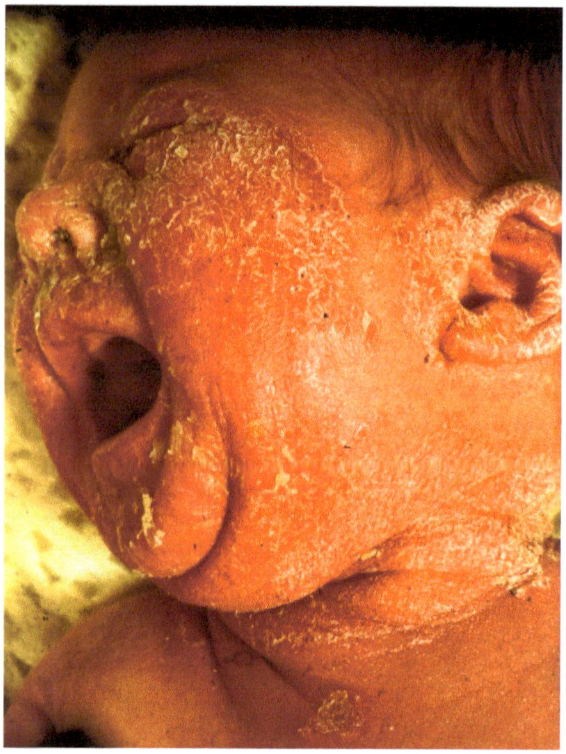

FIGURE 111.1 Staphylococcal scalded skin syndrome in FST1 newborn. (Courtesy Dr. Richard Ashton, UK.)

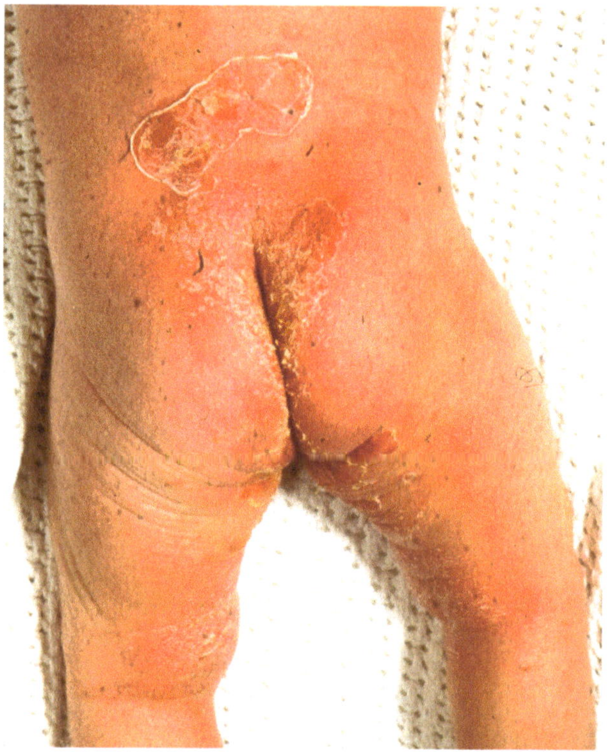

FIGURE 111.2 Staphylococcal scalded skin syndrome in FST1 newborn. (Courtesy Dr. Richard Ashton, UK.)

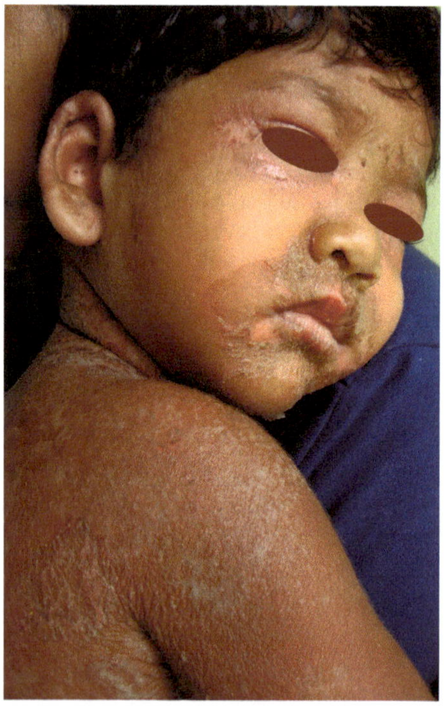

FIGURE 111.3 Staphylococcal scalded skin syndrome in a 3-year-old child FST5. Note predilection to the central part of the face. The skin is extremely tender to touch and children are very irritable, which are important signs in dark skin where erythema is masked.

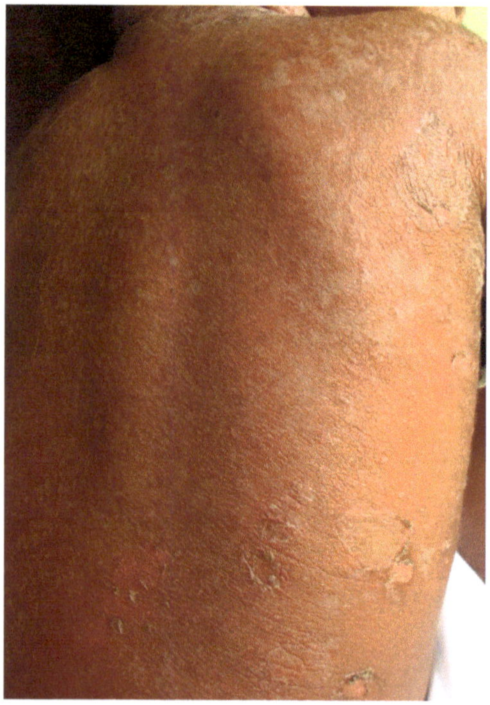

FIGURE 111.4 Staphylococcal scalded skin syndrome in a 3-year-old child FST5. Skin surface becomes wrinkled before starting to separate, leaving raw, red erosions. Note positive Nikolsky sign.

112
STEROID ACNE (ACNEIFORM ERUPTION)

Introduction

Monomorphic inflammatory lesions with an absence of comedones, often presenting acutely on sites not commonly affected by acne should alert the diagnosis. Corticosteroids may provoke an acneiform reaction regardless of their route of administration.

Epidemiology

Common in adolescence, teenagers, and in young men and women.

Associated diseases

May associate with bronchial asthma who use steroid inhalers.

Clinical characteristics in light skin (Fitzpatrick skin types I–III)

Steroid acne is mainly but not exclusively observed in patients during and after treatment with glucocorticosteroids, usually topical on large areas but also systemic (Figures 112.1 and 112.2). Small acneiform papules form that have no comedo. They are monomorphic and barely inflammatory. With long-term steroid application, steroid atrophy, erythema, and telangiectasiae are seen. Whereas steroid acne disappears after withdrawal of the steroid, steroid atrophy does not or only very slowly.

There are a number of other drugs that cause similar acneiform eruptions.

Clinical characteristics in dark skin (Fitzpatrick skin types IV–V)

Monomorphic inflammatory lesions appear on the sites not commonly affected by acne such as anterior and back of the trunk (Figure 112.3). The most common cause in young females we observe is using skin-bleaching agents containing steroids (whitening creams). In young males, abuse of androgenic anabolic steroids, synthetic derivatives of testosterone, and testosterone salts in the form of milk powders, or tablets are the most common triggering factors as well as using over-the-counter bleaching creams.

Investigations

This is a clinical diagnosis.

Treatments

Treatment is same as in acne vulgaris. Find out the causative factors individually, educate patients on how they acquire the problem and to avoid triggering factors.

Further reading

Bhargava K, Christou E, Tziotzios C (2024). Acquired Non-Infective Disorders of the Pilosebaceous Unit. In: Griffiths C, et al. (eds). *Rook's Textbook of Dermatology*, 10th ed. John Wiley & Sons Ltd., UK; 91.2.

Gammanpila RR, Kannangara AP (2024). Skin Problems in Adolescents and Puberty in FST 5. In: Gammanpila RR, Kannangara AP (eds). *Paediatric Cases in Coloured Skin*. CRC Press, UK; 145.

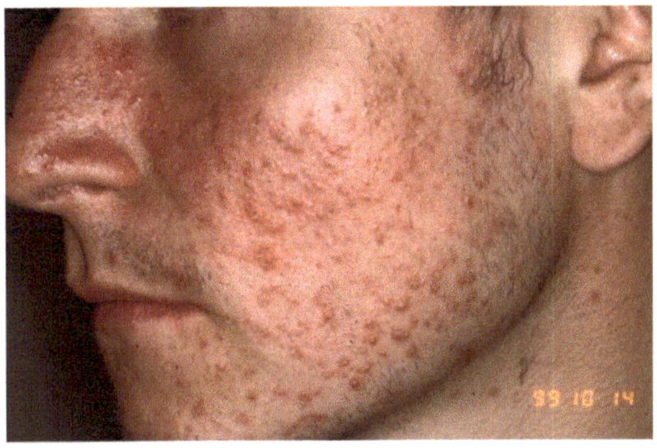

FIGURE 112.1 Steroid-induced acneiform eruption FST1. (Courtesy Dr. Richard Ashton, UK.)

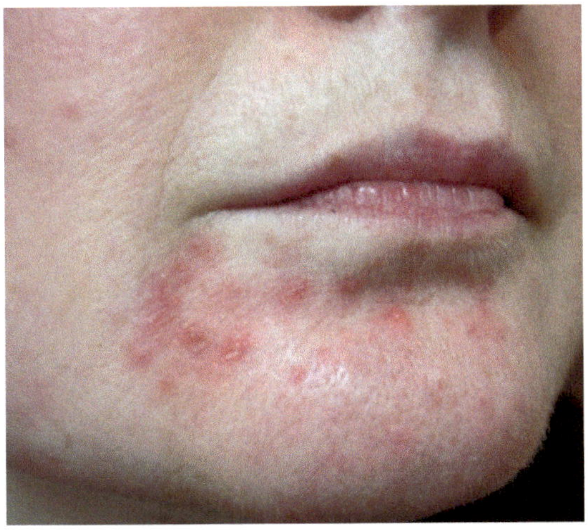

FIGURE 112.2 Perioral dermatitis due to topical steroids FST1. (Courtesy Prof. Ian Coulson, UK.)

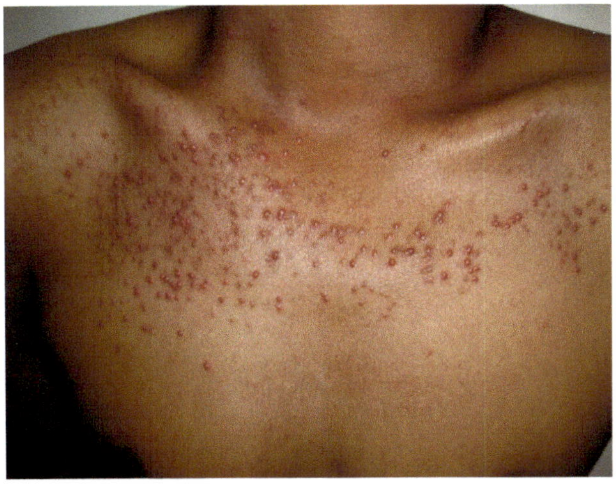

FIGURE 112.3 Steroid acne (acneiform eruption) in an 18-year-old man FST5 who has applied topical clobetasol ointments as bleaching creams.

DOI: 10.1201/9781003479512-112

113
STEROID PURPURA

Introduction

Purpura is the discoloration of the skin or mucous membranes due to the extravasation of red blood cells.

Purpura and bruising may occur as isolated phenomena or as part of a systemic disorder. Purpura is the hallmark of vasculitis affecting smaller vessels of the skin. Purpura is also commonly seen due to platelet and coagulation disorders and may be idiopathic or drug-induced.

Corticosteroid purpura is due to a lack of support in blood vessels. It has the same pattern whether due to topical, oral, endogenous (Cushing syndrome), or even inhaled corticosteroids. They are usually asymptomatic and vary in size from a few millimeters to several centimeters. They are usually not palpable and may persist for several weeks.

Epidemiology

This can occur in anyone of age who is on a high dose or long-term corticosteroids, but it is more common in old age.

Associated diseases

May be associated with Cushing syndrome.

Clinical characteristics in light skin (Fitzpatrick skin types I–III)

After long-term application of potent steroids, bleeding into the atrophic dermis may occur. The mechanism is atrophy of the perivascular connective tissue with vessel fragility and consequent blood extravasation. This is often associated with actinic purpura, but may occur also in other chronically steroid-treated areas.

Clinical characteristics in dark skin (Fitzpatrick skin types IV–V)

Non-palpable purpura on hands, forearms, or on the legs (Figure 113.1). They are mostly a few millimeters in size and uniform in color, size, and appearance. In dark skin, these are clearly seen on the medial aspects of arms, forearms, and thighs. These areas are lighter in complexion than the sun-exposed extensor aspect, which may mask the purpuric lesions.

Investigations

This is a clinical diagnosis.

Regular hematology screening to exclude platelet disorders.

Treatments

Resolve spontaneously after the withdrawal of corticosteroids.

Further reading

Levell NJ (2024). Purpura. In: Griffiths C, et al. (eds). *Rook's Textbook of Dermatology*, 10th ed. John Wiley & Sons Ltd., UK; 99.2.

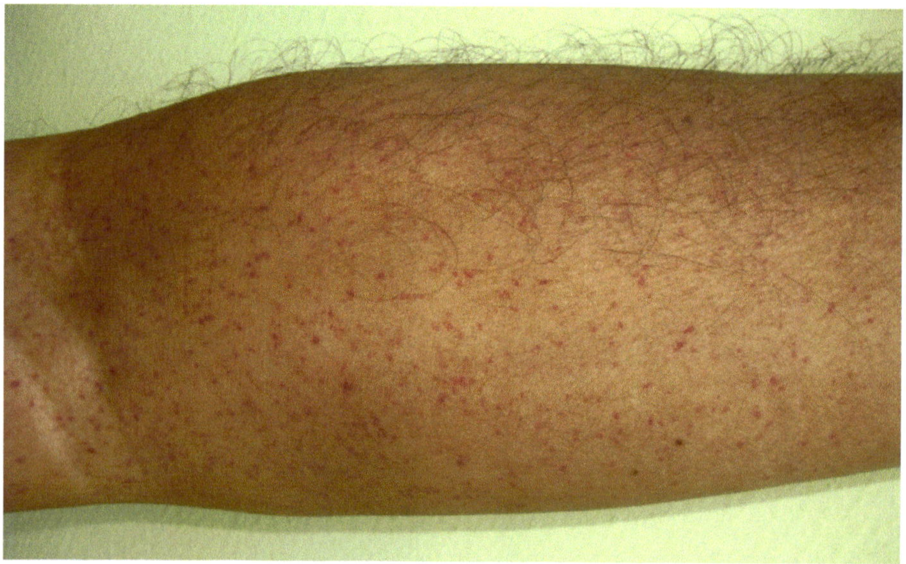

FIGURE 113.1 Steroid purpura FST5. Non-palpable purpura, a few millimeters in size, uniform in color, size, and appearance. In dark skin these are clearly visible on medial aspect or sunlight-covered body areas where the skin color is lighter.

DOI: 10.1201/9781003479512-113

114
STEVENS–JOHNSON SYNDROME

Introduction

Stevens–Johnson syndrome (SJS) is defined as epidermal detachment of less than 10% body surface area (BSA), plus widespread purpuric macules or flat atypical target lesions. In SJS, there is mucous membrane involvement and cutaneous blistering. There is overlap SJS and toxic epidermal necrolysis (TEN) when the detachment is 10–30% BSA, plus widespread purpuric macules or flat atypical targets. At the less severe end of the spectrum, differentiation of SJS from erythema multiforme major (EMM) is difficult. In both EMM and SJS, there is mucous membrane involvement and cutaneous blistering with epidermal detachment of less than 10% BSA. However, in EMM, the lesions consist of typical targets or raised atypical targets, predominantly localized on the limbs and extremities, while in SJS, the lesions are atypical targets with predilection for the torso. EMM is mostly related to herpes simplex virus reactivation and rarely to drugs, while SJS and TEN are usually triggered by a drug.

Epidemiology

SJS can occur in any age group. There is an increased incidence in the elderly and in women.

Associated diseases

There is an increased risk of SJS and TEN in HIV and systemic lupus erythematosus (SLE).

Clinical characteristics in light skin (Fitzpatrick skin types I–III)

SJS is a serious and potentially life-threatening disease involving up to 10% of the body surface, including the oral, genital, and conjunctival mucosa, probably also the esophagus, as well as the palms and soles (Figure 114.1). It may develop from erythema multiforme major or directly. Most cases are due to an allergic reaction, either to drugs or viral, bacterial, and mycoplasma infections; however, up to 20% remain idiopathic. The patient feels severely ill with fever, malaise, and headache. Usually starting on the upper trunk and spreading to the extremities, atypical target lesions rapidly develop from confluent red macules. The flaccid blister roof detaches and leaves red erosions.

When more than 10% are affected, this is called Stevens–Johnson/toxic epidermal necrolysis overlap; more than 30% is called TEN.

Clinical characteristics in dark skin (Fitzpatrick skin types IV–V)

A patient with SJS is unwell with malaise, fever, and, usually, prostration. The earliest skin lesions are atypical targets or purpuric macules anywhere on the body. Involvement of the palms and soles with target lesions is often prominent. These erythematous or purpuric macular early-stage lesions may go unnoticed in darker skin, which can lead to higher morbidity and mortality in inexperienced settings. Later, vesicles or fluid-filled blisters develop within lesional skin. Involvement of the mucous membranes of the eyes, mouth, nose, and genitalia is usually an early feature and leads to erosive and hemorrhagic mucositis (Figures 114.2 to 114.6).

Investigations

This is a clinical diagnosis. Routine investigations are performed to assess and monitor the systemic involvement.

Treatments

- Withdraw the culprit drug.
- If epidermal loss is >10% BSA, transfer to a specialist unit (intensive care unit or burns unit).
- Institute a supportive care package, with particular attention to:
    - Heated environment.
    - Fluid replacement.
    - Nutritional regimen.
    - Analgesia.
    - Preventing and treating infection.
    - Specialist skin care nursing is essential for the delivery of topical therapy/dressings.
    - Severe SJS is managed as TEN.

Further reading

Creamer D, Walsh S, Lee HY (2024). Severe Cutaneous Adverse Reactions to Drugs. In: Griffiths C, et al. (eds). *Rook's Textbook of Dermatology*, 10th ed. John Wiley & Sons Ltd., UK; 118.12.

Roujeau JC, Bastuji-Garin S (2011). Systematic Review of Treatments for Stevens-Johnson Syndrome and Toxic Epidermal Necrolysis Using the SCORTEN Score as a Tool for Evaluating Mortality. *Ther Adv Drug Saf*;2(3):87–94.

Shekhar M, Iqbal O, Dharan A, et al. (2024). The Role of NLRP3 Inflammasome in the Pathogenesis of Stevens-Johnson Syndrome/Toxic Epidermal Necrolysis. *Med Res Arch*;12(1):10.18103/mra.v12i1.4939.

DOI: 10.1201/9781003479512-114

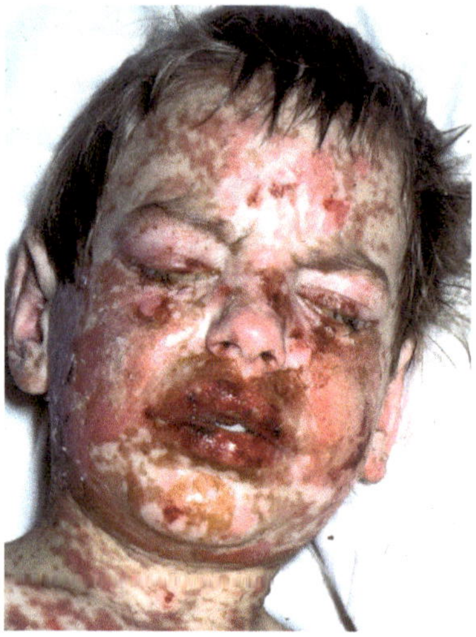

FIGURE 114.1 Stevens–Johnson syndrome FST1. (Courtesy Prof. Ian Coulson, UK.)

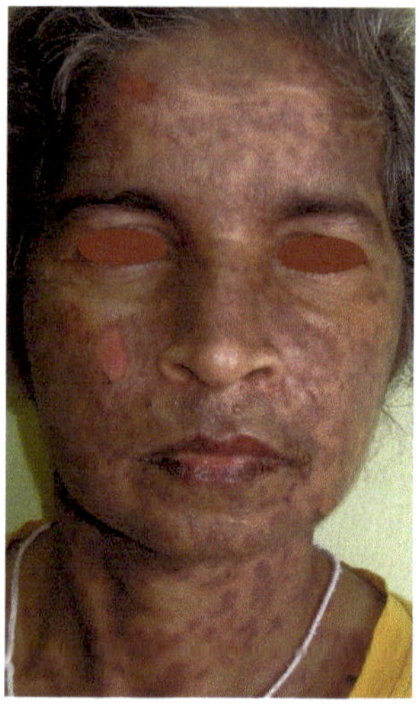

FIGURE 114.2 Stevens-Johnson syndrome FST5.

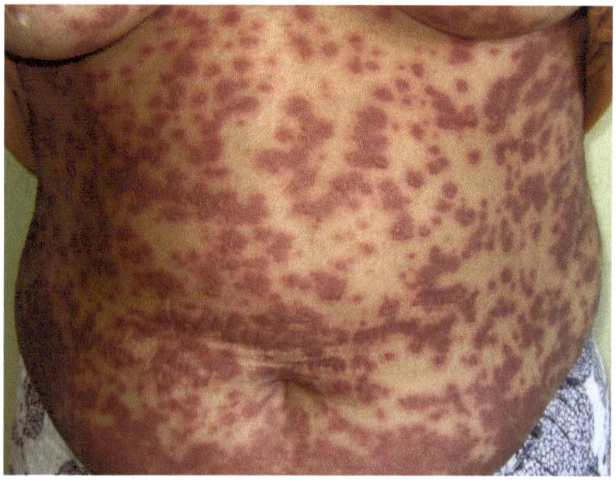

FIGURE 114.3 Stevens–Johnson syndrome in a 43-year-old woman FST5; widespread erythematous atypical target lesions and blisters involving 10–30% BSA.

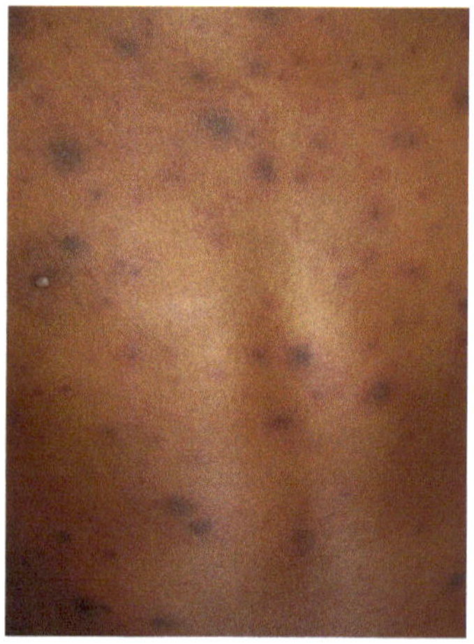

FIGURE 114.4 Stevens–Johnson syndrome; atypical target lesions in a 14-year-old boy with a history of drug allergy. Note erythema is concealed in dark skin leading to delayed diagnosis.

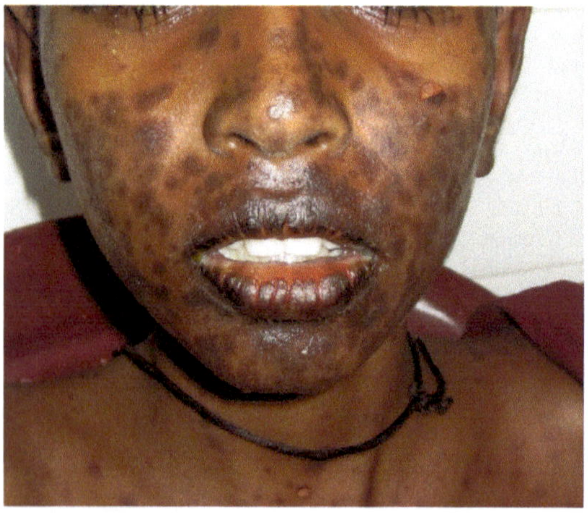

FIGURE 114.5 Stevens–Johnson syndrome in a 14-year-old boy. He had very dark skin where erythema was hidden and hyperpigmentation was marked concealing the severity of the illness.

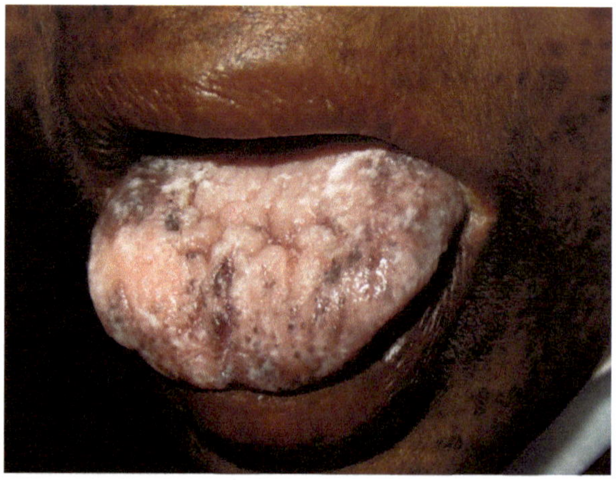

FIGURE 114.6 Stevens–Johnson syndrome in a 14-year-old boy with painful mucositis. This boy passed away 2 days later. Even in local settings, dark skin can disguise and deceive the severity assessment leading to a fatal outcome.

115
STRIAE OR STRETCH MARKS

Introduction

Striae (stretch marks) are visible linear subepidermal scars that form in areas of dermal damage produced by overstretching of the skin. They are characterized histologically by thinning of the overlying epidermis, with fine dermal collagen bundles arranged in straight lines parallel to the surface. Striae are associated with growth spurts, e.g., bodybuilding, puberty in males (adolescent striae), or pregnancy (striae gravidarum); more rarely they may reflect structural abnormalities of connective tissue such as Marfan syndrome or the effect of glucocorticoids (steroid striae) (Borrelli 2021). Striae are commonly absent in pregnancy in Ehlers–Danlos syndrome.

Epidemiology

Striae are very common and occur in most adult women at puberty or during pregnancy. Adolescent striae are common in adolescent boys.

Associated diseases

They may reflect structural abnormalities of connective tissue, such as in Marfan syndrome.

Striae are associated with Cushing syndrome and obesity.

Clinical characteristics in light skin (Fitzpatrick skin types I–III)

Striae distensae are due to overstretching of the skin (Figures 115.1 and 115.2). As mentioned above, there are particular events that render individuals prone to these stretch marks, such as rapid growth in boys, where the striae run parallel and horizontal. In pregnant women, striae are often red and very embarrassing. It takes some time for these striae rubrae to fade and turn whitish (striae albae). As they represent, in fact scars they will never completely disappear and sometimes leave very flaccid skin. Whether or not 'scar ointments' are really helpful is difficult to say. However, fractional CO_2 laser treatment has been proven to be beneficial.

Clinical characteristics in dark skin (Fitzpatrick skin types IV–V)

The appearance of striae differs in different situations (Figures 115.3 to 115.5):

- *Pubertal growth striae* that appear in adolescent boys are all asymptomatic and horizontally arranged right across the back. They are either skin-colored or mildly hypopigmented. After some years, they fade and become inconspicuous.
- In *obesity-related striae*, the most common sites are the outer aspect of the thighs and the lumbosacral region in boys, and the thighs, buttocks, and breasts in girls, also the inner aspect of the upper arms. Early lesions may be raised and irritable, but they soon become flat, smooth, and livid red. Their surface may be finely wrinkled. In darker skin, the redness may not be apparent, and they are generally paler than the surrounding skin.
- *Pregnancy-induced striae* are common in all childbearing women and are sometimes itchy, red, and hyperpigmented. They persist throughout as wrinkled skin.
- *Steroid-induced striae* are thick, erythematous, and very angry-looking. Even when steroids are withdrawn, the striae persist, changing the erythematous color to dark or light brown.
- Young men engaging in bodybuilding develop *skin-colored or pallor striae* on their shoulders, closer to the upper arms.

Investigations

This is a clinical diagnosis.

Treatments

- There are no proven preventive measures for striae gravidarum.
- In the case of common adolescent striae, the patient may be reassured that, in time they will become less conspicuous.
- Striae gravidarum generally improve after delivery, but wrinkled skin marks last for many years.
- Even corticosteroid-induced striae may disappear or become less conspicuous when the treatment is stopped.
- After reviewing 151 studies, it was concluded that the highest rates of complete response were injection-based devices for striae distensae (7%; n = 12/172), CO_2 lasers for striae alba (4%; n = 12/341), and platelet-rich plasma injections for striae rubra (31%; n = 4/13) (Zhu

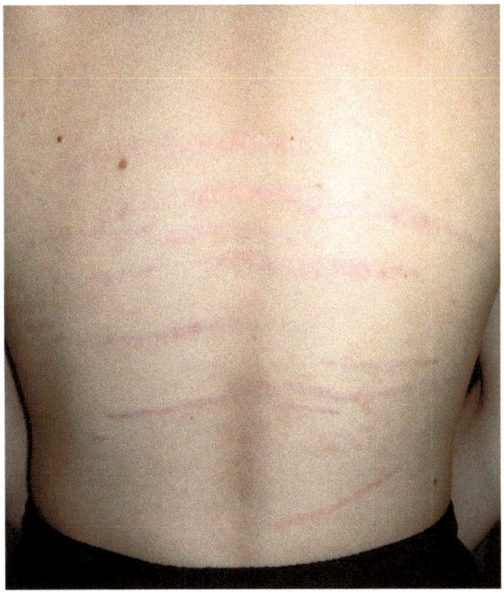

FIGURE 115.1 Adolescent striae in a 15-year-old boy FST1. (Courtesy Prof. Ian Coulson, UK.)

et al. 2024). Non-ablative lasers are preferred in darker skin tones due to a lower risk of post-inflammatory hyperpigmentation.

Further reading

Ayuningsih S, Jusuf NK, Putra IB (2024). Efficacy of Green Tea (*Camellia sinensis* Linn) 3% Extract Cream on Improvement of Striae Distensae. *F1000Res*;13:208.

Fahy CMR, Lovell CR (2024). Acquired Disorders of Dermal Connective Tissue. In: Griffiths C, et al. (eds). *Rook's Textbook of Dermatology*, 10th ed. John Wiley & Sons Ltd., UK; 94.9.

Gammanpila RR (2023) Skin Problems in Adolescent and Puberty in FST 5. In: Gammanpila RR, et al. (eds). *Paediatric Cases in Coloured Skin*. CRC Press, UK; 142–161.

Madegowda SB, Rajegowda HM, Kalegowda D, et al. (2023). Efficacy of Fractional Carbon Dioxide Laser versus Fractional Carbon Dioxide Laser with Platelet-Rich Plasma in Treatment of Striae Distensae in a Tertiary Care Center: A Comparative Study. *J Cutan Aesthet Surg*;16(3):178–185.

Zhu CK, Mija LA, Koulmi K, et al. (2024). A Systematic Review on Treatment Outcomes of Striae. *Dermatol Surg*;50(6):546–552.

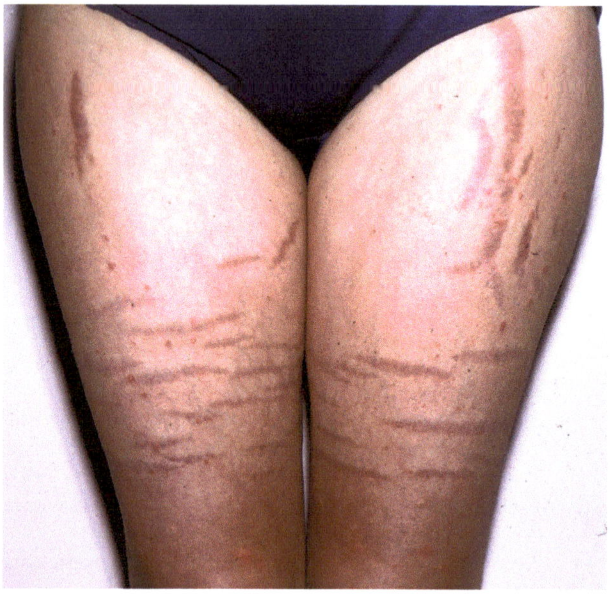

FIGURE 115.2 Striae FST1. (Courtesy Dr. Richard Ashton, UK.)

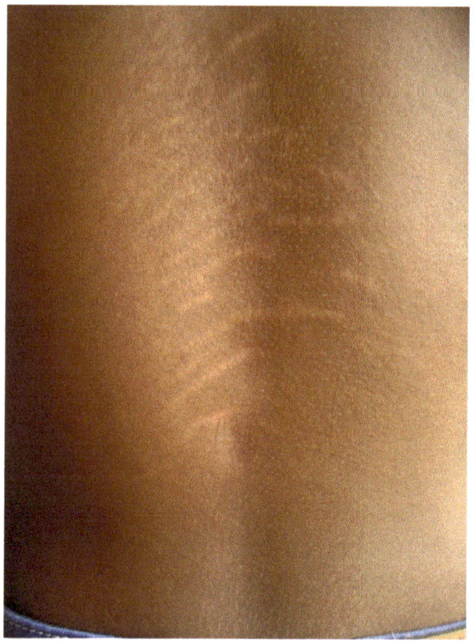

FIGURE 115.3 Adolescent striae in a 14-year-old boy FST5.

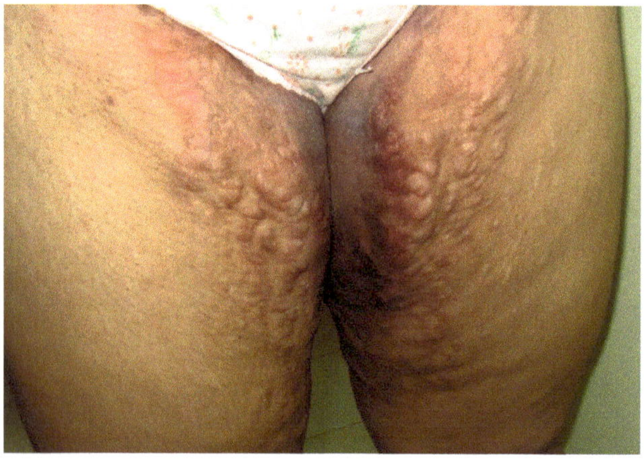

FIGURE 115.4 Steroid striae in a 38-year-old woman FST5 who had used clobetasol ointment as a bleaching cream on groin.

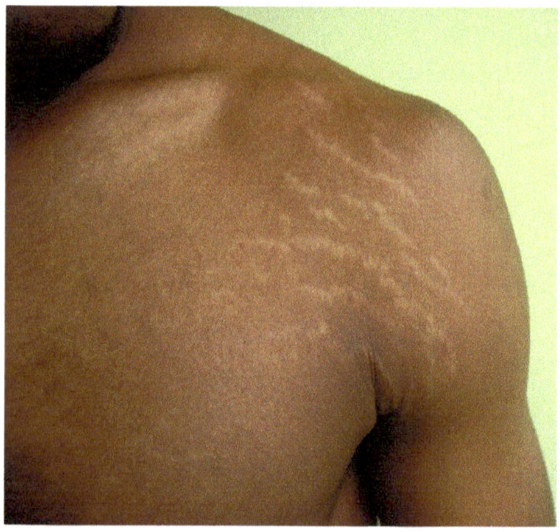

FIGURE 115.5 Bodybuilder's striae in 21-year-old man FST5.

116
SWEET SYNDROME

Introduction

Sweet syndrome (SS) is also known as acute febrile neutrophilic dermatosis. SS may be categorized into three subtypes: Classic, malignancy-associated, and drug-induced.

- *Classic SS* – This is characterized by the abrupt onset of painful erythematous plaques or nodules in association with constitutional symptoms like fever and arthralgia. Many clinical variants of cutaneous lesions may be pustular, bullous, cellulitis-like, or necrotizing lesions on any part of the body. Targetoid lesions have been reported in some patients.
- *Malignancy-associated SS* – In old age, vesiculo-bullous morphology is associated with leukopenia, anemia, thrombocytopenia, elevated erythrocyte sedimentation rate (ESR), and the absence of arthralgia are seen in this type of SS.
- *Drug-induced SS* – About 1–27% of cases of SS are due to drugs. Granulocyte colony-stimulating factor (G-CSF) is the drug most often associated with SS; however, numerous other medications can cause it, e.g., propylthiouracil, novel antineoplastic, and immunologic agents.

Diagnostic criteria for SS: Two major criteria are (1) acute onset of typical lesions, and (2) histopathological findings consistent with SS. Four minor criteria are (1) fever >38°C, (2) association with malignancy, inflammatory disorder, or pregnancy, or antecedent respiratory or gastrointestinal infection, (3) excellent response to systemic corticosteroids or potassium iodide, and (4) abnormal laboratory values at presentation (three of four required: ESR >20 mm; leukocytes >8000; neutrophils >70%; elevated C-reactive protein).

Epidemiology

It can affect any age, but typically affects those between the ages of 30 and 60 years, and is more common in women.

Associated diseases

A wide range of malignancies is described in association with SS, e.g., hematologic malignancies and myeloproliferative or myelodysplastic disorders, most notably acute myeloid leukemia and myelodysplastic syndrome.

Clinical characteristics in light skin (Fitzpatrick skin types I–III)

Patients may present with acute fever, leucocytosis, general malaise, headache, arthritis, and myalgias. The skin shows tender red to purple papules and nodules extending to plaques (Figures 116.1 and 116.2). They often present with very edematous lesions that give the impression of vesiculation immediately under the epidermis. Some lesions clear centrally, resulting in an annular or even targetoid aspect. A particular aspect of SS is pathergy, where lesions appear at sites of previous trauma or can be elicited by wounding the skin (similar to Behçet syndrome). Neutrophilic panniculitis, giant cellulitis-like, and necrotizing variants have been observed.

Several internal organs may be involved, such as the heart, central nervous system, spleen, bones, oral mucosa, eyes, and inner ear.

Healing may take weeks, although the disease rapidly responds to steroid treatment.

There are many diseases that may occur before, during, or after SS; however, it is not always clear whether they are independent or just internal manifestations of SS. Leukemia cutis may be differentiated histopathologically by the almost exclusive occurrence of mature neutrophils in SS.

Clinical characteristics in dark skin (Fitzpatrick skin types IV–V)

The classical appearance is of tender red papules, nodules, and eventually plaques distributed over the head, neck, upper trunk, and upper arms (Figure 116.3). The plaques are often edematous, and as the process develops, they may become studded with pseudovesicles or pseudopustules. Patients often have a fever and feel unwell.

Central nervous system involvement in SS, neuro–Sweet's syndrome (NSS), is rare and reported especially among Asian patients. The initial presentation is usually with the typical SS skin lesions followed by neurological involvement.

Investigations

Skin biopsy: The classical and diagnostic histopathological features are a dense infiltrate of neutrophils in the dermis and prominent dermal papillary edema. True vasculitis is not seen, although leukocytoclasis is a common finding, and endothelial swelling without fibrinoid necrosis is also observed.

Routine blood tests, full blood count (FBC), liver function test (LFT), renal function, C-reactive protein (CRP), and erythrocyte sedimentation rate (ESR).

FBC shows peripheral leukocytosis (>8000), > 70% neutrophils.

Elevated CRP and ESR >20 are common.

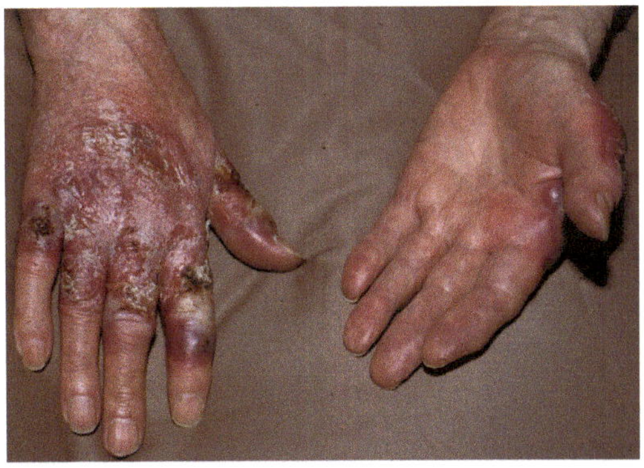

FIGURE 116.1 Bullous hemorrhagic Sweet syndrome FST2. (Courtesy Prof. Ian Coulson, UK.)

DOI: 10.1201/9781003479512-116

Additional tests should be guided by the clinical findings and may include thyroid function tests, rheumatoid factor, and antistreptolysin O antibody titers.

All patients should receive age-appropriate malignancy screening.

Treatments

- Treatment should be tailored to the individual patient.
- Systemic corticosteroids are the standard for SS. The response to corticosteroids is usually rapid.
- Steroid-sparing systemic agents include dapsone, colchicine, and potassium iodide and may be needed in some cases.
- Without treatment, the disease will often resolve within 3 months. Approximately one-third of cases will recur.

Further reading

Aydemir H, Oztoprak N, Celebi G, et al. (2008). Pulmonary and Central Nervous System Involvement in Sweet's Syndrome: A Very Rare Case Report. *Intern Med*;47(16):1481–1484.

Drago F, Ciccarese G, Agnoletti AF, et al. (2017). Neuro Sweet Syndrome: A Systematic Review. A Rare Complication of Sweet Syndrome. *Acta Neurol Belg*;117(1):33–42.

Hampton PJ, Ball S (2024). Neutrophilic Dermatoses. In: Griffiths C, et al. (eds). *Rook's Textbook of Dermatology*, 10th ed. John Wiley & Sons Ltd., UK; 49.3.

Moreno-Artero E, Torrelo A (2024). Pediatric Neutrophilic Dermatoses. *Dermatol Clin*;42(2):267–283.

Vongsachang H, Chiou CA, Azad AD, et al. (2024). Periorbital Necrotizing Sweet Syndrome: A Report of Two Cases Mimicking Necrotizing Soft Tissue Infections. *Am J Ophthalmol Case Rep*;34:102033.

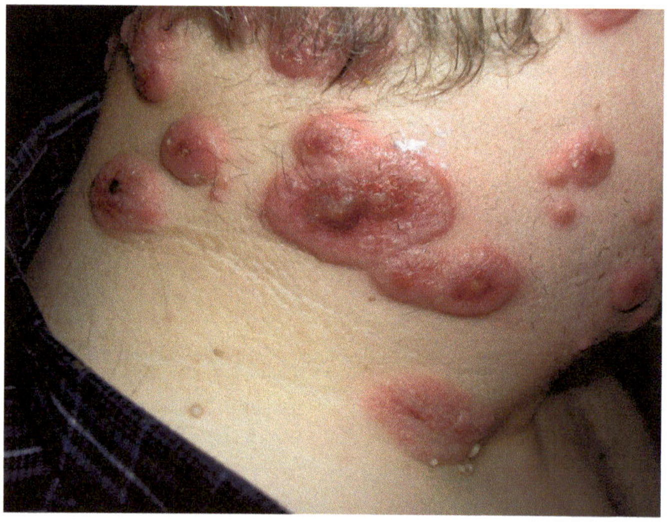

FIGURE 116.2 Classical Sweet syndrome FST1. (Courtesy Prof. Ian Coulson, UK.)

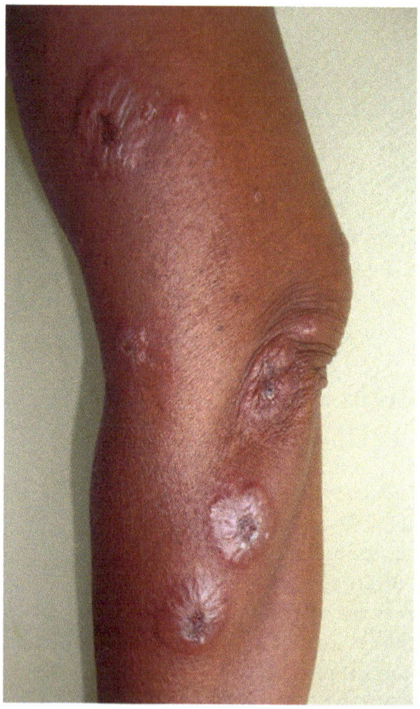

FIGURE 116.3 Classical Sweet syndrome in a 65-year-old woman FST5.

117
TINEA BARBAE

Introduction

This is ringworm of the beard and mustache areas of the face, with the invasion of coarse hairs. It is thus a disease of adult males. Causative organisms are animal species of *Trichophyton verrucosum* and *T. mentagrophytes.*

Epidemiology

This affects male adults.

Clinical characteristics in light skin (Fitzpatrick skin types I–III)

Tinea barbae used to be called *trichophytia profundae barbae* (Figure 117.1 and 117.2). It is an infection of beard hair by dermatophytes of the *Trichophyton* spp., most commonly by zoophilic species that cause an intense inflammatory host response. Starting with single follicular papules, these turn rapidly to pustules with putrid discharge. This may be a source of autoinoculation. Left untreated, the infection may destroy the hair follicles and result in cicatricial alopecia; however, it is sometimes astonishing how much of the hair can regrow over a longer period of time.

The involved beard hair can easily be extracted, and direct microscopy shows ectothrix fungi.

Although principally very similar, kerion Celsi is a disease of children and usually heals spontaneously after puberty; however, it can cause irreversible scarring alopecia and should therefore be treated as early as possible.

Clinical characteristics in dark skin (Fitzpatrick skin types IV–V)

Highly inflammatory, pustular folliculitis, often showing all the features of a kerion or sycosis barbae (Figure 117.3). Hairs of the beard or mustache regions are surrounded by red inflammatory papules or pustules.

Investigations

For culture specimens, if dermatophytosis is suspected, the hairs should be removed with the roots intact; cut hairs are unsuitable. The affected hairs may be recognized because they are dull and broken but, if not, the fact that they slip out easily with fine forceps is in favor of this diagnosis.

For routine examination, specimens are usually mounted in 10–30% potassium hydroxide; the higher the percentage, the faster the specimen will clear. For skin scrapings and nails, warming gently over the pilot light of a Bunsen burner will speed up the process, but boiling should be avoided. The cover slip should be pressed down firmly to obtain a monolayer of cells before microscopic observation.

Large-spored ectothrix invasion with the spores in chains is observed in direct microscopy.

Treatments

- Griseofulvin: 500–1000 mg/day for 6–12 weeks
- Terbinafine: 250 mg/day for 4–6 weeks
- Oral itraconazole: 200 mg/day for 4–6 weeks

Fairly long-term follow-up is recommended, and late recurrences can occur.

- Early diagnosis and prompt treatment of the individual patient and the encouragement of high standards of hygiene in the livestock industry are recommended.

Further reading

Hay RJ (2024). Fungal Infections. In: Griffiths C, et al. (eds). *Rook's Textbook of Dermatology,* 10th ed. John Wiley & Sons Ltd., UK; 32.40.

Ranawaka RR (2021). Superficial Fungal Infections. In: Ranawaka RR, et al. (eds). *Atlas of Dermatoses in Pigmented Skin.* Springer, Singapore; 336.

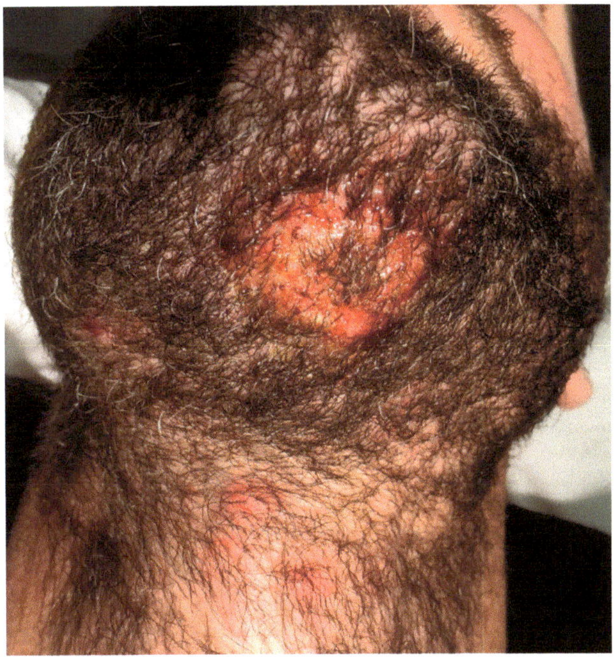

FIGURE 117.1 Tinea barbae FST1. (Courtesy Dr. Richard Ashton, UK.)

DOI: 10.1201/9781003479512-117

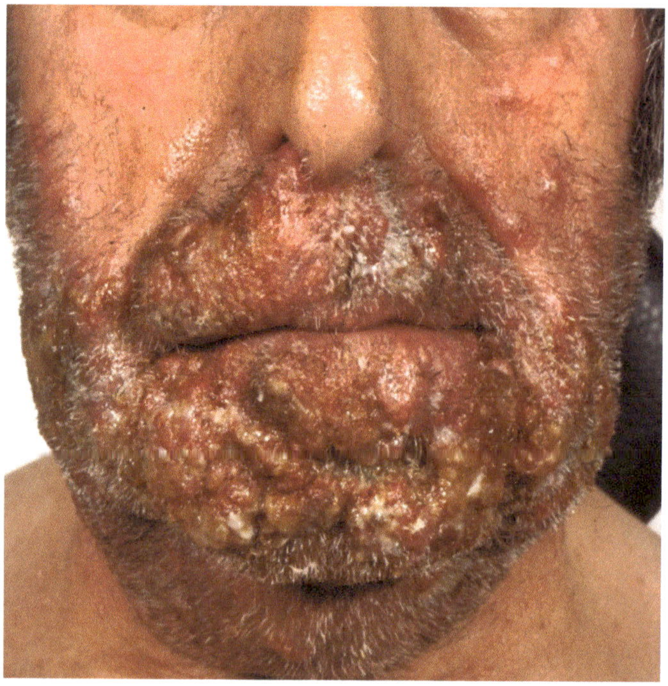

FIGURE 117.2 Tinea barbae FST1. (Courtesy Dr. Richard Ashton, UK.)

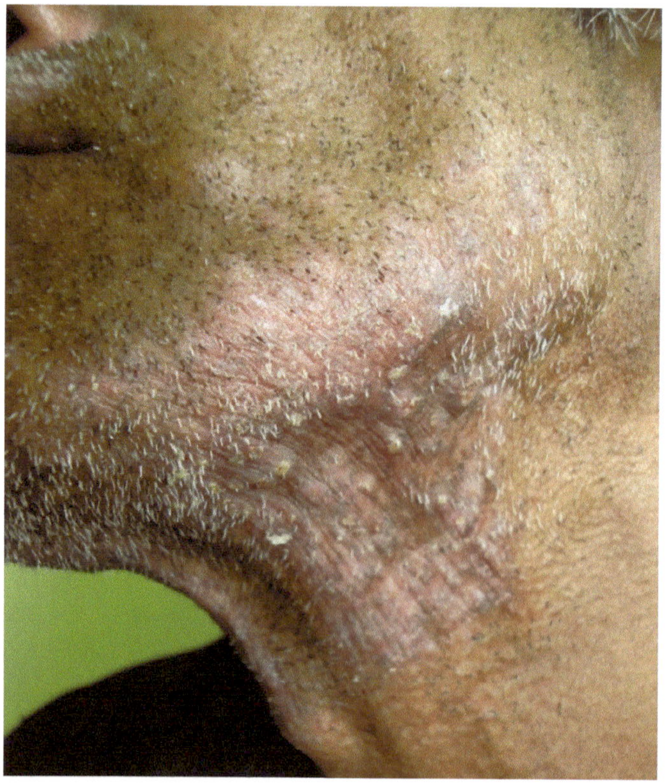

FIGURE 117.3 Tinea barbae in a 67-year-old farmer FST5. Differentiate from sycosis barbae is not possible clinically. Poor response to systemic antibiotics warrants further investigations for fungal etiology.

118
TINEA CORPORIS

Introduction

Tinea corporis is ringworm of the body skin. The clinical manifestations result from the invasion and proliferation of the causal fungi in the stratum corneum. Common organisms are *Trichophyton rubrum*, *T. mentagrophytes*, *T. tonsurans*, and *Microsporum canis*.

Epidemiology

Tinea corporis can occur in any climate, although it is more common in the tropics. It is common in all ages except in infants.

Clinical characteristics in light skin (Fitzpatrick skin types I–III)

In Europe and North America, the most common etiological fungi of tinea corporis are *Trichophyton rubrum*, *T. mentagrophytes*, *Microsporum canis*, and *Epidermophyton floccosum*, although many other dermatophytes may sometimes be isolated. The infection may occur anywhere on the hairy skin of the body and extremities (Figure 118.1). Starting with a slightly itchy red papule, this may extend and then form rings with central clearing and marginal inflammatory plaques with slight scaling. New inflammatory papules may arise in the center of the rings. The groin and intercrural skin are the most commonly infected. In the gluteal region, very large areas may be involved.

As the tinea becomes itchier with time, inappropriate use of corticosteroids is frequent and may mask the original disease, a condition called tinea incognita. It is up to the diagnostic skills of the dermatologist to make the correct diagnosis in these cases.

The diagnosis is confirmed with direct microscopy of skin scrapings from the margin of the rings after clearing with 20% potassium hydroxide (KOH) and mycological culture. Histopathology has frequently demonstrated a tinea in unsuccessfully steroid-treated inflammatory dermatoses.

Clinical characteristics in dark skin (Fitzpatrick skin types IV–V)

Very itchy, sharply marginated circular lesions with a raised edge (Figure 118.2). Central resolution is common. Post-inflammatory hyperpigmentation is common in dark skin and persists for years even after a complete cure. Resistant and extensive tinea corporis is common in our setting due to the inappropriate use of topical steroids in tinea infection. This might have been responsible for the emergence of resistant dermatophytes, particularly *T. indotineae*.

Investigations

This is a clinical diagnosis.

Skin scrapings are performed in doubtful cases and for research purposes. Skin scrapings are used for both light microscopic examination and cultures.

To obtain skin scrapings, disposable blunt scalpel blades of the solid type, held vertically to the skin, are used to obtain scrapings. If the lesion has a definite edge, the material should be taken from the active margin. The scrapings for culture should be collected and transported in folded paper, which keeps the specimen dry, thus preventing overgrowth of bacterial contaminants. Squares of brightly colored paper card are ideal. Dermatophytes in skin scrapings may remain viable for months, and yeasts for several weeks.

For microscopy examination, specimens are usually mounted in 10–30% potassium hydroxide; the higher the percentage, the faster the specimen will clear. For skin scrapings and nails, warming gently over the pilot light of a Bunsen burner will speed up the process, but boiling should be avoided. The coverslip should be pressed down firmly to obtain a monolayer of cells before microscopic observation.

Direct examination of skin scrapings will show fungal hyphae.

Treatments

Tinea corporis is normally treated with topical agents such as azole creams, allylamines, ciclopirox, or amorolfine. In cases of widespread or recalcitrant tinea corporis, oral antifungal drugs should be considered.

Localized disease, recent onset

- Topical azole creams (clotrimazole, ketoconazole, oxiconazole, econazole, miconazole) should be applied once or twice daily for 2–4 weeks.
- Topical allylamines (terbinafine cream) twice daily for 2–4 weeks

Widespread disease

- Oral terbinafine: 250 mg/day for 3–4 weeks
- Itraconazole: 100 mg/day for 3–4 weeks
- Griseofulvin: 500 mg to 1 g/day for 4 weeks

Resistant and extensive tinea corporis needs prolonged and higher doses of an oral antifungal. A particular problem is the appearance of terbinafine-resistant strains of *T. mentagrophytes*, now called *T. indotineae*. Sensitivity testing is therefore indicated in terbinafine-resistant tinea of any type.

Further reading

Ranawaka RR (2021). Superficial Fungal Infections. In: Ranawaka RR, et al. (eds). *Atlas of Dermatoses in Pigmented Skin*. Springer, Singapore; 330.

Shaw D, Dogra S, Singh S, et al. (2024). Prolonged Treatment of Dermatophytosis Caused by *Trichophyton indotinea* with Terbinafine or Itraconazole Impacts Better Outcomes Irrespective of Mutation in the Squalene Epoxidase Gene. *Mycoses*; 67(8):e13778.

Sonego B, Corio A, Mazzoletti V, et al. (2024). *Trichophyton indotineae*, an Emerging Drug-Resistant Dermatophyte: A Review of the Treatment Options. *J Clin Med*;13(12):3558.

DOI: 10.1201/9781003479512-118

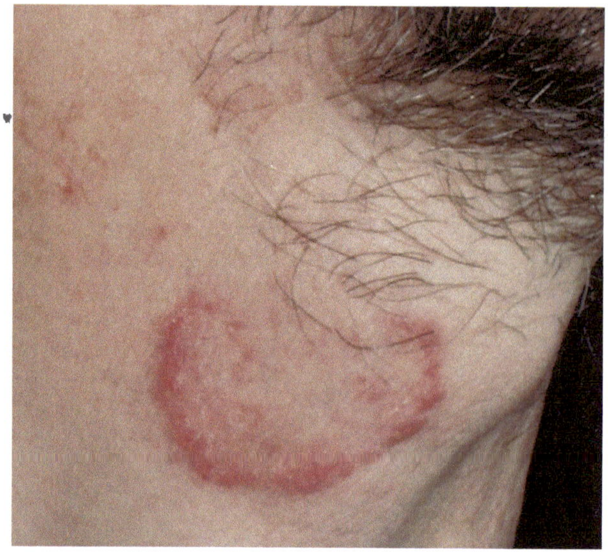

FIGURE 118.1 Tinea infection on the neck FST1. (Courtesy Prof. Ian Coulson, UK.)

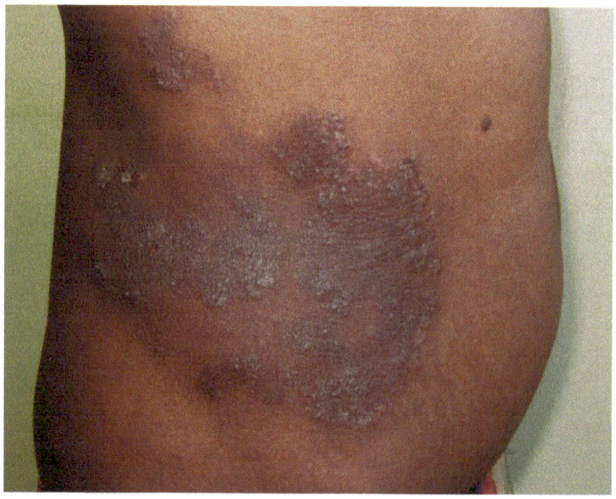

FIGURE 118.2 Tinea corporis in a 45-year-old man FST5. Post-inflammatory hyperpigmentation is very common in dark skin which may last for many years after cure.

119
TINEA CRURIS

Introduction

Tinea cruris is an infection of the groin by a species of dermatophyte. *Trichophyton rubrum* is the main cause; *Trichophyton interdigitale* and *Epidermophyton floccosum* also account for some cases. Inappropriate use of topical steroids may mask the active inflammatory edge, leading to misdiagnosis.

Epidemiology

Commoner in adults and in both sexes. The sharing of towels and clothing is an important predisposing factor, and it is more common in hot, humid climates.

Clinical characteristics in light skin (Fitzpatrick skin types I–III)

Tinea cruris is a variant of tinea corporis localized in the groin and intercrural folds, including the adjacent genital and perineal skin (Figure 119.1). Here, the particular microclimate of moisture and heat favors fungal growth. In the obese patient, itch in the groin and perigenital skin is common, and the skin lesions are often only noted late by the patient, who cannot look into the skin folds. There is a ring of inflammatory papules with slight scaling in the dry skin, which is not seen directly in the folds as this is rubbed away due to friction of the skin. In contrast, intertriginous candidosis forms red plaques without a raised margin. Post-inflammatory pigmentation is not common in light-skinned individuals.

Clinical characteristics in dark skin (Fitzpatrick skin types IV–V)

Itching is a predominant feature. A distinct raised margin differentiates tinea infection from candida intertrigo (Figures 119.2 and 119.3). Erythematous lesions start at the groin and extend down the thighs, curved with sharp margins. Post-inflammatory hyperpigmentation is marked and common in darker skin, persisting for years even after a complete cure.

Investigations

This is a clinical diagnosis.

Skin scales are taken from skin scrapings at the active edge of the lesion. Skin scales are mounted in 30% potassium hydroxide (KOH) solution, which shows hyphae in direct microscopy. The hyphae are very even in diameter and regularly septate. Cultures are used for species identification.

Treatments

Mild tinea cruris is treated by topical agents such as azole creams, allylamines, ciclopirox, or amorolfine. In the case of widespread or recalcitrant tinea cruris, oral antifungal drugs should be considered.

Localized disease, recent onset

- Topical azole creams (clotrimazole, ketoconazole, oxiconazole, econazole, miconazole) once or twice daily for 2–4 weeks.
- Topical allylamines (terbinafine cream) twice daily for 2–4 weeks.

Widespread disease

- Oral terbinafine: 250 mg/day for 3–4 weeks
- Itraconazole: 100 mg/day 3–4 weeks
- Griseofulvin: 500 g/day for 4 weeks

Resistant and extensive tinea cruris needs prolonged and higher doses of an oral antifungal as well as sensitivity testing.

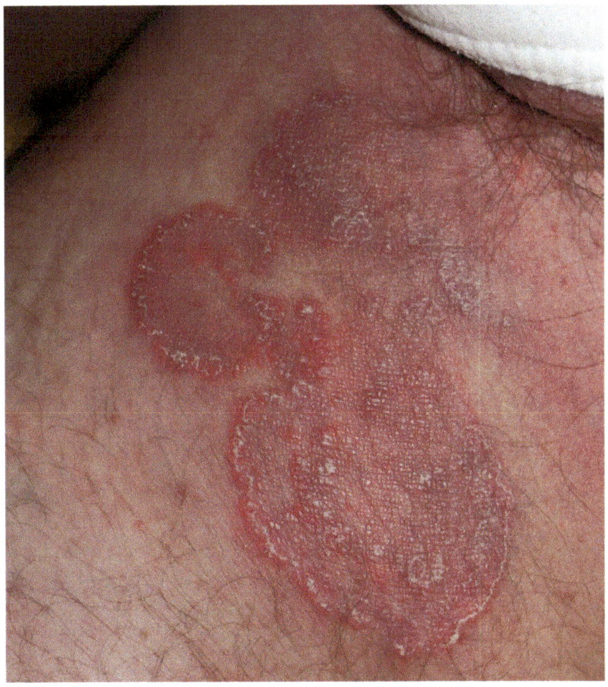

FIGURE 119.1 Tinea cruris FST1. (Courtesy Prof. Ian Coulson, UK.)

DOI: 10.1201/9781003479512-119

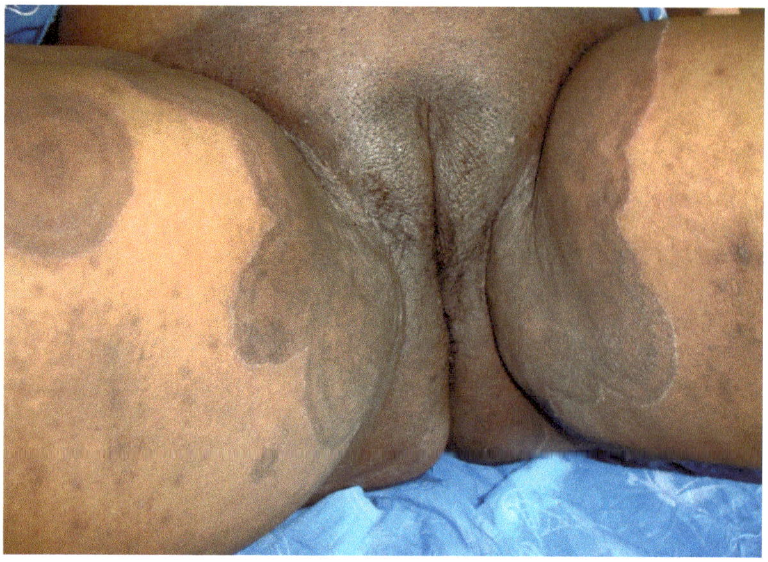

FIGURE 119.2 Tinea cruris in an obese woman FST5. Post-inflammatory hyperpigmentation is very common in dark skin, which may last for many years after cure. Note the distinctive raised edge of the active inflammatory margin.

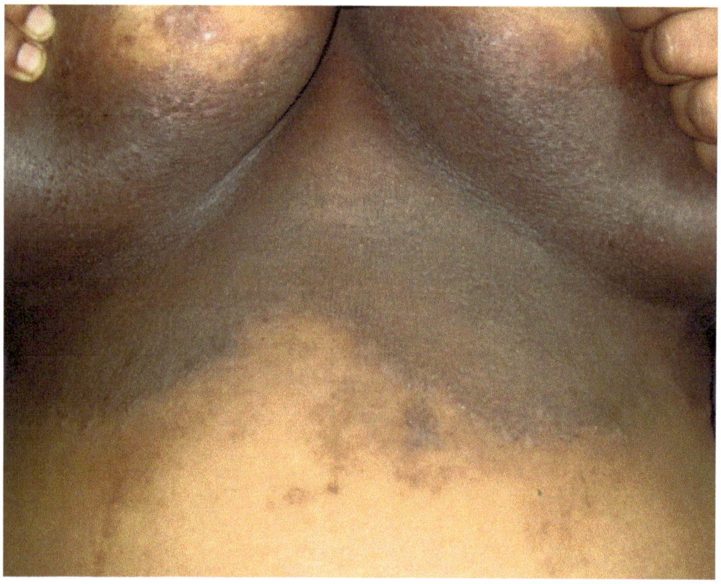

FIGURE 119.3 Tinea corporis in the submammary area in a woman FST5. Note the marked post-inflammatory hyperpigmentation which may persist for years. The active inflammatory margin is obscured in this woman, possibly following partial antifungal treatments or topical steroids.

120
TINEA NIGRA

Introduction

Tinea nigra is an asymptomatic, superficial fungal infection caused by *Hortaea werneckii*. It is more common in tropical climates. The palms are most commonly affected, but other areas of the body such as the soles, neck, and trunk have been reported.

Epidemiology

It can occur at any age. It occurs sporadically in many parts of the world, including the Americas and the Caribbean, South Africa, Australia, Europe, and the Far East.

Clinical characteristics in light skin (Fitzpatrick skin types I–III)

Tinea nigra is a rare fungal infection in people living in temperate and cold climates. The author observed a patient who had acquired the infection in tropical South America. He noticed the gray spot on his sole several months ago and tried to wash and later rub it away with pumice in vain. Histopathology showed typical pigmented fungal filaments of large caliber. Treatment with topical clotrimazole was successful.

Clinical characteristics in dark skin (Fitzpatrick skin types IV–V)

This is not a common infection even in the tropics. The lesions are macular, sharply defined, and not scaly. The most distinctive feature is the dark brown or black color (Figure 120.1).

Investigations

This is a clinical diagnosis.

Microscopy of infected epidermal scales in potassium hydroxide (30% KOH) and/or culture will show fungal hyphae.

Treatments

- Topical azole creams (clotrimazole, ketoconazole, oxiconazole, econazole, miconazole) until complete clearance.
- Topical application of fungicidal preparations such as butenafine.
- Benzoic acid compound ointment is also effective.

Further reading

Haneke E, Kienlein-Kletschka B (1983). Histologie und Elektronenmikroskopie der Tinea nigra [Histopathology and electron microscopy of tinea nigra]. *Mykosen*;26(10):514–520.

Ranawaka RR (2021). Superficial Fungal Infections. In: Ranawaka RR, et al. (eds). *Atlas of Dermatoses in Pigmented Skin*. Springer, Singapore; 319–359.

Sarawgi D, Sen S (2023). Tinea Nigra Palmaris. *Indian Pediatr*;60(11):964–965.

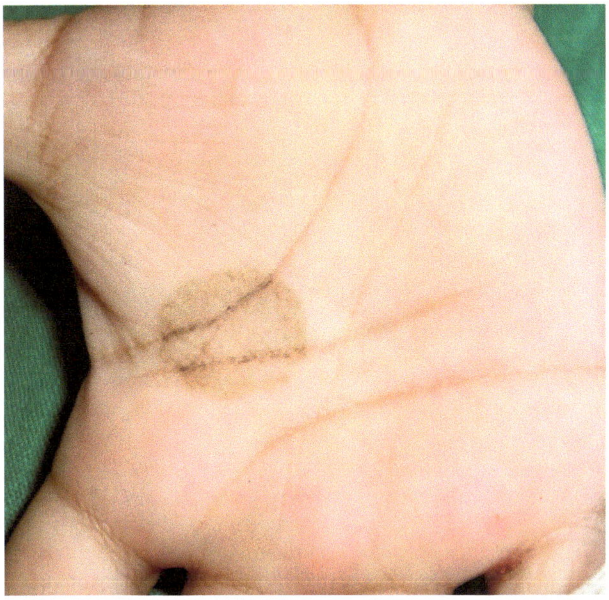

FIGURE 120.1 Tinea nigra FST5. Well-circumscribed asymptomatic dark brown or black patch that gradually enlarges over time.

DOI: 10.1201/9781003479512-120

121
TOXIC EPIDERMAL NECROLYSIS

Introduction

Toxic epidermal necrolysis (TEN) is primarily a drug-induced phenomenon, with a culprit drug being demonstrated in approximately 85% of cases. The disease is characterized by widespread epithelial keratinocyte necrosis of both skin and mucous membranes, a process initiated by drug-induced cytotoxic T-lymphocytes.

Extensive epidermal detachment in TEN is complicated by deranged thermoregulatory control, leading to hypothermia or hyperthermia. Epidermal detachment leads to a water loss of 2–3 L/day from exudation and evaporation, which result in end organ hypoperfusion leading to acute kidney injury. Hypoalbuminemia, hyperglycemia, anemia, leucopenia, bronchial erosions and airway obstruction, and septicemia are common complications. Overall mortality in TEN is approximately 30%. The cause of death is usually septicemia-induced multiorgan failure.

Epidemiology

TEN occurs in all age groups, including infants and children. There is an increased incidence in the elderly and in women.

Associated diseases

There is an increased risk of TEN in HIV and systemic lupus erythematosus (SLE).

Clinical characteristics in light skin (Fitzpatrick skin types I–III)

TEN is a rare life-threatening disease of the skin and mucous membranes with a serious impact on the entire organism (Figure 121.1). It is a widespread necrosis of keratinocytes induced by cytotoxic T-lymphocytes and proinflammatory cytokines, particularly granulysin. Areas of the skin redden, and the erythema rapidly spreads to form large patches with flaccid blisters and large areas of epidermal detachment. This process begins on the upper trunk and spreads to the entire body, including palms and soles, nails, oral mucosa, etc. The necrotic epidermis lies on the denuded dermis like a wet towel. The Nikolsky sign is positive. Roughly 80% of the cases are due to a drug reaction, and immediate withdrawal of the culprit is essential. In the full-blown disease, the patient looks like a second-degree burn patient and needs treatment as such. The skin is denuded and red, losing water, electrolytes and proteins with the consequence of hypovolemia and decreased end-organ blood supply. The mortality rate is about 30% and is higher in older patients. Healing may occur with sequelae such as nail dystrophy, corneal scarring, etc.

Clinical characteristics in dark skin (Fitzpatrick skin types IV–V)

Early erythema that develops within 1–5 days of drug exposure may go unnoticed in darker skin in inexperienced settings, which lead to higher morbidity and mortality (Figure 121.2).

Detachable epidermis is demonstrated by a positive Nikolsky sign (i.e., gentle lateral pressure causes lesional epidermis to slide over the dermis) which appears later. Nikolsky sign is a helpful clinical indicator of epidermal necrolysis. Involvement of the mucous membranes of the eyes, mouth, nose, and genitalia is usually an early feature and leads to erosive and hemorrhagic mucositis. Post-inflammatory dyspigmentation (either hypo or hyper) may persist in darker-skinned patients from months to years.

Investigations

This is a clinical diagnosis. Routine investigations are performed to assess and monitor the systemic involvement.

Treatments

- Withdraw the culprit drug.
- If epidermal loss is >10% body surface area (BSA), transfer to a specialist unit (intensive care unit or burns unit).
- Institute a supportive care package, with particular attention to:
  - Heated environment.
  - Fluid replacement.
  - Nutritional regimen.
  - Analgesia.
  - Preventing and treating infection.
- Specialist nursing skin care is essential for the delivery of topical therapy and dressings.
- In the early stages of the acute phase, consider using:
  - IVIG (0.5–1 g/kg daily for 3–4 consecutive days), *or*
  - Systemic corticosteroid (e.g., prednisolone 0.5–1 mg/kg daily for 10 days, and tapered; or IV methylprednisolone 500 mg on 3 consecutive days), *or*
  - Ciclosporin (3 or 4 mg/kg/day in divided doses for 10 days, then tapered).

Further reading

Creamer D, Walsh S, Lee HY (2024). Severe Cutaneous Adverse Reactions to Drugs. In: Griffiths C, et al. (eds). *Rook's Textbook of Dermatology*, 10th ed. John Wiley & Sons Ltd., UK; 118.21.

Puccio J, Kirven RM, Kaffenberger BH, et al. (2024). Toxic Flexural Epidermolysis in Hospitalized Patients. *Arch Dermatol Res*; 316(7):416.

Shekhar M, Iqbal O, Dharan A, et al. (2024). The Role of NLRP3 Inflammasome in the Pathogenesis of Stevens-Johnson Syndrome/Toxic Epidermal Necrolysis. *Med Res Arch*;12(1): 10.18103/mra.v12i1.4939.

Wijenayake, BKS (2021). Cutaneous Adverse Reactions to Drugs. In: Ranawaka RR, et al. (eds). *Atlas of Dermatoses in Pigmented Skin*. Springer, Singapore; 1017–1048.

DOI: 10.1201/9781003479512-121

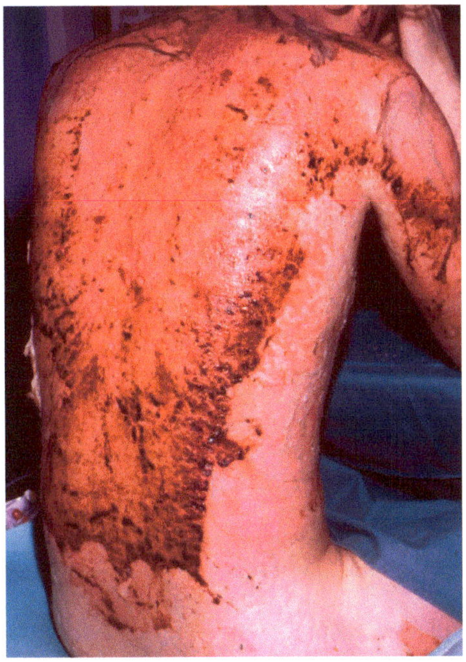

FIGURE 121.1 Toxic epidermal necrolysis FST1. (Courtesy Prof. Ian Coulson, UK.)

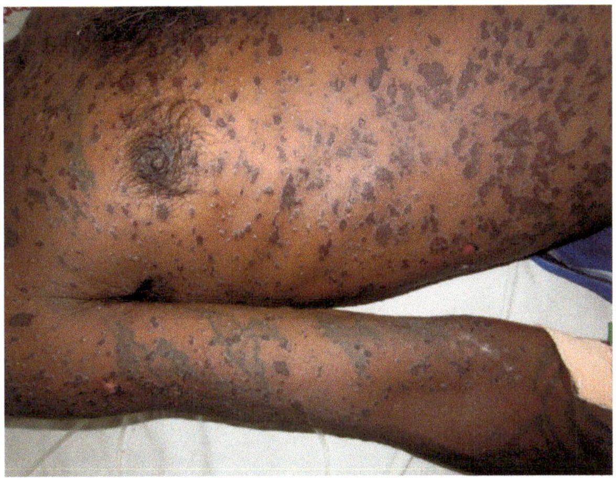

FIGURE 121.2 Toxic epidermal necrolysis in a 32-year-old man FST5. Note generalized erythema, blistering and detachable skin involving more 30% of body surface area.

122
URTICARIA AND DERMOGRAPHISM

Introduction

Urticaria is short-lived itchy or non-itchy wheals, angioedema, or both. It may be spontaneous or inducible. Urticaria may be acute (the disease resolving in less than 6 weeks) or chronic (continuous disease lasting for 6 weeks or more).

Dermographism is a type of inducible urticaria. The triple response of local erythema (due to capillary vasodilatation), followed by edema and a surrounding flare (due to axon reflex-induced dilatation of arterioles) after stroking the skin is characteristic.

Simple dermographism is physiological and not itchy.

Symptomatic dermographism (factitious urticaria) is accompanied by severe itching. This can occur at any age, but the greatest incidence is in young adults. Patients complain of whealing and itching at sites of trauma, friction with clothing, or scratching the skin.

Cholinergic dermographism is seen in some patients with cholinergic urticaria, whose dermographic response consists of an erythematous line studded with punctate wheals characteristic of cholinergic wheals. This occurs in response to sweating caused by an increase in core temperature and can also be triggered by emotional and gustatory sweating.

Red dermographism is a much less common form of dermographism where repeated rubbing is necessary to induce small punctate weals.

Delayed dermographism is rare. After the normal fading of the triple response or an immediate dermographic response, a weal returns in the same site, but is usually tender and persists for up to 48 hours.

It should be noted that not all forms of dermographism are urticaria.

White dermographism, which is not an urticaria (due to capillary vasoconstriction following light stroking of the skin), occurs normally but is particularly pronounced in atopic eczema.

Black dermographism is discoloration of the skin after pressure from a metallic object, also not urticaria.

Epidemiology

Dermographism may occur at any age, and there are no sex differences.

Associated diseases

May appear with food or drug allergies.

Clinical characteristics in light skin (Fitzpatrick skin types I–III)

Urticaria is a frequent condition (Figures 122.1 to 122.3). It may be allergic, due to intolerance to aspirin, non-steroidal anti-inflammatory agents, and other drugs like angiotensin-converting enzyme inhibitors (bradykinin-mediated angioedema), toxic, temperature- and solar light-dependent, vibration, exercise-induced, aquagenic, or mechanical as in urticarial dermographism and delayed pressure urticaria. In addition, a great number of other mechanisms may cause urticaria, e.g., urticarial vasculitis.

The common type of wheal is a rapidly developing raised lesion, red in the beginning, often blanching within a certain time due to internal pressure of the wheal on the capillaries, and then usually a red halo develops. Itch may be very intense. Wheals from nettles characteristically burn. Jellyfish nettles may cause extensive urticaria, sometimes becoming bullous and leaving hyperpigmentation even in light skin. Cholinergic urticaria demonstrates myriads of small round hard papular wheals on a red base; they may be first red and then blanch.

'Deep urticaria' is a less well-demarcated swelling thought to be due to the same mechanism of histamine release with subsequent vessel dilatation and fluid extravasation; it is also called angioedema and can be life-threatening when obstructing the airways, e.g., a bee or wasp sting in the soft palate. If these lesions later turn bluish and are painful, the erythrocyte auto-sensitization syndrome of Gardner–Diamond should be suspected.

Acute urticaria is defined as an acute-onset condition of no longer than 6 weeks' duration. The wheals appear within minutes and disappear within a few hours while new ones continue to develop.

Chronic spontaneous urticaria lasts longer than 6 weeks. It is a relatively frequent condition whose cause very often remains enigmatic despite intensive search for its etiology.

Independent of their cause, the wheals look alike in almost all cases except for cholinergic urticaria.

Clinical characteristics in dark skin (Fitzpatrick skin types IV–V)

Mildly erythematous or skin-colored wheals (Figures 122.4 and 122.5).

Investigations

This is diagnosed clinically.

Obtaining a detailed medical history of the patient with comprehensive information about predisposing factors, drug intake, particular eating habits, and hobbies, as well as physical examination and provocation testing (challenge tests), is indispensable.

Treatments

- Explanation and non-specific measures including the wearing of loose-fitting clothing and application of soothing creams with menthol may be helpful (be aware of the sensitizing potential of menthol).
- Patients should minimize aggravating factors including overheating, stress, and alcohol.
- Aspirin, aspirin-containing compounds, and other non-steroidal anti-inflammatory drugs (NSAIDs) should be avoided.
- H1 antihistamines are the first-line treatment of all types: e.g., acrivastine, cetirizine, fexofenadine, loratadine, rupatadine.

DOI: 10.1201/9781003479512-122

- A combination of an H1 antihistamine with an H2 antagonist may be more effective in some, e.g., ranitidine.
- Oral corticosteroids are effective in severe urticaria at high doses, e.g., prednisolone 0.5 mg/kg/day, and may be used as rescue treatment over 1–3 days, but prolonged use should be avoided.
- Leukotriene receptor antagonists, doxepin (a tricyclic antidepressant), danazol, and narrow-band phototherapy have been tried in severe refractory cases.
- Plasmapheresis, intravenous immunoglobulin (IVIG) infusions, ciclosporin, mycophenolate mofetil, and omalizumab (anti-IgE) have been tested on severe unremitting spontaneous urticaria not responding to conventional therapy.

Further reading

Grattan CEH, Sears AV (2024). Urticaria. In: Griffiths C, et al. (eds). *Rook's Textbook of Dermatology*, 10th ed. John Wiley & Sons Ltd., UK; 42.1.

Maurer M, Bonnekoh H, Grekowitz E, et al. (2024). An Algorithm for the Diagnosis and Treatment of Chronic Inducible Urticaria, 2024 Update. *Allergy*;Sep;79(9):2573–2576.

Soegiharto R, Alizadeh Aghdam M, Sørensen JA, et al. (2024). Multinational Drug Survival Study of Omalizumab in Patients with Chronic Urticaria and Potential Predictors for Discontinuation. *JAMA Dermatol*;Sep 1;160(9):927–935.

Zuberbier T, Ensina LF, Giménez-Arnau A, et al. (2024). Chronic Urticaria: Unmet Needs, Emerging Drugs, and New Perspectives on Personalised Treatment. *Lancet*;404(10450):393–404.

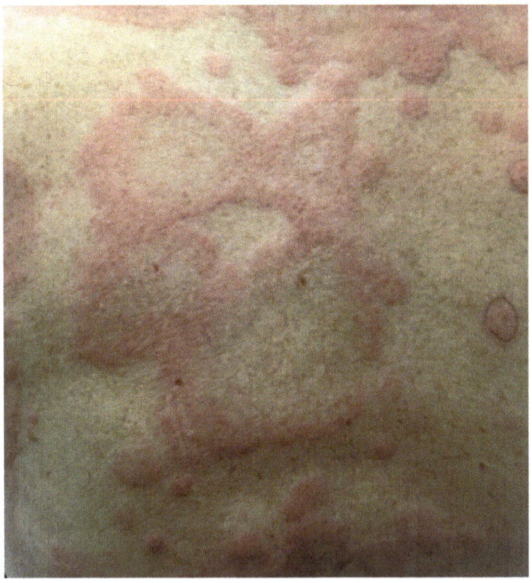

FIGURE 122.1 Acute urticaria FST1. (Courtesy Dr. Richard Ashton, UK.)

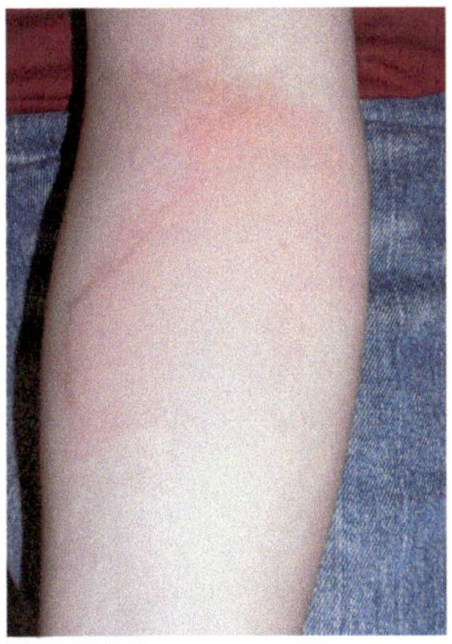

FIGURE 122.2 Cold urticaria showing ice cube test FST1. (Courtesy Prof. Ian Coulson, UK.)

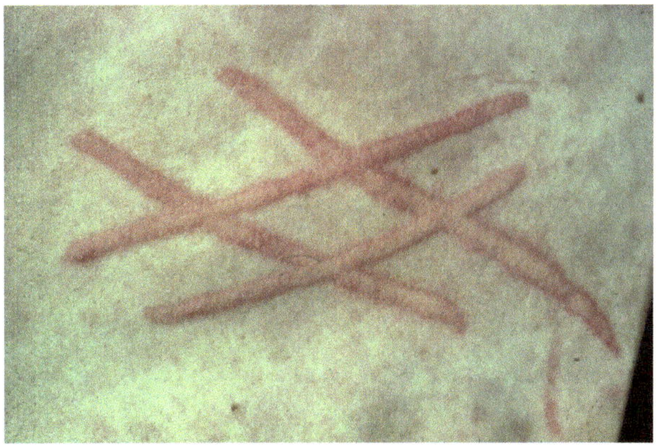

FIGURE 122.3 Dermographism FST1. (Courtesy Dr. Richard Ashton, UK.)

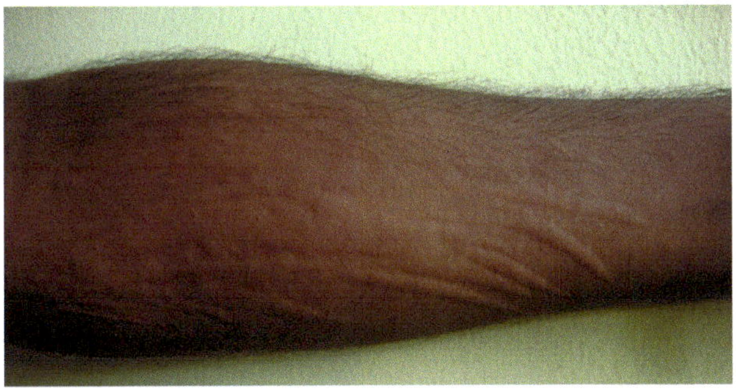

FIGURE 122.4 Urticarial dermographism in a man FST5.

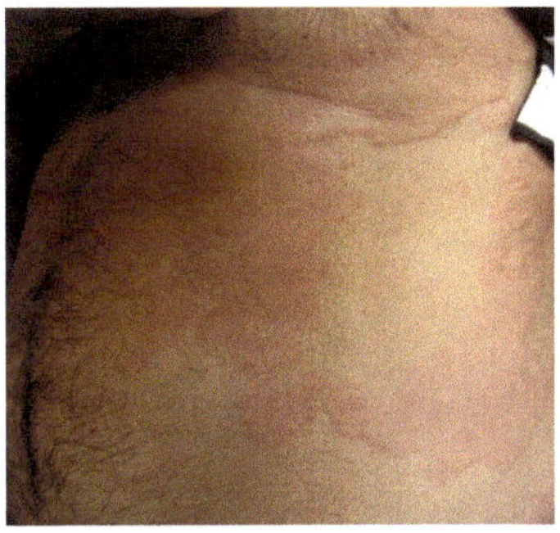

FIGURE 122.5 Acute urticaria FST5. Note erythema may be hidden in darker skin.

123
URTICARIAL VASCULITIS

Introduction

Urticarial vasculitis is a rare disease characterized by continued whealing associated with histopathological evidence of leucocytoclastic vasculitis. These weals are recurrent, and are typically painful rather than itchy, last longer than 24 hours, and leave residual hyperpigmentation.

Distinguishing between hypocomplementemic (HUVS) and normocomplementemic urticarial vasculitis (NUVS) is important since the former may have multisystem involvement, including nephritis, whereas the latter usually runs a benign and, ultimately, self limiting course.

In addition to wheals, other cutaneous signs in urticarial vasculitis may include livedo reticularis, Raynaud phenomenon, and very occasionally bullous lesions. Joint involvement is common; usually arthralgia and joint stiffness, and rarely, arthritis or synovitis. Associated gastrointestinal features are nausea, vomiting, abdominal pain, intestinal bleeding, or diarrhea. Pulmonary symptoms may include cough, dyspnea, or hemoptysis. In HUVS, chronic obstructive pulmonary disease or laryngeal angioedema can be a life-threatening complication.

Epidemiology

Urticarial vasculitis occurs with peak incidence in the fourth to fifth decades of life. Both forms are rare in children.

Associated diseases

HUVS has a high risk for the development of systemic lupus erythematosus.

Clinical characteristics in light skin (Fitzpatrick skin types I–III)

Cutaneous leucocytoclastic vasculitis is a typical type III immunological reaction mediated by complement (Figures 123.1 and 123.2). Clinically, different variants are seen that have the same histopathological characteristics, although with variable expression. In light-skinned persons, hemorrhagic vasculitis involving the small vessels of the upper reticular dermis is the most common type. The palpable hemorrhagic lesions start as small points on the lower leg and enlarge while extending onto the thighs and lower trunk. A generalized rash is rare.

Urticarial vasculitis is much less common in the author's experience. Wheals that do not come and go are typical.

Biopsy of a fresh lesion shows perivascular immunoglobulin and complement deposition, whereas neutrophilic infiltrates with vessel wall necrosis come a bit later.

Clinical characteristics in dark skin (Fitzpatrick skin types IV–V)

Urticarial vasculitis is very rare in our setting. Even though the weals are obvious, erythema may be obscured in darker skin (Figure 123.3).

Investigations

Lesional skin biopsy is the cornerstone of the diagnosis of urticarial vasculitis. Urticarial vasculitis affects predominantly post-capillary venules in the superficial dermis.

Full blood count, blood biochemistry, erythrocyte sedimentation rate, urinalysis (microscopic hematuria or proteinuria),

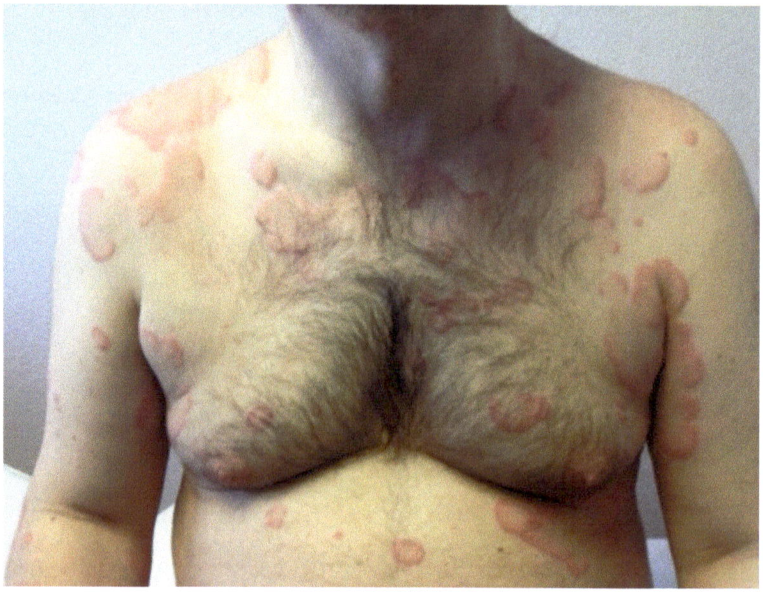

FIGURE 123.1 Urticarial vasculitis FST1. (Courtesy Dr. Carlo Enrico Urbani, Italy.)

DOI: 10.1201/9781003479512-123

and liver function tests are essential in the laboratory work-up for systemic involvement.

Complement profile (CH50, C3, C4, and anti-C1q antibodies) is important for differentiating between NUVS and HUVS.

Antinuclear antibodies, antibodies against extractable nuclear antigens, rheumatoid factor, and circulating immune complexes.

Testing for hepatitis B and C is important; chronic viral infections (hepatitis B and C) are important co-morbidities in urticarial vasculitis.

Treatments

- In most patients, urticarial vasculitis is a self-limiting disease, but in some it may last for years.
- First-line treatment is H1 antihistamines and non-steroidal anti-inflammatory drugs (NSAIDs).
- Second-line therapies are dapsone 75–100 mg/day, colchicine 1.0–1.5 mg/day, and/or hydroxychloroquine 400 mg/day. In unresponsive patients, corticosteroids (prednisolone at doses of 40 mg/day or more) can then be considered for short-term management.
- For severe refractory cases, immunosuppressive agents (cyclophosphamide, azathioprine), ciclosporin, mycophenolate mofetil, and biologics may be beneficial. Intravenous immunoglobulins, methotrexate, intramuscular gold, and plasmapheresis have also been used.

Further reading

Krause K, Grattan CEH (2024). Urticarial Vasculitis. In: Griffiths C, et al. (eds). *Rook's Textbook of Dermatology*, 10th ed. John Wiley & Sons Ltd., UK; 44.1

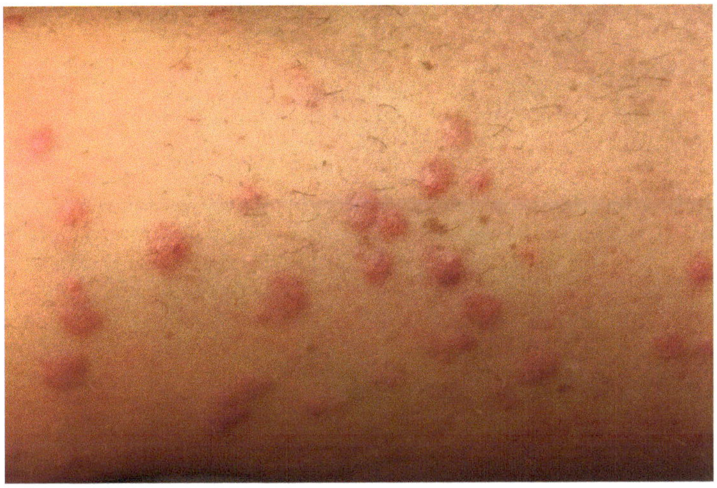

FIGURE 123.2 Urticarial vasculitis FST2. (Courtesy Prof. Eckart Haneke, Germany.)

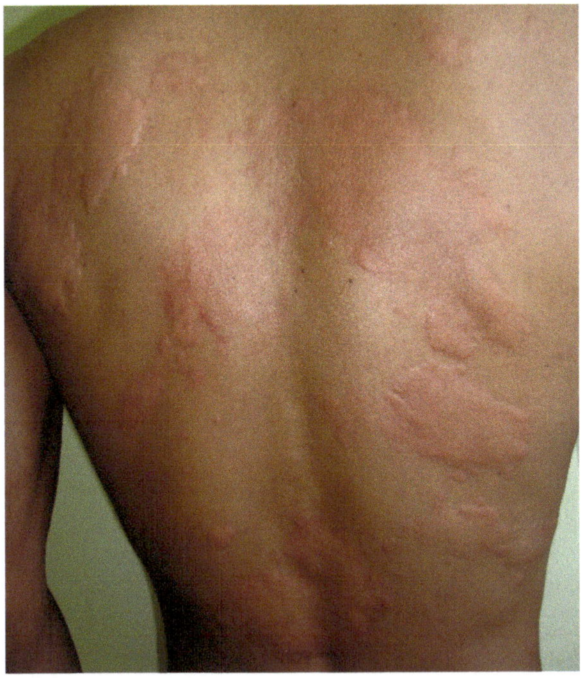

FIGURE 123.3 Urticarial vasculitis FST5. Urticaria and urticarial vasculitis is clinically indisguisable except individual urticarial vasculitic lesions last more than 24 hours and when it heals leaves post-inflammatory hyperpigmentation. Skin biopsy is essential to differentiate.

124
CUTANEOUS SMALL-VESSEL VASCULITIS

Introduction

Cutaneous vasculitis is inflammation of the blood vessel walls, usually resulting in palpable purpura. Vasculitis is a multisystem disorder. Its diagnosis is based on a detailed history and careful examination. Since cutaneous vasculitis presents with varied clinical manifestations, only cutaneous small-vessel vasculitis (CSVV), which is the most common, is discussed here. CSVV is also called cutaneous leukocytoclastic vasculitis.

CSVV is a single-organ vasculitis producing leukocytoclastic angiitis of the cutaneous vasculature. However, it may be the first manifestation of a more generalized vasculitis, therefore, ongoing surveillance is important. Mostly idiopathic, a small number of cases may be related to bacterial infections or drugs.

Epidemiology

The mean age at onset is between 36 and 56 years, but it may extend from the second to eighth decade of life. It affects both sexes equally.

Associated diseases

CSVV may be a precursor for other systemic vasculitides.

Clinical characteristics in light skin (Fitzpatrick skin types I–III)

CSVV is a very obvious condition in light-skinned people (Figure 124.1). Starting in the distal area of the lower legs, it may slowly – rarely rapidly – extend to more proximal parts of the body, but virtually always predominantly on dependent skin areas; this points to the important role of gravitation and undisturbed blood flow. The single lesion starts with a point of bleeding in the skin that enlarges and is typically palpable. Depending on the severity, the lesions may range from pinpoint size to ecchymoses of several centimeters in diameter. In the latter case, they may merge. Rarely, the lesions may take on a pustular, bullous, or ulcerative aspect. Healing may take 2–6 weeks.

Clinical characteristics in dark skin (Fitzpatrick skin types IV–V)

CSVV is very common in our patients, too (Figures 124.2 to 124.5). Palpable purpura sizes range from 1 mm to several centimeters and commonly start on ankles and lower legs. They may later progress into papules, nodules, vesicles, plaques, bullae, or pustules, with secondary findings of ulceration or necrosis. These usually heal without any sequelae. These erythematous purpura lesions may be inconspicuous on dark or black skin.

Investigations

This is diagnosed clinically, and investigations are tapered to history and examination findings. A vasculitis screen should not be done routinely for all the patients. Investigations are necessary for two main purposes. First, it is important to establish if the vasculitis is primary or secondary. Investigations should be directed to identify underlying rheumatological disease, malignancy, infection, or a primary vasculitis. Second, investigations should be carried out to demonstrate the presence of vasculitis involving internal organs; for example, urinalysis to exclude renal disease is useful in most patients.

Skin biopsy for histopathology should be taken from a fresh lesion less than 48 hours old. Older lesions would show secondary thrombosis leading to misdiagnosis of a thrombo-occlusive disorder.

A skin biopsy from an early lesion for direct immunofluorescence should be taken if IgA vasculitis (Henoch–Schonlein purpura [HSP]) is suspected.

Treatments

- The management of vasculitis depends on the diagnosis and the severity and presence of systemic vasculitis. Most cases of CSVV may be self-limiting.
- If a triggering agent is identified, such as a drug or infection, it should be removed or treated.
- Minimize stasis, such as the use of compression hosiery and the elevation of dependent areas.
- Non-steroidal anti-inflammatory drugs (NSAIDs) and antihistamines may reduce symptoms.
- In more severe cases, oral prednisolone 30–80 mg is taken once daily, tapered over 2–3 weeks.
- Colchicine 0.6 mg twice daily or dapsone 50–150 mg daily are second-line therapies.

Further reading

Cassisa A, Cima L (2024). Cutaneous Vasculitis: Insights into Pathogenesis and Histopathological Features. *Pathologica*;116(2): 119–133.

Levell NJ, Mukhtyar C (2024). Cutaneous Vasculitis. In: Griffiths C, et al. (eds). *Rook's Textbook of Dermatology*, 10th ed. John Wiley & Sons Ltd., UK; 100.5.

Wijenayake BKS (2021). Cutaneous Vasculitis. In: Ranawaka RR, et al. (eds). *Atlas of Dermatoses in Pigmented Skin*. Springer, Singapore; 547–561.

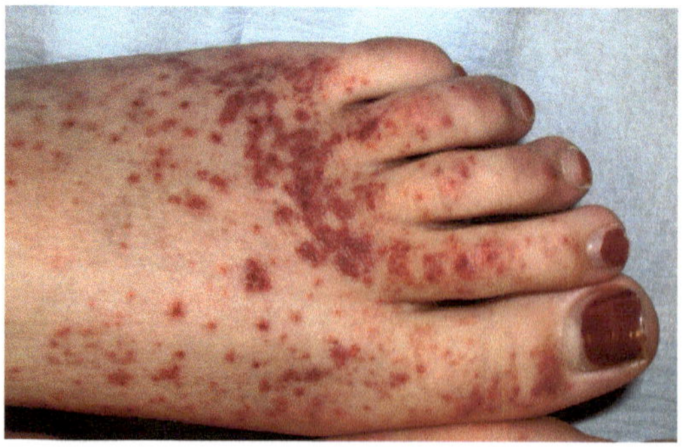

FIGURE 124.1 Henoch–Schonlein purpura or IgA vasculitis FST1. (Courtesy Prof. Ian Coulson, UK.)

DOI: 10.1201/9781003479512-124

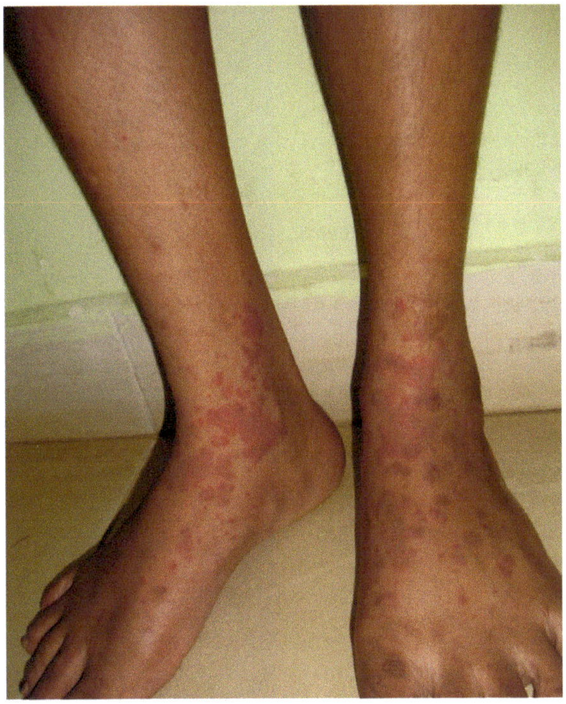

FIGURE 124.2 Cutaneous small-vessel vasculitis starts around the ankle, FST5.

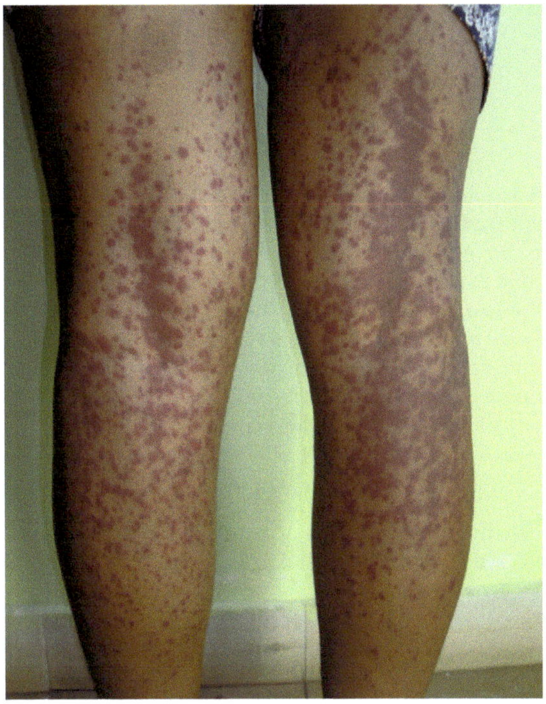

FIGURE 124.3 Extensive cutaneous small-vessel vasculitis in a 32-year-old woman. Even though the skin involvement was extensive she did not develop systemic vasculitides, FST5.

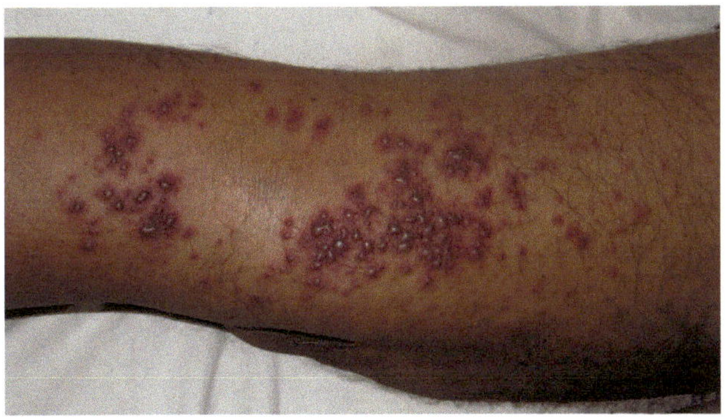

FIGURE 124.4 Cutaneous small-vessel vasculitis showing hemorrhagic vesicles. Necrosis is not a major feature in cutaneous small-vessel vasculitis, FST5.

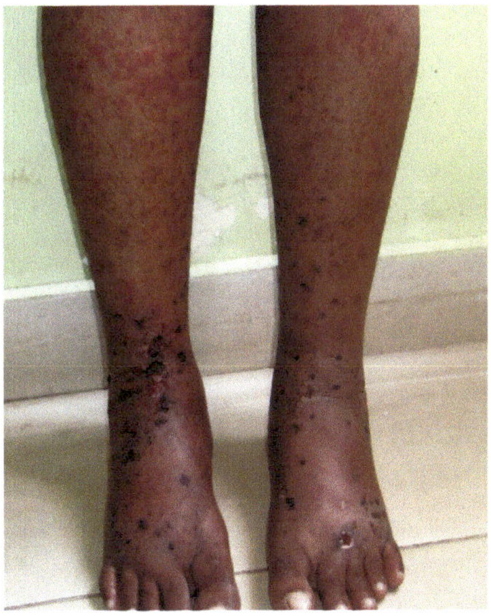

FIGURE 124.5 Ulcerated lesions in cutaneous small-vessel vasculitis, FST5.

125
VENOUS (GRAVITATIONAL) ECZEMA OR STASIS DERMATITIS

Introduction

Stasis dermatitis or eczema relates to the skin changes that result from reduced lower leg venous flow and venous hypertension. An exudative eczematous eruption is usually seen around the ankle and lower leg in a patient with varicose veins. These can be bilateral if varicosities are bilateral, but mostly they are unilateral. The eczema is often accompanied by other manifestations of venous hypertension, including dilation or varicosity of the superficial veins, edema, purpura, hemosiderosis, ulceration, or atrophie blanche.

Epidemiology

Usually in middle-aged or elderly individuals, there is an increased incidence in females.

Associated diseases

This may be associated with allergic contact dermatitis.

Clinical characteristics in light skin (Fitzpatrick skin types I–III)

Stasis dermatitis is a very frequent condition, particularly in overweight patients with varicosis or lower leg edema (Figures 125.1 and 125.2). The skin is erythematous, often discolored by erythrocyte extravasation and their degradation to hemosiderin (purpura jaune d'ocre), as well as increased melanin pigmentation due to the iron in the dermis that stimulates melanocytes. With time, the skin starts oozing, and the erythema intensifies. Typical eczema papules and vesicles may occur; however, as these patients often get a variety of topical drugs, it is not easy to distinguish this from allergic contact dermatitis. Depending on the degree of stasis, shallow ulcerations may appear that develop into varicose or post-thrombotic ulcers. These, again, are often treated with neomycin-containing creams, causing an allergy. In addition, atrophie blanche may occur, which is usually tender or frankly painful.

Clinical characteristics in dark skin (Fitzpatrick skin types IV–V)

Stasis dermatitis is common in men in our setting (Figure 125.3). They are mostly farmers and manual laborers and are non-obese. Venous dermatitis is situated around the medial malleolus; post-inflammatory hyperpigmentation is marked in dark skin.

Investigations

Investigations are performed to assess varicose veins.

Ankle brachial pressure index (ABPI) measurement is required prior to the consideration of compression therapy. An ABPI of more than 0.8 indicates suitability for graduated compression bandages.

Treatments

- Obese patients should be urged to lose weight.
- Any underlying venous hypertension and/or pedal edema should be controlled. Well-fitted support stockings or firm bandages can be helpful if worn regularly.
- Mild topical steroids may be used to relieve irritation. The use of potent corticosteroids should be limited to short periods of a few days, as they may cause cutaneous atrophy and increase the risk of ulceration.
- Referral to a vascular surgeon to consider surgical intervention.

Further reading

Awad N, Hetzel JD, Bhupalam V, et al. (2024). Stasis Dermatitis: Pathophysiology, Current Treatment Paradigms, and the Use of the Flavonoid Diosmin. *J Clin Aesthet Dermatol*;17(1):15–23.

Ranawaka RR (2021). Leg Ulcers. In: Ranawaka RR, et al. (eds). *Atlas of Dermatoses in Pigmented Skin*. Springer, Singapore; 529.

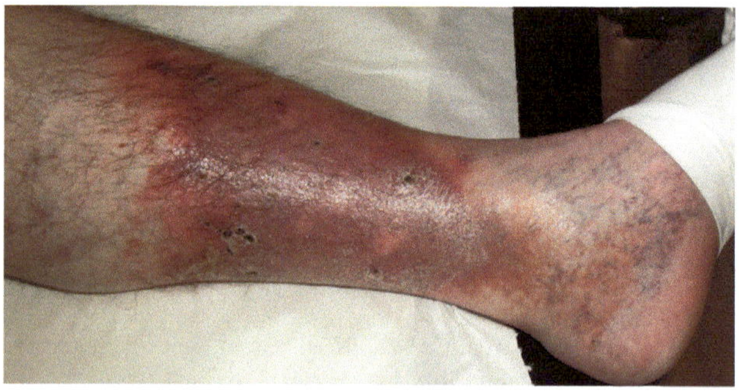

FIGURE 125.1 Lipodermatosclerosis in stasis dermatitis FST1. (Courtesy Prof. Ian Coulson, UK.)

DOI: 10.1201/9781003479512-125

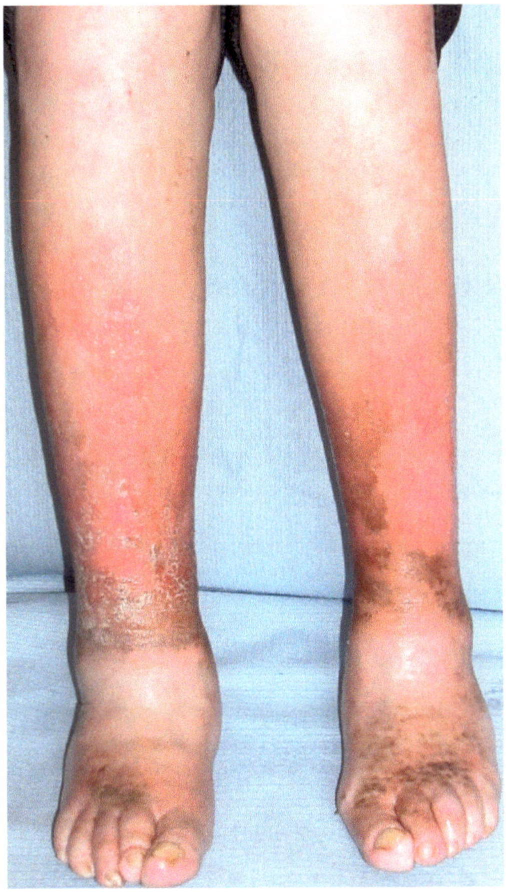

FIGURE 125.2 Stasis dermatitis FST1. (Courtesy Prof. Ian Coulson, UK.)

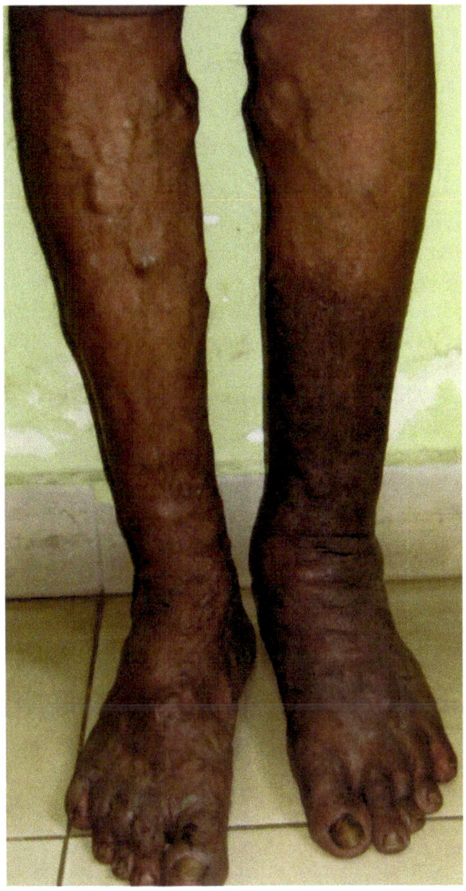

FIGURE 125.3 Stasis dermatitis in a 67-year-old male farmer FST5. Note he is not an obese person. Hyperpigmentation due to hemosiderosis and post-inflammation is common in dark skin.

126
VENOUS LEG ULCERS OR STASIS ULCERS

Introduction

Venous leg ulcers are chronic skin ulcers in the gaiter area that result from chronic peripheral venous hypertension. They affect 1% of the population, and the prevalence increases with age. They are the most extreme manifestation of chronic venous insufficiency (CVI). CVI results from chronic peripheral venous hypertension caused by venous reflux and/or obstruction, or by neuro-musculoskeletal dysfunction of the leg. Nearly half of all venous ulcers are associated with deep-vein valvular incompetence or post-thrombotic damage, while the remainder result from incompetence of the superficial or communicating veins.

Patients present with skin changes attributed to chronic venous insufficiency: Stasis dermatitis, lipodermatosclerosis, hyperpigmentation, induration, and leg shape of an inverted champagne bottle.

Epidemiology

Prevalence increases with age and is more common in females. Obesity and reduced levels of physical activity are predisposing factors.

Associated diseases

Venous thromboembolism, superficial venous thrombophlebitis, varicose veins, CVI, stasis dermatitis, lipodermatosclerosis, acroangiodermatitis, obesity, ankle joint ankylosis, rheumatoid arthritis, and neuromuscular diseases are associated with stasis ulcers.

Clinical characteristics in light skin (Fitzpatrick skin types I–III)

Venous ulcers are extremely common, particularly in overweight women (Figure 126.1). CVI is graded in corona phlebectatica (grade I), pigmentary disturbances and edema (purpura jaune d'ocre, grade II), and venous ulcer (grade III). Edema is an important early sign, which is first seen in the evening, then becomes more and more stable. The serum extravasation contains proteins which lead to dermato- and dermatoliposclerosis. Finally, the skin thickens, called pachydermia. Either the swelling alone or the topical treatment may lead to stasis dermatitis and secondary allergic contact eczema. In patients with varicose veins, a superficial thrombophlebitis may develop which, when extending to the sapheno-femoral junction, may require immediate ligation to prevent ascending thromboembolism. Around the inner ankle, capillaritis alba may develop from a short initial inflammatory phase. When this ulcerates, pain is often intense. Well-demarcated violet-to-brown plaques may indicate acroangiodermatitis. Eventually, a venous ulcer may appear that can reach enormous sizes. Their treatment is skilled compression. Antibiotics should not be used or should be used very sparingly as the risk of sensitization is very high.

Clinical characteristics in dark skin (Fitzpatrick skin types IV–V)

Venous ulcers are equally common in both sexes in our setting (Figure 126.2). Men are mostly farmers and manual laborers and are non-obese. In obese women, reduced physical activity is a common feature. Venous ulcers start around the medial malleolus; they are chronic, large, and relatively painless. Hyperpigmentation is marked in dark skin. Recurrences are common as patients are reluctant to continue wearing compression stockings in a hot, humid climate.

Investigations

Assessment of systolic ankle blood pressure and calculation of the ankle brachial pressure index to assess peripheral arterial disease.

Doppler ultrasound to assess superficial venous reflux.

Duplex ultrasound to assess deep venous reflux/obstruction and/or post-thrombotic findings.

Treatments

- Compression therapy, either using bandages or stockings, is the mainstay in the treatment of venous leg ulcers.
- Approximately half of the patients with venous leg ulcers suffer from superficial venous reflux, which can be abolished by flush ligation and stripping, endovenous thermoablation, and foam sclerotherapy, whereas patients with predominantly deep venous reflux have less or no benefit from superficial vein surgery.
- Refractory venous leg ulcers can be treated with skin equivalents or tangential fibrosectomy with split-skin grafts.
- Topical negative pressure (vacuum) significantly enhances the healing of superinfected chronic leg ulcers with substantial tissue loss.
- Venous leg ulcer recurrence is common, with 30% in 12 months. Consistent compression therapy and the elimination of superficial venous reflux are keys to prevention.
- Endovenous ablation of superficial venous incompetence in combination with compression improves leg ulcer healing when compared with compression alone (Cai et al. 2023).

DOI: 10.1201/9781003479512-126

Further reading

Cai PL, Hitchman LH, Mohamed AH, et al. (2023). Endovenous Ablation for Venous Leg Ulcers. *Cochrane Database Syst Rev*;7(7):CD009494.

Hafner J, Rabe E (2024). Ulceration Resulting from Disorders of the Veins and Arteries. In: Griffiths C, et al. (eds). *Rook's Textbook of Dermatology*, 10th ed. John Wiley & Sons Ltd., UK; 102.1.

Ranawaka RR (2021). Leg Ulcers. In: Ranawaka RR, et al. (eds). *Atlas of Dermatoses in Pigmented Skin*. Springer, Singapore; 529.

Shi C, Dumville JC, Cullum N, et al. (2021). Compression Bandages or Stockings versus No Compression for Treating Venous Leg Ulcers. *Cochrane Database Syst Rev*;Jul 26:7(7):CD013397.

Zheng G, Xie H, Lai M, et al. (2024). Comparison of Two Ablation Procedures Combined with High Ligation and Foam Sclerotherapy and Compression Therapy for Patients with Venous Leg Ulcers. *Postgrad Med*;Jun;136(5):514–522.

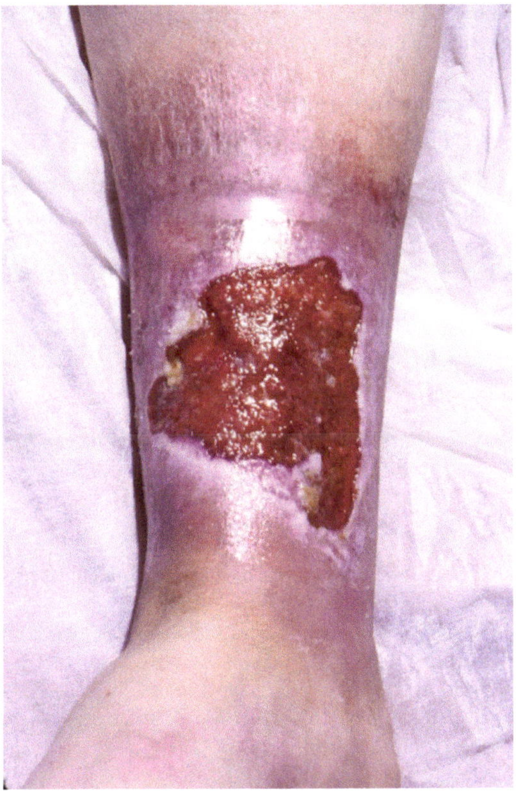

FIGURE 126.1 Stasis/venous ulcer FST1. (Courtesy Dr. Richard Ashton, UK.)

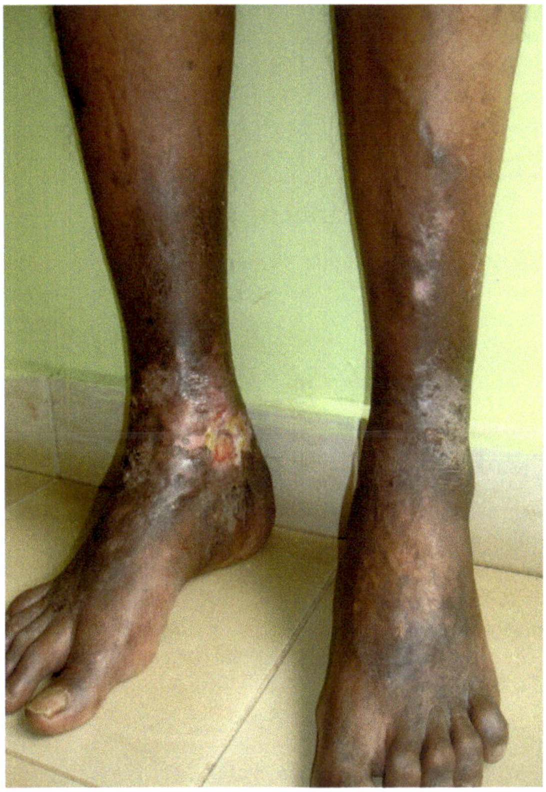

FIGURE 126.2 Stasis ulcer in a non-obese woman FST5. Note stasis dermatitis and hyperpigmentation in both legs.

127
VIRAL WARTS (COMMON WART/VERRUCA VULGARIS, PLANE WART/VERRUCA PLANA)

Introduction

Human papilloma virus (HPV) infection.

Viral warts on the skin may present in a number of different morphological forms, dependent on virus type, body site, immunological status of the patient, and environmental influences: 70% are common warts (verruca vulgaris), 24% plantar warts, 3.5% plane warts, 2% filiform warts, 0.5% anogenital warts, and periungual warts. New viral warts may form at sites of trauma: Koebner-like isomorphic phenomenon.

Epidemiology

Viral warts are common throughout the world. Cutaneous viral warts occur at any age, but are unusual in infancy and early childhood.

Associated diseases

Warts are more common and more persistent in immune-compromised statuses; inherited, acquired, or drug-induced.

Epidermodysplasia verruciformis is an inherited disorder in which there is widespread and persistent infection with HPV, giving rise to a characteristic combination of plane warts, pityriasis versicolor-like lesions, and reddish plaques. Malignant change is very common in adult life in these patients. They present in childhood with rapidly developing numerous warts on the trunk, limbs, the sides of the fingers, and on the palms and soles, as well as small warts on the vermilion border of the lips.

Clinical characteristics in light skin (Fitzpatrick skin types I–III)

Warts are contagious, virus-induced benign tumors (Figures 127.1 to 127.5). They are said to have a lifespan of approximately 2 years; however, in this period, they may give rise to many so-called daughter warts. Thus, having viral warts may be a long-term problem.

Most common warts are localized on acral skin where the body temperature is lower, over the knees and elbows, but also on the face. They are hard, keratotic papules and nodules with a diameter of 5 to 10 mm that occasionally merge to form larger conglomerates. Their rough surface has a dirty aspect. Areas of pressure may be painful.

Palmar and plantar warts are often less raised. Their surfaces are darker, sometimes fissured. Plantar warts come in two variants: Deep-reaching warts and multiple aggregated warts.

Plane warts are sometimes called juvenile warts. They often occur in large numbers, predominantly on the face, are distributed in scratch lines. The more a patient has, the more difficult their treatment.

Despite their banal nature, one thing all warts have in common is that their treatment may be very tedious.

Clinical characteristics in dark skin (Fitzpatrick skin types IV–V)

Firm, skin-colored, or hyperpigmented papules with a rough, horny surface (Figures 127.6 to 127.12). They range in size from less than 1 mm to over 1 cm in diameter and may occur anywhere on the skin. In darker skin, the palmar and plantar warts may be hyperpigmented. Plane warts are smooth, flat, or slightly elevated, usually skin-colored or dark brown. They are round or polygonal in shape and vary in size from 1 to 5 mm.

Investigations

This is a clinical diagnosis.

Treatments

- Spontaneous clearance of warts can occur at any time, from a few months to years.
- The 16–40% salicylic acid lotion or creams, and liquid nitrogen cryotherapy are widely used to treat common warts on the skin, palms, and soles.
- Topical podophyllotoxin, imiquimod, or cryotherapy are used for anogenital warts.

Further reading

Ajagbe OA, Ayandipo OO, Afuwape OO, et al. (2024). Surgical Treatment of Perineal Giant Condylomata Acuminata (Buschke Lowenstein Tumor): Case Series from a Developing Country. *Int J Surg Case Rep*;Aug;121:109994.

Gammanpila RR, Kannangara AP (2024). Infections in Children with FST 5. In: *Paediatric Cases in Coloured Skin*. CRC Press, UK; 44, 45.

Gharib K, Taha A, Elradi M (2024). Intralesional Acyclovir Versus Intralesional Hepatitis-B Vaccine in Treatment of Resistant Plantar Warts: A Randomized Controlled Trial. *Arch Dermatol Res*;316(6):325.

Martin A, Thatiparthi A, Nourmohammadi N, et al. (2022). Emerging Intralesional Treatments for Plantar Warts: A Systematic Review. *J Drugs Dermatol*;21(12):1322–1329.

Rajendiran P (2021). Viral Infections. In: Ranawaka RR, et al. (eds). *Atlas of Dermatoses in Pigmented Skin*. Springer, Singapore; 308–311.

DOI: 10.1201/9781003479512-127

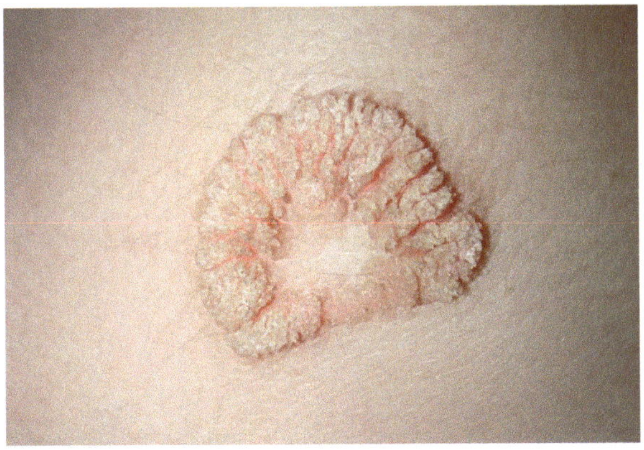

FIGURE 127.1 Doughnut wart FST1. (Courtesy Prof. Ian Coulson, UK.)

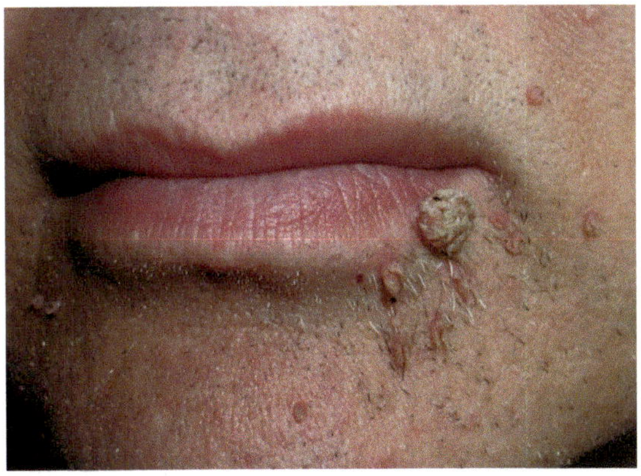

FIGURE 127.2 Filiform warts FST1. (Courtesy Prof. Ian Coulson, UK.)

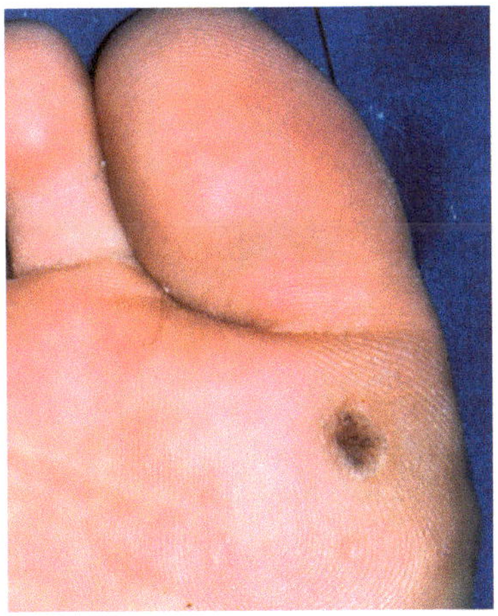

FIGURE 127.3 Plantar wart FST1. (Courtesy Prof. Ian Coulson, UK.)

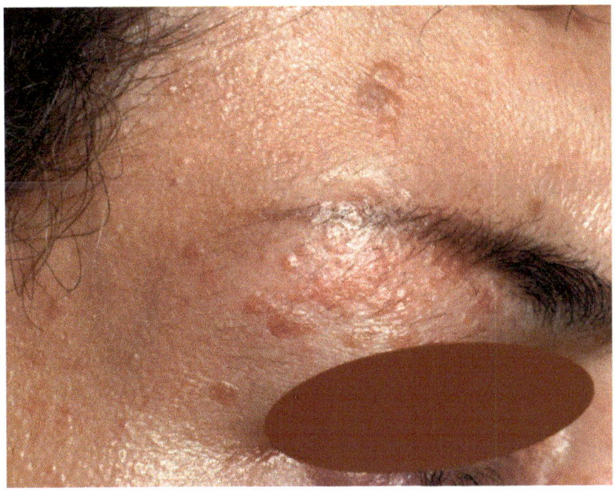

FIGURE 127.4 Plane warts or verruca plana FST1.

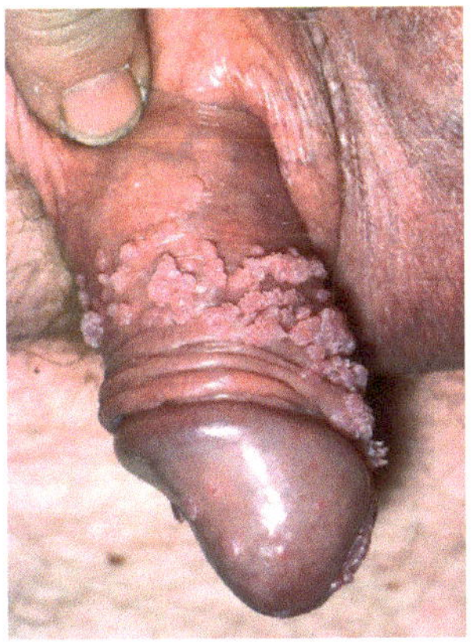

FIGURE 127.5 Penile warts FST1. (Courtesy Prof. Ian Coulson, UK.)

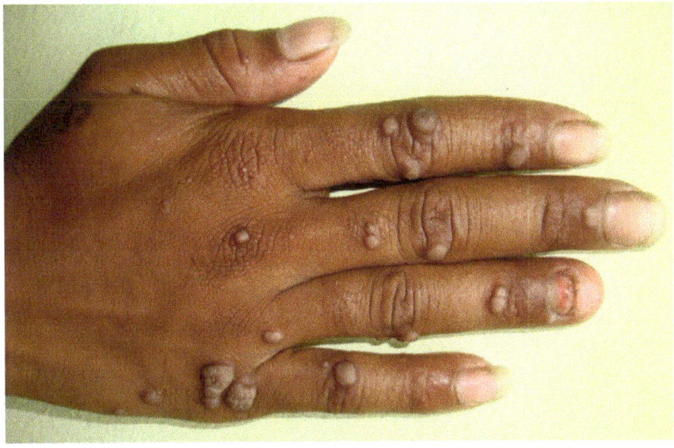

FIGURE 127.6 Common warts or verruca vulgaris FST5.

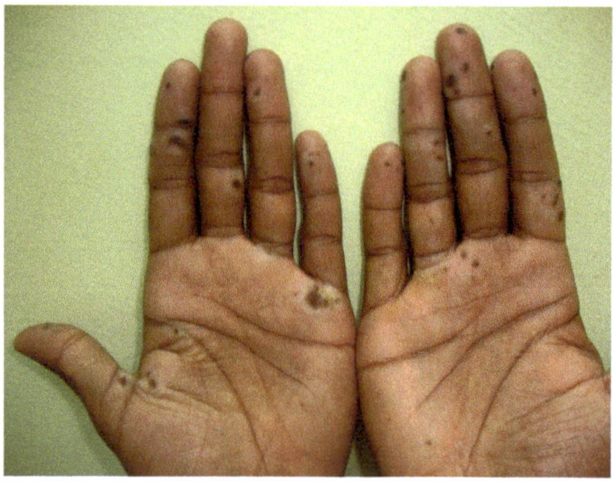

FIGURE 127.7 Palmar warts FST5.

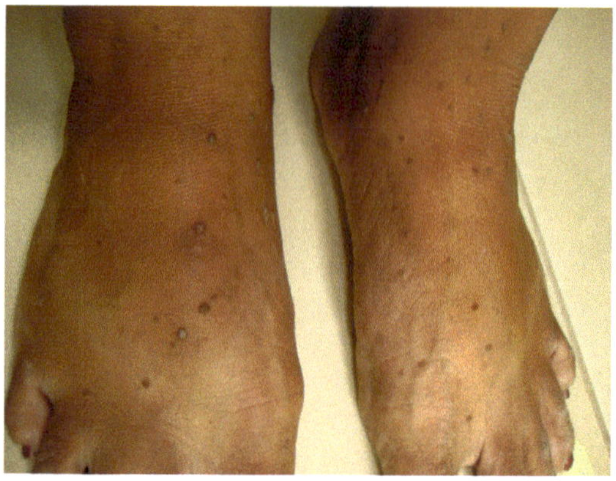

FIGURE 127.8 Plane warts or verruca plana FST5

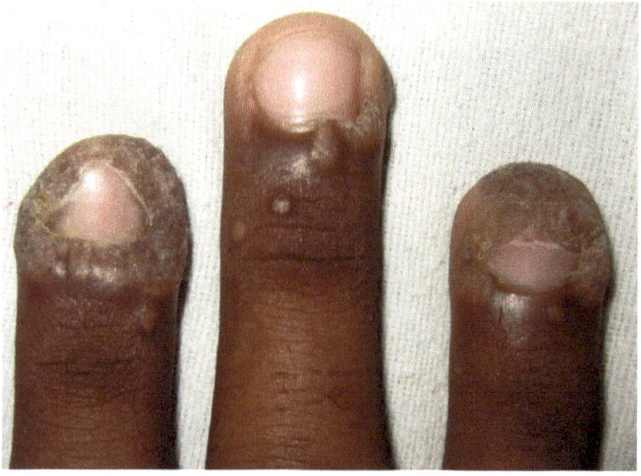

FIGURE 127.9 Periungual verruca vulgaris FST5.

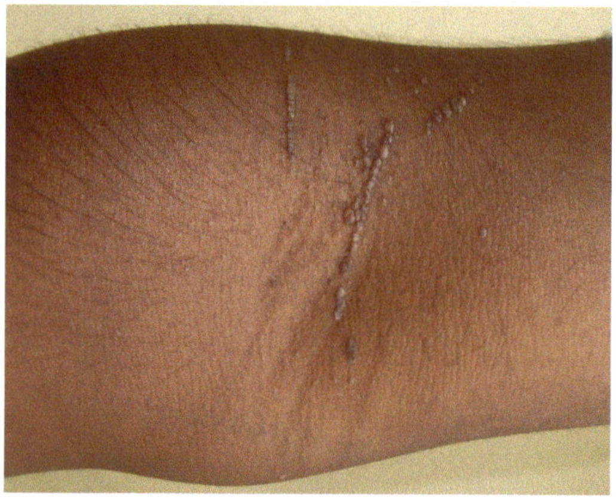

FIGURE 127.10 Koebner phenomenon in viral warts FST5.

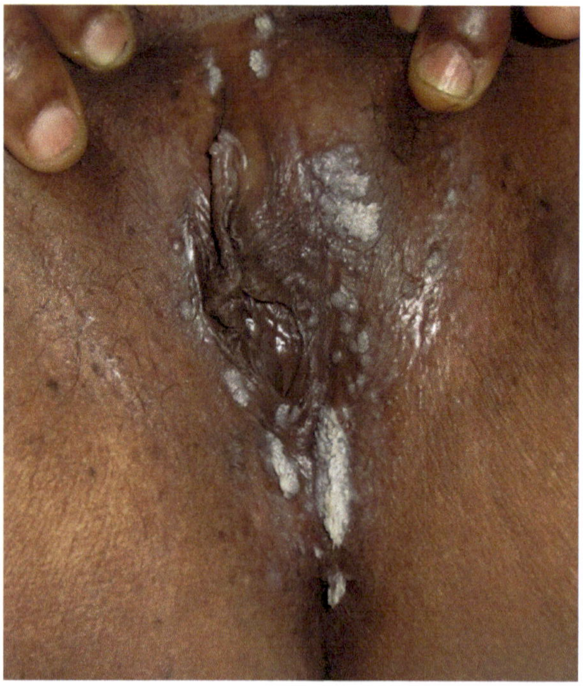

FIGURE 127.11 Genital warts (condylomata acuminata) in a woman FST5.

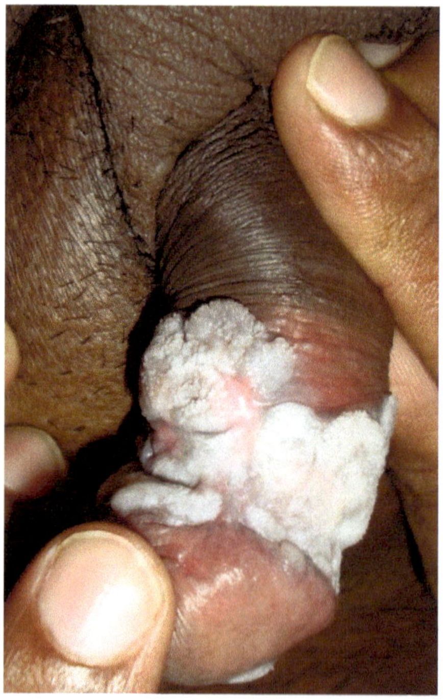

FIGURE 127.12 Penile warts FST5.

128
VITILIGINOUS DEPIGMENTATION ON SHINS

Introduction

These unexplained spotty vitiliginous patches on shins are common in our setting. They are asymptomatic, bilateral, may not be symmetrical, and patients seek treatments due to fear of vitiligo. It starts as spotty depigmentation that slowly increases over many years. It does not spread beyond the shins and remains spotty, and does not coalesce to large vitiligo patches. It is not associated with vitiligo on other areas of the body or other autoimmune diseases. There is no association with eczema, dermatitis, or any other skin diseases except post-inflammatory depigmentation. Further studies have not been done on these vitiliginous patches.

We have observed similar but extensive vitiliginous patches on the shins in middle-aged and elderly women following mild dermatitis or eczema in the area. These are itchy or started as itchy dermatitis. However, these vitiliginous patches are more extensive and prolonged than the dermatitis they have. The associated dermatitis is mild and not the major complaint in these women. Whether this is the same entity exacerbated by itching is not elucidated. These vitiliginous patches are more extensive, extend beyond the dermatitis, and are more deeply white than post-inflammatory depigmentation.

Epidemiology

Only women seek treatment; therefore, this was not observed in men. Women are of middle age and elderly, 40 years and above. Accurate epidemiological studies have not been done in our settings.

Associated diseases

No association with vitiligo or other autoimmune diseases.

Clinical characteristics in light skin (Fitzpatrick skin types I–III)

Although this might possibly be due to age-related melanocyte exhaustion (as in hypomelanosis guttata idiopathica), this is not (?) seen in patients with fair skin.

Clinical characteristics in dark skin (Fitzpatrick skin types IV–V)

Asymptomatic spotty depigmentation on shins (Figures 128.1 to 128.3). Both shins are affected equally and simultaneously. These patches do not spread beyond the shins and remain spotty, and do not coalesce into large vitiligo patches. This is a major cosmetic issue in middle-aged and elderly women in our setting.

Investigations

This is diagnosed clinically.

Treatments

- If associated with dermatitis, diluted topical steroids are prescribed with antihistamines. The dermatitis responds to treatments, whereas depigmentation persists.
- If not associated with dermatitis, only reassurance is needed.
- Topical tacrolimus ointment has been tried on worried patients, but the response has been unsatisfactory.

Further reading

No published data found. We discussed this entity in:

Ranawaka RR (2021). Vitiligo. In: Ranawaka RR, et al. (eds). *Atlas of Dermatoses in Pigmented Skin*. Springer, Singapore; 823–836.

DOI: 10.1201/9781003479512-128

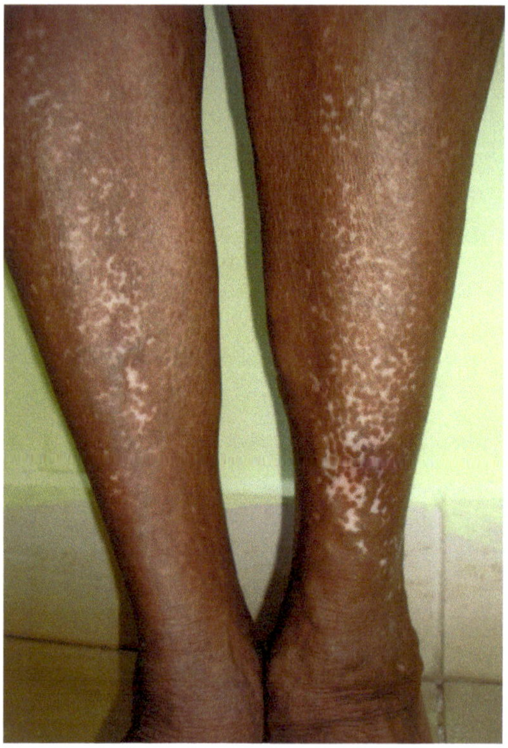

FIGURE 128.1 Bilateral (may not be symmetrical) spotty vitiliginous patches on the shins in a 57-year-old woman FST5. Note absence of associated dermatitis.

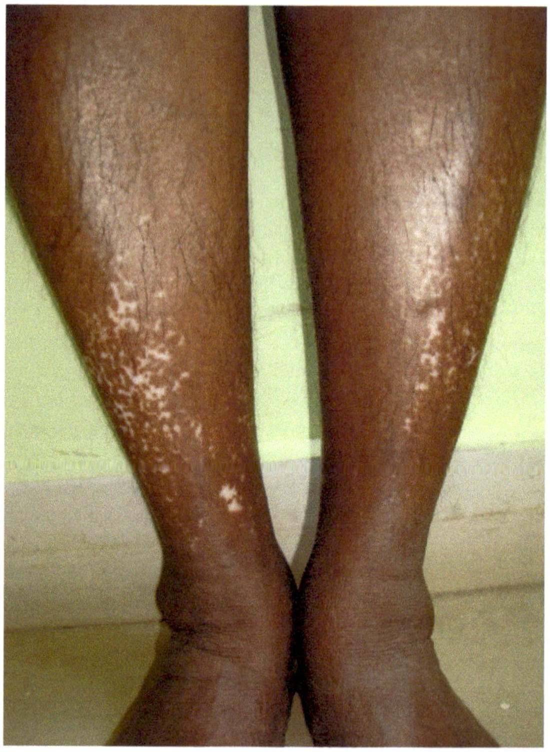

FIGURE 128.2 Bilateral spotty vitiliginous patches on the shins in a 47-year-old woman FST5. Note no associated dermatitis.

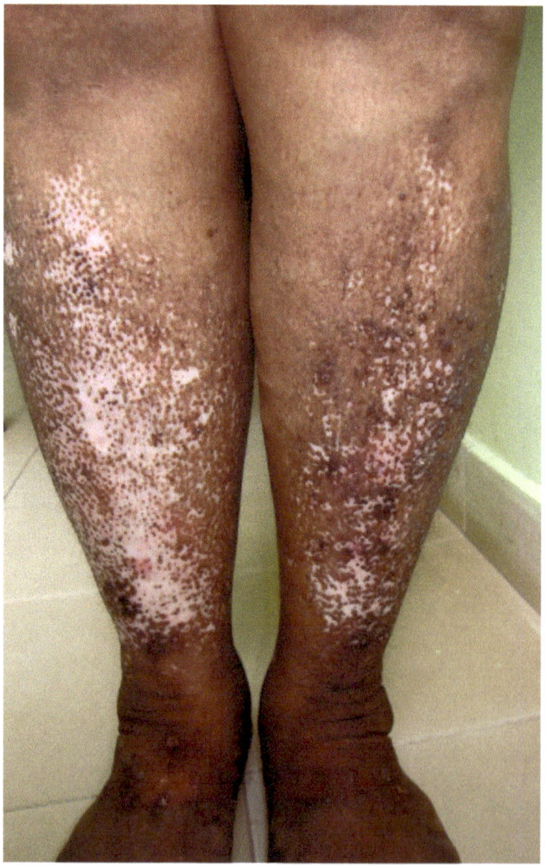

FIGURE 128.3 Bilateral spotty vitiliginous patches on the shins in a 55-year-old woman associated with dermatitis FST5. Note wider spread of depigmentation compared to the dermatitis which is milder.

129
VITILIGO

Introduction

Vitiligo is a common form of localized depigmentation. It is an acquired condition resulting from the progressive loss of melanocytes. Various theories have been suggested for the etiology of vitiligo; the autoimmune/autoinflammatory theory is currently the leading hypothesis and is supported by strong evidence.

Vitiligo is classified into two major forms: Segmental vitiligo and non-segmental vitiligo (NSV). The distribution of the lesions is usually symmetrical in NSV, while in the segmental subtype it is usually unilateral and band-shaped. The Koebner phenomenon is well known in vitiligo (also called an isomorphic response). There can be complete vitiligo (universalis), trichrome vitiligo when the pigment loss may be partial, or hairs in the patches depigment (poliosis/leukotrichia).

Epidemiology

It is stated that vitiligo affects 0.5–1% of the world's population and can begin at any age. Vitiligo affects all races but is a major cosmetic issue in darker skin.

Associated diseases

Vitiligo is associated with other autoimmune diseases; the strongest association is with thyroid disease. The association between vitiligo and halo nevi is well established (31%). Areas of depigmentation sometimes develop in patients with melanoma. Vitiligo with inner ear affection is called Vogt–Koyanagi syndrome.

Clinical characteristics in light skin (Fitzpatrick skin types I–III)

Vitiligo is probably as common in light skin as in dark skin; however, as it is much less obvious and light-skinned people live more in areas where leprosy was/is not a major health issue anymore, its psychosocial impact is considerably lower (Figures 129.1 to 129.3). White skin areas of variable size and configuration are usually distributed in a symmetrical fashion. The lighter the patients' skin, the less their vitiligo embarrasses them.

A Wood's lamp may be useful for detecting vitiligo of the palms and soles.

Clinical characteristics in dark skin (Fitzpatrick skin types IV–V)

It is characterized by milky-white, sharply demarcated macules and is a major cosmetic problem in darker skin (Figures 129.4 to 129.6).

Hypochromic vitiligo (vitiligo minor) is a form of NSV that seems to be limited to dark-skinned individuals. The term 'minor' refers to the partial defect in pigmentation.

Investigations

This is a clinical diagnosis in dark skin. A Wood's lamp examination is helpful in white skin, but not necessary for dark skin.

Treatments

- Response to treatment of vitiligo varies between individuals but is often unsatisfactory, especially for acral lesions.
- Use of sunscreen is advised on vitiligo patches.
- Providing ways of coping with vitiligo could also benefit patients while this disease has no cure.
- Treatment of vitiligo may be divided into pharmacological, physical, and surgical, which can sometimes be combined.

1. **Pharmacological treatment**

- Topical corticosteroid therapy is considered a first-line treatment for vitiligo, since it is low cost and easy to apply. It is limited by the risk of local adverse effects, such as atrophy, striae, and telangiectasias and also systemic side effects.
- Calcineurin inhibitors – topical tacrolimus has no risk of atrophy, but is expensive.

Topical tacrolimus ointment 0.03% or pimecrolimus cream 1% has efficacy for vitiligo in infants, which serves to achieve an appropriate level of safety and tolerability during the 6-month period of applications. No sign of immunosuppression was found among infants treated intermittently with 1% pimecrolimus cream for up to 2 years; they demonstrated normal immune responses to vaccinations and did not show increases in the incidence of systemic infections or skin infections over time.

- Systemic corticosteroid therapy is used in cases of disseminated vitiligo lesions with rapid progression. Minipulses have been used in order to minimize adverse events.
- Janus kinase inhibitors are of great promise and are now even available as topical preparations.

2. **Physical treatment** – ultraviolet (UV) radiation, both in the UVA and UVB spectrum. Narrow-band UVB (311 nm) is considered a first-line option for vitiligo.

- **Phototherapy with UVA and psoralens (PUVA therapy)** in the forms 8-methoxypsoralen, 5-methoxypsoralen or trimethylpsoralen which may be used in their oral and topical presentations.

3. **Surgical treatment** – surgical melanocyte transplantation for patients with stable disease who failed to respond to classical therapies. Punch grafting is the easiest and lowest cost technique, although it is generally limited to treating small areas. Suction blister epidermal grafting, split-thickness skin grafts.

DOI: 10.1201/9781003479512-129

4. **Depigmenting treatment** – in those patients with extensive vitiligo and only a few residual areas of pigmentation, skin bleaching with laser therapy (e.g., Q-switched alexandrite 755 nm, Q-switched ruby 694 nm), cryotherapy, or creams (e.g., 20% monobenzylether of hydroquinone) may be used.
5. **Cosmetic camouflage** may be the only option for many.

Further reading

Maghfour J, Bardhi R, Huggins R, et al. (2023). Recipient-to-Donor Ratios in the Surgical Treatment of Vitiligo, Leukoderma, and Piebaldism: A Retrospective Review. *Dermatology*;239(5):828–831.

Ranawaka RR (2021). Vitiligo. In: Ranawaka RR, et al. (eds). *Atlas of Dermatoses in Pigmented Skin*. Springer, Singapore; 823–836.

Silpa-Archa N, Griffith JL, Huggins RH, et al. (2017). Long-Term Follow-Up of Patients Undergoing Autologous Noncultured Melanocyte-Keratinocyte Transplantation for Vitiligo and Other Leukodermas. *J Am Acad Dermatol*;77(2):318–327.

van Geel N, Speeckaert R (2024). Acquired Pigmentary Disorders. In: Griffiths C, et al. (eds). *Rook's Textbook of Dermatology*, 10th ed. John Wiley & Sons Ltd., UK; 86.34.

Yamaguchi Y, Peeva E, Duca ED, et al. (2024). Ritlecitinib, a JAK3/TEC Family Kinase Inhibitor, Stabilizes Active Lesions and Repigments Stable Lesions in Vitiligo. *Arch Dermatol Res*;316(7):478.

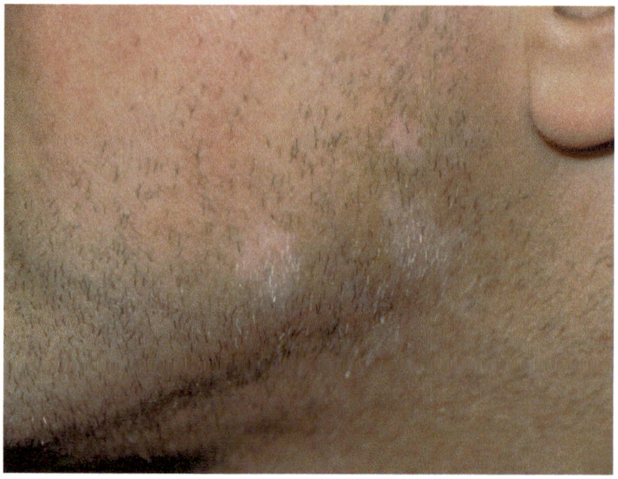

FIGURE 129.1 Vitiligo and poliosis FST2. (Courtesy Prof. Ian Coulson, UK.)

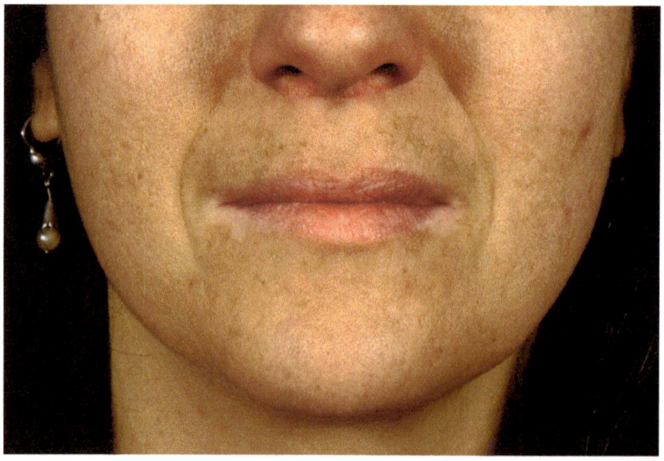

FIGURE 129.2 Vitiligo around the mouth FST2.

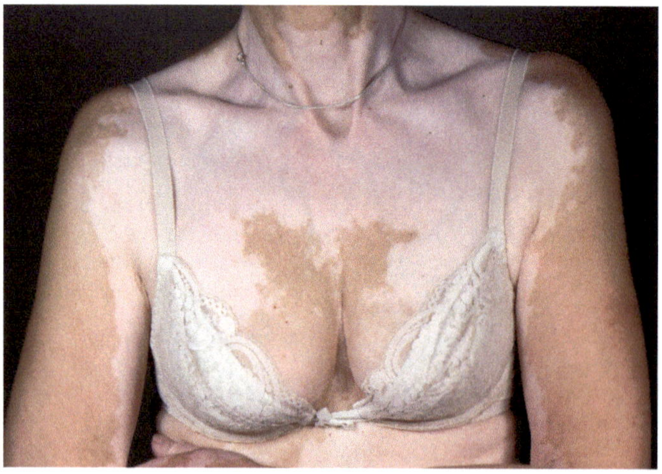

FIGURE 129.3 Vitiligo FST2. (Courtesy Dr. Richard Ashton, UK.)

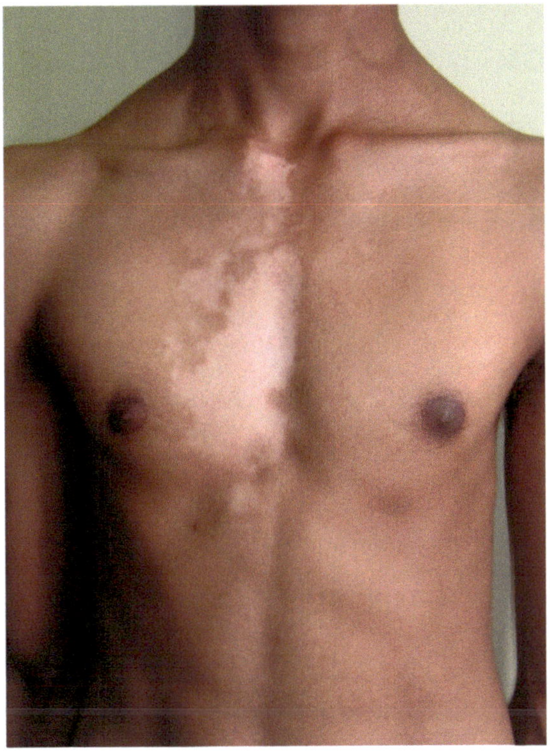

FIGURE 129.4 Segmental vitiligo in a 17-year-old boy FST5.

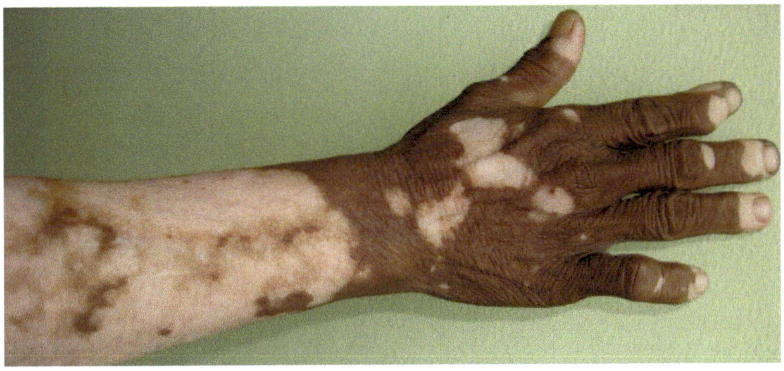

FIGURE 129.5 Generalized vitiligo (non-segmental) in a 65-year-old woman FST5.

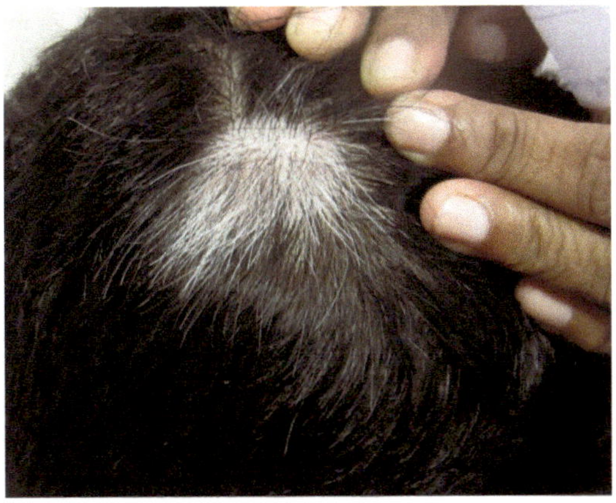

FIGURE 129.6 Poliosis or leukotrichia following vitiligo on scalp FST5.

130
XANTHOMAS AND XANTHELASMA PALPEBRARUM

Introduction

Xanthomas are cutaneous lipid deposits. All xanthomas contain macrophages loaded with cholesterol and cholesterol esters ('foam cells').

In xanthoma, there are a number of clinical types; some are associated with hyperlipidemias.

1. *Tendon xanthoma* – subcutaneous nodules or papules in relation to tendons (over the knuckles and in the Achilles tendon). They are most frequently seen in familial hypercholesterolemia (FH) and rare lipid disorders, such as cerebrotendinous xanthomatosis and sitosterolemia.
2. *Tuberous xanthoma/tubero-eruptive xanthoma* – firm nodules that occur over sites of pressure, commonly the elbows and knees. Usually indicate the presence of type III hyperlipoproteinemia.
3. *Eruptive xanthoma* – multiple small papules over extensor surfaces, and are associated with hypertriglyceridemia.
4. *Dyslipidemic plane xanthomas* consist of three types:

   - *Xanthelasma* – plane xanthomas that develop around the eyes (xanthelasma palpebrarum).
   - *Plane xanthoma* – flat, smear-like lesions that can occur anywhere on the body, can be a feature of homozygous FH.
   - *Palmar xanthoma* – appear in palmar creases and are pathognomonic of type III hyperlipoproteinemia.

Epidemiology

Commonly seen in middle-aged women.

Associated diseases

Xanthelasmata are seen in FH, type III hyperlipoproteinemia, and chronic cholestasis (especially primary biliary cirrhosis), but are also often seen in people with normal circulating lipid levels and after thyroidectomy.

Clinical characteristics in light skin (Fitzpatrick skin types I–III)

Xanthelasma, which literally means yellow plaque, is frequently localized in the medial aspect of the lower and upper eyelids (Figure 130.1). They are characterized by cholesterol-accumulating histiocytes in the upper dermis, giving them a foam-like aspect. Xanthelasmata can occur with and without hyperlipidemia; however, in both variants, lowering the blood cholesterol level reduces their size and sometimes makes them disappear.

Diffuse papular xanthomas are very often associated with hypertriglyceridemia. They are predominantly located on the buttocks; they spread to the remaining trunk and proximal extremities. In the beginning, they are pink to salmon-colored before they turn more and more yellow.

Rigorous diet with lowering of blood fat levels is the treatment of choice.

Clinical characteristics in dark skin (Fitzpatrick skin types IV–V)

Xanthelasma most commonly affects the upper eyelids and the area around the medial canthus (Figure 130.2). They are relatively soft on palpation and range from pale yellow to yellow-orange in color. Some are hyperpigmented in dark-skinned individuals.

Investigations

Full lipid profile and liver function tests.

Treatments

- If LDL cholesterol levels are high, then treatment to lower the LDL cholesterol (e.g., with a statin).
- Xanthelasmas are often a cosmetic problem. Treatments include surgical excision, electrocautery, topical trichloroacetic acid (TCA) or lasers.
  - Erbium:YAG laser, ablation was more effective and had fewer recurrences than 50% TCA (Arora et al. 2024).

Further reading

Arora A, Mohta A, Mehta RD, et al. (2024). A Clinical and Dermatoscopic Perspective of the Efficacy and Safety of Erbium: YAG Laser Ablation versus 50% Trichloroacetic Acid for the Management of Xanthelasma Palpebrarum. *J Cutan Aesthet Surg*;17(1):1–6.

Flynn PD (2024). Xanthomas and Abnormalities of Lipid Metabolism and Storage. In: Griffiths C, et al. (eds). *Rook's Textbook of Dermatology*, 10th ed. John Wiley & Sons Ltd., UK; 60.4.

DOI: 10.1201/9781003479512-130

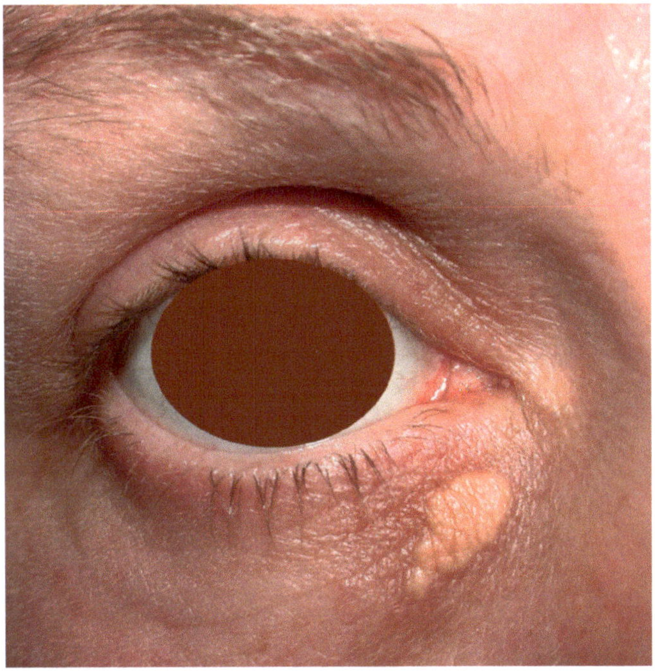

FIGURE 130.1 Xanthelasmata palpebrum FST1. (Courtesy Prof. Ian Coulson, UK.)

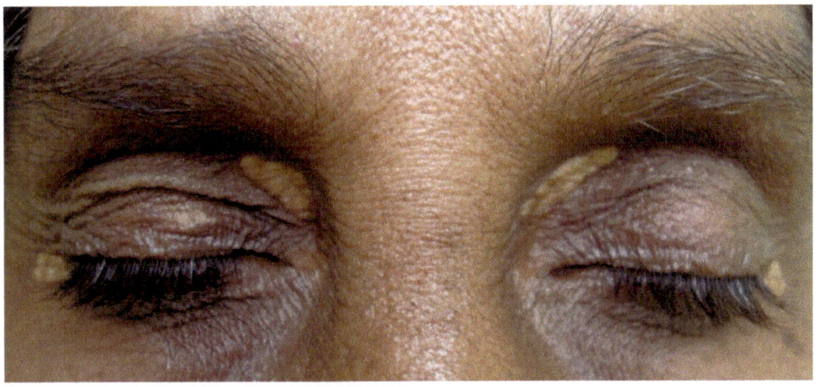

FIGURE 130.2 Xanthelasmata palpebrum in a 50-year-old woman FST5. Her lipids were within normal limits.

INDEX

I

J

K

L

M

N

O

P